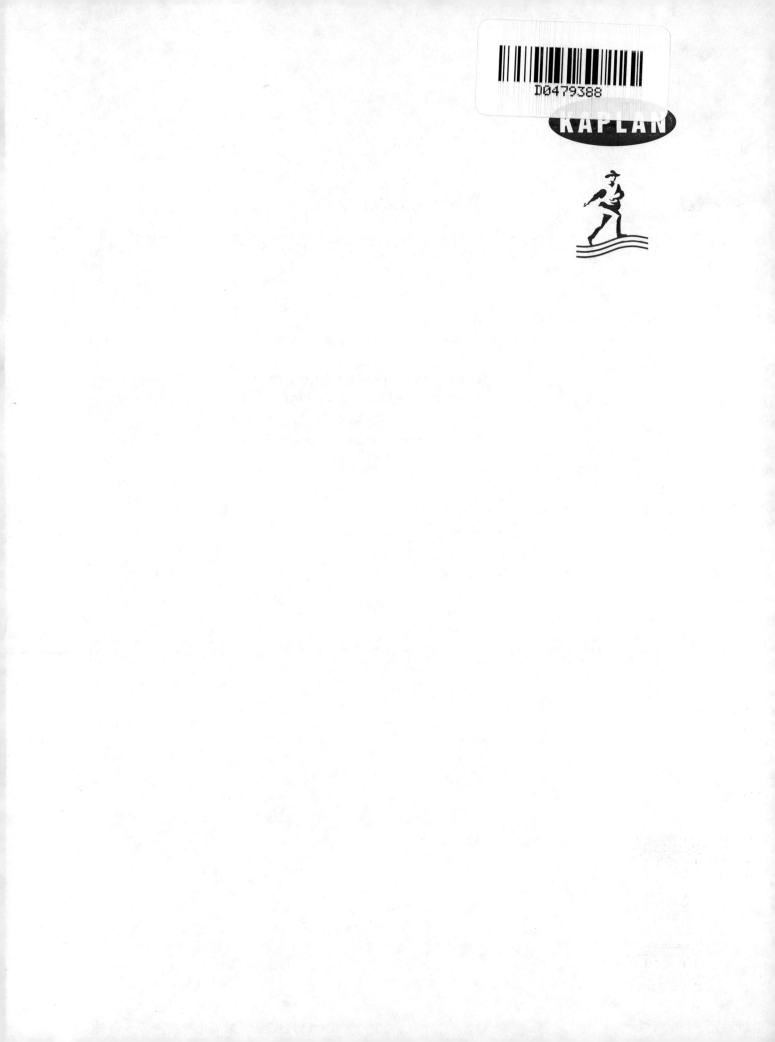

**Other Kaplan Books Relating to
Medical School Admissions**

Get Into Medical School
MCAT Comprehensive Review
MCAT 45

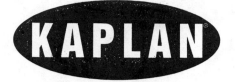

MCAT®
Practice Tests
Fourth Edition

By the Staff of Kaplan, Inc.

Simon & Schuster

New York · London · Sydney · Toronto

Kaplan Publishing
Published by Simon & Schuster
1230 Avenue of the Americas
New York, NY 10020

Excerpt from "Maya Beginning Extended Back at Belize Site," by Bruce Bower, reprinted with permission from *Science News*, the weekly newsmagazine of science, copyright © 1994 by Science Service.

Excerpt from "The Complexity Problem," by John Sedgwick, reprinted with permission from John Sedgwick.

Excerpt from *The First New Nation* by Seymour Martin Lipset, reprinted with permission from Transaction Publishers.

Excerpt from "Selective Incapacitation: A Sheep in Wolf's Clothing?" by Brian Forst, reprinted with permission from Brian Forst.

Excerpt from *Secrets* by Sissela Bok, copyright © 1982 by Sissela Bok. Used by permission of Pantheon Books, a division of Random House, Inc.

Excerpt from *The Future Eaters* by Tim Flannery, reprinted with permission from Grove/Atlantic Press.

Contributing Editor: Albert Chen
Editor: Larissa Shmailo
Cover Design: Cheung Tai
Production Artist: Hugh Haggerty
Production Editor: Angela Cress
Production Manager: Michael Shevlin
Managing Editor: Déa Alessandro

Manufactured in the United States of America
Published simultaneously in Canada

February 2004

10   9   8   7   6   5   4   3

ISBN: 0-7432-4111-8

Contents

SECTION ONE: MCAT Strategies

SECTION TWO: Full-Length Practice Tests

About the Authors

Tessa Cigler
B.A. (Biochemistry), Harvard University
M.D., Duke University

Richard Cohen, Ph.D.
B.S. (Physics), Brown University
Ph.D. (Physics), University of Maryland

William Dracos
B.A. (Biology), Duke University
M.B.A., Duke University

Sascha Dublin
B.A. (Renaissance Studies), Brown University
M.D./Ph.D., University of Washington
School of Medicine

Richard Friedland, D.P.M.
B.A. (Biology), Ithaca College
D.P.M., Pennsylvania College of Podiatric Medicine

Sharon Klotz
B.S. (Physics), Massachusetts Institute of Technology

Andy Koh, M.D.
B.A. (Biology), Harvard University
B.A. (English Literature), Oxford University
M.D., Harvard Medical School

Karl Lee, M.A.
B.A. (Chemistry), Amherst College
M.A. (Physical Chemistry), Harvard University

Alan Levine, M.S.
B.A. (Mathematics), Rice University
M.S. (Chemistry), University of Houston

Michael Manley, M.D.
B.S. (Psychobiology), University of California,
Los Angeles
M.D., University of California, San Diego

Leslie Manley, Ph.D.
B.A. (Biochemistry & Cell Biology),
University of California, San Diego
Ph.D. (Physiology & Pharmacology),
University of California, San Diego

Eileen A. McDonnell
B.A. (English Literature), CUNY
J.D., Fordham University

Ingrid Multhopp
B.A. (English Literature), University of Chicago

Amjed Mustafa
B.S. (Cell Biology & Neuroscience, Cognitive Science),
Rutgers University
Ph.D. (In Progress), UMDNJ/Rutgers University

Stacie Orell
B.A. (Biology), University of Pennsylvania

Rochelle Rothstein, M.D.
B.A. (Biology), Princeton University
M.D., University of California, San Diego

Evan Skowronski, Ph.D.
B.S. (Chemistry), Duke University
Ph.D. (Microbiology), Loma Linda University

Andrew Taylor
B.A. (Biology), Boston University

How to Use
This Book

Congratulations on buying the best MCAT workbook available: *MCAT Practice Tests*. Kaplan's *MCAT Practice Tests* provides you with key subject-specific MCAT strategies and two full-length practice tests followed by thorough, detailed explanations.

Before you start practicing with the MCAT-style tests in this book, it's important that you have a fundamental understanding of the science material tested on the MCAT, including college-level biology, general chemistry, organic chemistry, and physics. In addition, you should be familiar with the format and style of the MCAT.

If you already have a strong understanding of the sciences tested and the format of the MCAT, you're ready to begin practicing with the *MCAT Practice Tests*. However, if you feel that you need more extensive content review, consider using Kaplan's *MCAT Comprehensive Review,* a companion to this book that covers all the science necessary for the MCAT, and provides practice sets and strategies for every area of the test, as well as an additional full-length MCAT complete with explanations.

Here's how to use the various components of *MCAT Practice Tests:*

STEP ONE: READ THE MCAT STRATEGIES SECTION

Kaplan's live MCAT course has helped more people get into medical school than all the other courses combined. In this section, we've distilled the main techniques and approaches from our course in a clear, easy-to-grasp format. We'll introduce you to the idiosyncrasies of the MCAT and show you how to take control of the test-taking experience on all levels:

Test Material
Specific methods and strategies for tackling MCAT passages and questions in all subjects.

Test Expertise
Item-specific techniques, as well as advice on how to pace yourself on each section, and how to decide when to answer questions and when to guess. We'll teach you how the peculiarities of a standardized test can be used to your advantage.

Test Mentality
The proper attitude for executing all you've learned and for facing the MCAT with confidence.

STEP TWO: TAKE KAPLAN'S FULL-LENGTH PRACTICE MCATS

After you've learned valuable test strategies, take the full-length practice tests—timed, simulated MCATs—as a test run for the real thing. The explanations for every question on the tests are included in this book so you can understand your mistakes. Try not to confine your review to the explanations for the questions you've gotten wrong. Instead, read all the explanations, to reinforce key concepts and sharpen your skills.

STEP THREE: REVIEW TO SHORE UP WEAK POINTS

If you find your performance was weak in any area, go back to the section in which that material was tested and review the explanations.

FOR MORE PRACTICE

Kaplan's MCAT content review book, *MCAT Comprehensive Review,* features in-depth review of all the science topics covered on the MCAT, as well as additional practice sets and another full-length practice test. You can use it independently or in conjunction with this book. You can also contact the Association of American Medical Colleges to receive the MCAT practice tests it publishes:

AAMC
MCAT Section
2450 N Street, NW
Washington, DC 20037-1127
Phone: (202) 828-0690
www.aamc.org

Different people have different learning styles. If after spending some time with this book, you feel that a live course with more individualized instruction and extensive opportunity for practice is what you need, consider taking a Kaplan MCAT course.

Our live MCAT course gives students personal attention, as well as unparalled opportunities to practice, including a library filled with subject-specific topical tests, practice tests similar to those contained in this book, and five simulated MCAT examinations, each accompanied by computer-assisted feedback. All the classes are taught by expert teachers who have undergone Kaplan's extensive National Teacher Training Program. Another option is for you to take one of Kaplan's MCAT STAT online courses.

If you would like more information on Kaplan's MCAT prep courses, please call us at 1-800-KAP-TEST. You can also contact us on the Web at **kaptest.com**.

A Special Note for International Students

Gaining admission to a U.S. medical school can be especially challenging if you are not a U. S. citizen. In recent years, fewer than one percent of first-year med students were non–U.S. citizens. Most of these students attended college in the United States prior to applying to medical school.

If you are an international student hoping to attend medical school in the United States, Kaplan can help you explore your options. Here are some things to think about.

- If English is not your first language, most medical schools will require you to take the TOEFL (Test of English as a Foreign Language) or provide some other evidence that you are proficient in English.

- Plan to take the MCAT; most U.S. medical schools require it.

- Begin the process of applying to medical schools at least 18 months before the fall of the year you plan to start your studies. Most programs will have only September start dates.

- You will need to obtain an I-20 Certificate of Eligibility from the school you plan to attend if you intend to apply for an F-1 Student Visa to study in the United States.

- If you've already completed medical training outside the United States, get information about taking the United States Medical Licensing Exam (USMLE).

KAPLAN ENGLISH PROGRAMS

If you need more help with the complex process of medical school admissions, assistance preparing for the MCAT, USMLE, NCLEX or TOEFL, or help building your English language skills, you may be interested in Kaplan's programs for international students. These programs were designed to help students and professionals from outside the United States meet their educational and career goals. At locations throughout the United States, international students are improving their academic and conversational English skills, raising their scores on standardized exams, and gaining admission to the schools of their choice. Our staff and instructors give you the individualized attention you need to succeed. Here are some brief program descriptions:

GENERAL INTENSIVE ENGLISH

This class is designed to help you improve your skills in all areas of English and to increase your fluency in spoken and written English. Classes are available for beginning to advanced students, and the average class size is 12 students.

TOEFL AND ACADEMIC ENGLISH

This course provides you with the skills you need to improve your TOEFL score and succeed at an American school. It includes advanced reading, writing, listening, grammar, and conversational English. Your training will include use of Kaplan's exclusive computer-based practice materials.

ENGLISH LANGUAGE STRUCTURED-STUDY PROGRAM

This program allows you to improve your English at your own pace. The books, tapes, and videos provided are for students whose skills range from beginner to intermediate.

MCAT TEST PREPARATION COURSE

In addition to test preparation for the MCAT, Kaplan offers professional counseling and advice to help you better understand the American educational system—from choosing the right medical school, to writing your application, to preparing for an interview.

MEDICAL ENGLISH COMMUNICATION REVIEW COURSE

This program is for international doctors and medical professionals. Lessons include mastering pronunciation, building your medical vocabulary, and developing presentation and medical writing skills. Coursework also helps you develop the English skills you will need for the CSA exam, professional interviews, and interactions with patients.

OTHER KAPLAN PROGRAMS

Since 1938, more than three million students have come to Kaplan to advance their studies, prepare for entry to American universities, and further their careers. In addition to the above programs, Kaplan offers courses to prepare for the SAT, ACT, GMAT, GRE, LSAT, MCAT, DAT, USMLE, NCLEX, and other standardized exams at locations throughout the United States. For more information, contact us at:

KAPLAN ENGLISH PROGRAMS

700 South Flower, Suite 2900
Los Angeles, CA 90017
Phone outside of the USA: 213.452.5800
Phone inside of the USA: 800.818.9128
Fax: 213.892.1364
Website: www.kaplanenglish.com
Email: world@kaplan.com

Kaplan is authorized under federal law to enroll nonimmigrant alien students. Kaplan is accredited by ACCET (Accrediting Council for Continuing Education and Training). Test names are registered trademarks of their respective owners.

FREE Services for International Students

Kaplan now offers international students many services online—*free of charge*!
Students may assess their TOEFL skills and gain valuable feedback on their English language proficiency in just a few hours with Kaplan's TOEFL Skills Assessment.
Log onto www.kaplaninternational.com today.

Section One

MCAT Strategies

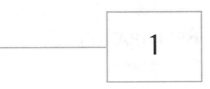

Introduction to the MCAT

HIGHLIGHTS

- Understand how the MCAT is structured and scored
- Learn to take control of the test using the MCAT Mindset

Take out a No. 2 pencil . . . . Do not make any stray marks on the grid . . . . What is the acceleration due to gravity of a penny thrown from the Empire State Building if . . . . You've faced these tests before, so you know the drill, right? Wrong.

The Medical College Admission Test, affectionately known as the MCAT, is different from any other test you've encountered in your academic career. It's not like the knowledge-based exams from high school and college, whose emphasis was on memorizing and regurgitating information. Medical schools can assess your academic prowess by looking at your transcript. The MCAT isn't even like other standardized tests you may have taken, where the focus was on proving your general skills.

Medical schools use MCAT scores to assess whether you possess the foundation upon which to build a successful medical career. Though you certainly need to know the content to do well, the stress is on thought process, because the MCAT is above all else a thinking test. That's why it emphasizes reasoning, critical and analytical thinking, reading comprehension, data analysis, writing, and problem-solving skills.

The MCAT's power comes from its use as an indicator of your abilities. Good scores can open doors. Your power comes from preparation and mindset, because the key to MCAT success is knowing what you're up against. And that's where this section of this book comes in. We'll explain the philosophy behind the test, review the sections one by one, show you sample questions, share some of Kaplan's proven methods, and clue you in to what the test makers are really after. You'll get a handle on the process, find a confident new perspective, and achieve your highest possible scores.

REGISTRATION

The only way to register for the MCAT is online. The registration site is:
www.aamc.org/mcat

You can access the site 8 to 12 weeks before your test date. Payment must be made by MasterCard, Visa, or E-payment.

Go to www.aamc.org/mcat/registration.htm and download *MCAT Essentials* for information about registration, fees, test administration, and preparation. For other questions, contact:

MCAT Program Office
P.O. Box 4056
Iowa City, IA 52243
(319) 337-1357
(Monday–Friday, 8:30 A.M.–4:30 P.M., central daylight time)
www.aamc.org
Email: mcat@aamc.org

Don't drag your feet gathering information. You'll need time not only to prepare and practice for the test, but also to get all your registration work done.

ANATOMY OF THE MCAT

Before mastering strategies, you need to know exactly what you're dealing with on the MCAT. Let's start with the basics: The MCAT is, among other things, an endurance test. It consists of four and three-quarter hours of multiple-choice testing plus one hour of writing sample. Add in the administrative details at both ends of the testing experience, plus three breaks (including lunch), and you can count on being in the test room for well over six hours.

It's a grueling experience, to say the least. If you can't approach it with confidence and stamina, you'll quickly lose your composure. That's why it's so important that you take control of the test.

The MCAT consists of four timed sections: Physical Sciences, Verbal Reasoning, the Writing Sample, and Biological Sciences. Later in this section of the book, we'll take an in-depth look at each MCAT section, including sample question types and specific test-smart hints, but here's a general overview:

PHYSICAL SCIENCES

Time	100 minutes
Format	77 multiple-choice questions:
	approximately 10–11 passages with 4–8 questions each; 15 stand alone questions (not passage-based)
What it tests	basic general chemistry concepts, basic physics concepts, analytical reasoning, data interpretation

VERBAL REASONING

Time	85 minutes
Format	60 multiple-choice questions:
	approximately 9–10 passages with 6–9 questions each
What it tests	critical reading

WRITING SAMPLE

Time	60 minutes
Format	2 essay questions (30 minutes per essay)
What it tests	critical thinking, intellectual organization, written communication skills

BIOLOGICAL SCIENCES

Time	100 minutes
Format	77 multiple-choice questions:
	approximately 10–11 passages with 4–8 questions each; 15 stand-alone questions (not passage-based)
What it tests	basic biology concepts, basic organic chemistry concepts, analytical reasoning, data interpretation

The sections of the test always appear in the same order:

Morning   Physical Sciences
[10-minute break]
Verbal Reasoning
[60-minute lunch break]

Afternoon   Writing Sample
[10-minute break]
Biological Sciences
[15 minute test-taker survey]

Be sure to bring at least three No. 2 pencils for the multiple-choice questions, and two ballpoint pens with black ink for the Writing Sample. You won't be allowed to use a calculator or scratch paper; use your test booklet to work out your answers.

International students: The MCAT is administered internationally as a computer-based exam (CBT). Lebanon and Qatar are the exceptions where a specially proctered MCAT is administered as a paper-and-pencil test.

SCORING

Each MCAT section receives its own score. Verbal Reasoning, Physical Sciences, and Biological Sciences are each scored on a scale ranging from 1–15, with 15 as the highest. You will also receive a "total score" for these three multiple-choice sections. The Writing Sample essays are scored alphabetically on a scale ranging from J to T, with T as the highest. The two essays are each evaluated by two official readers, so four critiques combine to make the alphabetical score.

The number of multiple-choice questions that you answer correctly per section is your "raw score." Your raw score will then be converted to yield the "scaled score"–the one that will fall somewhere in that 1–15 range. These scaled scores are what are reported to medical schools as your MCAT scores.

All multiple-choice questions are worth the same amount–one raw point–and *there's no penalty for guessing. That means that you should always fill in an answer for every question, whether you get to that question or not!* This is an important piece of advice, so pay it heed. Never let time run out on any section without filling in an answer for every question on the grid.

Your score report will tell you–and your potential medical schools–not only your scaled scores, but also the national mean score for each section, standard deviations, national scoring profiles for each section, and your percentile ranking. The same day scores are mailed they are posted on the Thx score reporting system on the aamc.org website.

WHAT'S A GOOD SCORE?

There's no such thing as a cut-and-dry "good score." Much depends on the strength of the rest of your application (if your transcript is first-rate, the pressure to strut your stuff on the MCAT isn't as intense) and on where you want to go to school (different schools have different score expectations). Here are a few interesting statistics:

For each MCAT administration, the average scaled scores are approximately 8s for Verbal Reasoning, Physical Sciences, and Biological Sciences, and N for the Writing Sample. You need scores of at least 10–11s to be considered competitive by most medical schools, and if you're aiming for the top, you've got to do even better, and score 12s and above.

You don't have to be perfect to do well. For instance, on the AAMC's Practice Test II, you could get as many as four questions wrong in Verbal Reasoning, 21 in Physical Sciences, and 16 in Biological Sciences and still score in the 80th percentile. To score in the 90th percentile, you could get as many as two wrong in Verbal Reasoning, 16 in Physical Sciences, and 11 in Biological Sciences. Even students who receive perfect scaled scores usually get a handful of questions wrong.

It's important to maximize your performance on every question. Just a few questions one way or the other can make a big difference in your scaled score. Here's a look at recent score profiles so you can get an idea of the shape of a typical score distribution.

Physical Sciences		
Scaled Score	Percent Achieving Score	Percentile Rank Range
15	0.1	99.9–99.9
14	1.3	98.7–99.9
13	2.1	96.6–98.6
12	4.4	92.2–96.5
11	7.2	85.0–92.1
10	13.9	71.1–84.9
9	11.7	59.4–71.0
8	18.6	40.8–59.3
7	14.0	26.8–40.7
6	13.4	13.4–26.7
5	8.5	04.8–13.3
4	3.4	01.4–04.7
3	1.2	00.3–01.3
2	0.1	00.1–00.2
1	0.0	00.0–00.0

Scaled Score
Mean = 8.1
Standard Deviation = 2.32

Verbal Reasoning		
Scaled Score	Percent Achieving Score	Percentile Rank Range
13–15	1.0	99.1–99.9
12	3.4	95.7–99.0
11	10.7	85.0–95.6
10	15.1	69.9–84.9
9	18.7	51.2–69.8
8	13.1	38.1–51.1
7	10.6	27.5–38.0
6	13.0	14.4–27.4
5	4.9	09.5–14.3
4	4.5	05.0–09.4
3	2.5	02.5–04.9
2	2.0	00.5–02.4
1	0.4	00.0–00.4

Scaled Score
Mean = 8.0
Standard Deviation = 2.43

Writing Sample		
Scaled Score	Percent Achieving Score	Percentile Rank Range
T	0.6	99.5–99.9
S	3.2	96.3–99.4
R	9.3	87.0–96.2
Q	12.1	74.9–86.9
P	12.1	62.8–74.8
O	13.1	49.7–62.7
N	12.7	37.1–49.6
M	21.3	15.8–37.0
L	9.5	06.3–15.7
K	4.0	02.3–06.2
J	2.2	00.0–02.2

75th Percentile = Q
50th Percentile = O
25th Percentile = M

Biological Sciences		
Scaled Score	Percent Achieving Score	Percentile Rank Range
15	0.1	99.9–99.9
14	0.5	99.5–99.8
13	2.4	97.2–99.4
12	4.3	92.9–97.1
11	8.8	84.1–92.8
10	16.0	68.1–84.0
9	15.5	52.6–68.0
8	16.0	36.6–52.5
7	12.6	24.0–36.5
6	9.9	14.1–23.9
5	6.3	07.8–14.0
4	4.6	03.2–07.7
3	2.2	01.0–03.1
2	0.7	00.3–00.9
1	0.2	00.0–00.2

Scaled Score
Mean = 8.2
Standard Deviation = 2.39

WHAT THE MCAT REALLY TESTS

It's important to grasp not only the nuts and bolts of the MCAT, so you'll know *what* to do on test day, but also the underlying principles of the test so you'll know *why* you're doing what you're doing on test day. We'll cover the straightforward MCAT facts later. Now it's time to examine the heart and soul of the MCAT, to see what it's really about.

THE MYTH

Most people preparing for the MCAT fall prey to the myth that the MCAT is a straightforward science test. They think something like this:

"It covers the four years of science I had to take in school: biology, chemistry, physics, and organic chemistry. It even has equations. OK, so it has Verbal Reasoning and Writing, but those sections are just to see if we're literate, right? The important stuff is the science. After all, we're going to be doctors."

Well, here's the little secret no one seems to want you to know: The MCAT is not just a science test; it's also a thinking test. This means that the test is designed to let you demonstrate your thought process, not only your thought content.

The implications are vast. Once you shift your test-taking paradigm to match the MCAT modus operandi, you'll find a new level of confidence and control over the test. You'll begin to work with the nature of the MCAT rather than against it. You'll be more efficient and insightful as you prepare for the test, and you'll be more relaxed on test day. In fact, you'll be able to see the MCAT for what it is rather than for what it's dressed up to be. We want your test day to feel like a visit with a familiar friend instead of an awkward blind date.

THE ZEN OF MCAT

Medical schools do not need to rely on the MCAT to see what you already know. Admission committees can measure your subject-area proficiency using your undergraduate coursework and grades. Schools are most interested in the potential of your mind.

In recent years, many medical schools have shifted pedagogic focus away from an information-heavy curriculum to a concept-based curriculum. There is currently more emphasis placed on problem solving, holistic thinking, and cross-disciplinary study. Be careful not to dismiss this important point, figuring you'll wait to worry about academic trends until you're actually in medical school. This trend affects you right now, because it's reflected in the MCAT. Every good tool matches its task. In this case the tool is the test, used to measure you and other candidates, and the task is to quantify how likely it is that you'll succeed in medical school.

Your intellectual potential—how skillfully you annex new territory into your mental boundaries, how quickly you build "thought highways" between ideas, how confidently and creatively you solve problems—is far more important to admission committees than your ability to recite Young's modulus for every material known to man. The schools assume they can expand your knowledge base. They choose applicants carefully because expansive knowledge is not enough to succeed in medical school or in the profession. There's something more. And it's this "something more" that the MCAT is trying to measure.

Every section on the MCAT tests essentially the same higher-order thinking skills: analytical reasoning, abstract thinking, and problem solving. Most test takers get trapped into thinking they are being tested strictly about biology, chemistry, etcetera. Thus, they approach each section with a new outlook on what's expected. This constant mental gear-shifting can be exhausting, not to mention counterproductive. Instead of perceiving the test as parsed into radically different sections, you need to maintain your focus on the underlying nature of the test: It's designed to test your thinking skills, not your information-recall skills. Each test section thus presents a variation on the same theme.

WHAT ABOUT THE SCIENCE?

With this perspective, you may be left asking the question: "What about the science? What about the content? Don't I need to know the basics?" The answer is a resounding *Yes!* You must be fluent in the different languages of the test. You cannot do well on the MCAT if you don't know the basics of physics, general chemistry, biology, and organic chemistry. We recommend that you take one year each of biology, general chemistry, organic chemistry, and physics prior to taking the MCAT, and that you review the content in this book thoroughly. Knowing these basics is just the beginning of doing well on the MCAT. That's a shock to most test takers. They presume that once they recall or relearn their undergraduate science, they are ready to do battle against the MCAT. Wrong! They merely have directions to the battlefield. They lack what they need to beat the test: a copy of the test maker's battle plan!

You won't be drilled on facts and formulas on the MCAT. You'll need to demonstrate ability to reason based on ideas and concepts. The science questions are painted with a broad brush, testing your general understanding.

TAKE CONTROL: THE MCAT MINDSET

In addition to being a thinking test, as we've stressed, the MCAT is a standardized test. As such, it has its own consistent patterns and idiosyncrasies that can actually work in your favor. This is the key to why test preparation works. You have the opportunity to familiarize yourself with those consistent peculiarities, to adopt the proper test-taking mindset.

The MCAT Mindset is something you want to bring to every question, passage, and section you encounter. Being in the MCAT Mindset means reshaping the test-taking experience so that you are in the driver's seat:

- Answer questions *when* you want to—feel free to skip tough but doable passages and questions, coming back to them only after you've racked up points on easy ones.
- Answer questions *how* you want to—use our shortcuts and methods to get points quickly and confidently, even if those methods aren't exactly what the test makers had in mind when they wrote the test.

The following are some overriding principles of the MCAT Mindset that will be covered in depth in the chapters to come:

- Read actively and critically.
- Translate prose into your own words.
- Save the toughest questions and passages for last.
- Know the test and its components inside and out.
- Do MCAT-style problems in each topic area after you've reviewed it.
- Allow your confidence to build on itself.
- Take full-length practice tests a week or two before the test to break down the mystique of the real experience.
- Learn from your mistakes—get the most out of your practice tests.
- Look at the MCAT as a challenge, the first step in your medical career, rather than as an arbitrary obstacle.

KAPLAN

And that's what the MCAT Mindset boils down to: Taking control. Being proactive. Being on top of the testing experience so that you can get as many points as you can as quickly and as easily as possible. Keep this in mind as you read and work through the material in this book and, of course, as you face the challenge on test day.

Now that you have a better idea of what the MCAT is all about, let's take a tour of the individual test sections. Although the underlying skills being tested are similar, each MCAT section requires that you call into play a different domain of knowledge. So, though we encourage you to think of the MCAT as a holistic and unified test, we also recognize that the test is segmented by discipline and that there are characteristics unique to each section. In the overviews, we'll review sample questions and answers and discuss section-specific strategies. For each of the sections—Verbal Reasoning, Physical/Biological Sciences, and the Writing Sample—we'll present you with the following:

- THE BIG PICTURE
  You'll get a clear view of the section and familiarize yourself with what it's really evaluating.

- A CLOSER LOOK
  You'll explore the types of questions that will appear and master the strategies you'll need to deal with them successfully.

- KAPLAN TIPS
  The key approaches to each section are outlined, for reinforcement and quick review.

Verbal Reasoning

2

- Practice "taking possession" of Verbal Reasoning passages by reading actively
- Learn strategies for answering each of the six Verbal Reasoning question types

THE BIG PICTURE

The Verbal Reasoning section is perhaps the most recognizable section of the MCAT, since it's similar to the reading comprehension sections of other standardized tests. It's 85 minutes long and typically consists of about 9 passages, with anywhere from 6 to 9 questions per passage, for a total of 60 multiple-choice questions. The passages, often complex, are drawn from the social sciences, philosophy, and other humanistic disciplines as well as from the natural sciences.

The Verbal Reasoning section tests your ability to:

- Read critically and actively
- "Possess" or truly comprehend written material
- Capture the essence of a passage by recognizing its main idea
- Intuit a writer's tone
- Draw inferences/conclusions

The passages you'll confront on test day probably won't be fun to read. Odds are, they'll be boring. If they're too engaging, check the cover. You may be taking the wrong test. As part of the challenge, you must be able to concentrate and glean meaning regardless of the nature of the text. This will involve working through your resistance to dry passages and overcoming any anxiety or frustration. The more control you can muster, the quicker you can move through each passage, through the questions, and to a higher score. Remember, Verbal Reasoning isn't there to entertain you or provide relief from the science, but to put you through a mental obstacle course.

DO YOU NEED TO STUDY FOR VERBAL REASONING?

Don't make the mistake that so many MCAT participants make in underestimating the challenge of the Verbal Reasoning section. Sometimes it falls under the shadow cast by the looming science sections. Also, students figure that there isn't anything to "study" for this section. Be aware that the scoring gradient for Verbal Reasoning is very steep. It's hard to get a good score, so you can't afford to be cavalier. Some medical schools add all your MCAT scores together for a composite score—if you blow off Verbal Reasoning, you could kill your composite. Practice Verbal Reasoning as you would the other test sections, and challenge yourself to acquire the specialized reading skills required on the MCAT.

HOW TO READ ACTIVELY

Usually we read for entertainment or information. Rarely do we read critically, to understand how the writer organizes ideas and uses detail to support themes. MCAT Verbal Reasoning requires that you abandon standard reading habits and take on the role of a critical, or active, reader. This means that you create a mental model of the passage while you're reading, capturing each idea the author constructs and making it part of your vision of the passage.

This can happen only if you resist feeling overwhelmed by the themes in the passage. If you're too awed by the author or bored by the subject matter, you won't be able to take possession of the passage. This notion of "taking possession" is the key to active reading. It means that you keep a distance from the words, and that you remain analytical rather than get emotional.

Your goal from the outset of the passage is to figure out what the author is saying and how the ideas are linked. Every passage contains one main idea. You can usually figure it out in the first few lines of the passage, and redefine your sense of it as you move through the passage. When you're done reading, you should be able to state the main idea in your own words. Being an active reader implies that you constantly ask yourself what the author intends and how that intention is conveyed and supported. Successfully answering the questions depends on your ability to quickly glean the author's point, to map out the passage in your mind, and to assess the inferences.

Pay Attention to Structure

The structure of each passage can help you organize a mental map. You know, for example, that each paragraph will explore a new angle of the main idea or provide detail associated with a key idea. The MCAT Verbal Reasoning passages are, for the most part, logical in their construction. They may contain complicated words or ideas, but their structure is very manageable, even predictable. Look for certain keywords (e.g., *consequently*) or phrases (e.g., *on the other hand*) that hold ideas together and can alert you as to what's ahead in the passage.

Some test takers feel more anchored as they read the passage if they've scoped out the questions first. As a rule, it won't save you time or effort to do so. Most of the questions will require that you demonstrate a general understanding of the passage's main idea and overall construction—neither of which can be derived from any particular section of the passage. You need to read for meaning and for organization whether or not you've reviewed the questions.

A CLOSER LOOK

Here's a chance to begin familiarizing yourself with Verbal Reasoning passages and questions, to learn how to approach them. You'll have more opportunities to practice this section in the practice tests in sections two and three of this book; for now we want to open your eyes to structure and strategy.

SAMPLE PASSAGE AND QUESTIONS

As you read through the MCAT-style passage below, try to articulate the main idea to yourself. Read actively and critically. Consider what the author is trying to say and how the ideas are communicated. You might want to pause between paragraphs to digest what you've read and put the ideas into your own words. In a real MCAT situation, you'll need to be time-conscious while you read. For now, just go at whatever pace feels comfortable to you. Keep in mind that the passages you'll see on the MCAT can come from history, philosophy, the arts, and other disciplines, and can vary in length and complexity. The passages are adapted from published sources (though the sources won't be identified on the page); this passage comes from *Smithsonian* magazine:

In 1948, *Look* magazine polled America's art critics and major artists, among them Edward Hopper, Stuart Davis, and Charles Burchfield, for a consensus on the creative spirit who could be pro-
Line nounced the best of the age. It is a fair measure of the art establish-
5 ment's limited attention span that a generation after John Marin was crowned prince of painters by his peers, his name had begun to fade. New styles raced in to seize the interest of the gallery and museum worlds; fashion embraced Abstract Expressionism, then thrilled to the distancing imagery of Pop Art and later, for about five minutes, went
10 gaga over a frail phenomenon labeled Op Art. To be sure, Marin's death in 1953 was the occasion for lavish obituary tributes. But mention him today to a reasonably literate American or a cultured, well-traveled European and, likely as not, the response will be a puzzled stare.

That is not only odd but hard to understand. Marin's legacy
15 embraces more than 3,000 works, many of them memorable. There are prime etchings, splendid if demanding oils and, in the main, watercol-ors—2,500 of them, amazing in color, design, and complexity. He seemed to have set down everything in a transport of excitement, as if he were recording themes for a fevered gavotte. Indeed, he once wrote
20 of the acts of drawing and painting as "a sort of mad wonder dancing."

Everything that came from Marin's loving hand radiated spontaneity. Here, it appeared, was a natural, creative spirit, a lucky man who was freed, rather than constrained, by his magnanimous imagination. In truth, hardly anything Marin turned out was unre-
25 hearsed. The paintings which hinted at the impetuosity of an artist

struggling to convey the "warring, pushing, pulling forces" of his surroundings were, as often as not, studio works. Even his letters, with
their blithe disregard for punctuation, were discovered to be the results
of many drafts.

30   As a husband and father, Marin lived a life of singular regu-
larity. He had one wife and, as far as anyone knows, no extramarital
entanglements. When he put away his paints at the end of his working day, Marin became a man of simple, harmless pleasures. Late pictures show a wiry-looking figure with a long, thin Yankee nose, the
35   parched skin of a farmer, and a humorous mouth that often held a cig-
arette. No one ever saw him down more drink than was good for his
speech or balance. His idea of fun was a good game of billiards.

The contrast between the art and the man who made it was
extreme, fascinating, and a trifle baffling. Marin's pictures were dar-
40   ing, the work of a sophisticated eye, an unfailing imagination, a vir-
tuoso hand; some of them verge on elegant abstraction, although he
looked down on abstract art. He hated efforts to interpret his art—or
for that matter anyone else's. The attitude is not uncommon to artists,
particularly American artists, but Marin's distrust of the critical and
45   academic establishments verged on the fanatic. "Intellectuals," he once
pronounced, "have in their makeup a form of Nazism."

1. The main point of the passage is to:

    A. explain why John Marin's work was virtually forgotten after his death.

    B. consider the contrast between Marin's artistic style and his personal life and habits.

    C. argue that the art establishment was unable to reach a consensus on the "best of the age" because of its limited attention span.

    D. suggest that Marin's vivacious watercolors were a reaction against Nazism in the art world.

2. Of the following, the author of the passage is most likely:

    A. a contemporary painter.

    B. a magazine art critic.

    C. an investigative reporter.

    D. a museum curator.

3. The author refers to Op Art (line 10) in order to:

   A. place Marin's art within a specific category or genre.

   B. identify the origins of Marin's artistic style.

   C. emphasize the fleeting popularity of artistic styles.

   D. compare Marin's stylistic simplicity with later psychedelic trends.

4. The author's attitude toward Marin may be described as one of:

   A. grudging approval.

   B. playful irreverence.

   C. flippant disrespect.

   D. reverent appreciation.

5. The passage discusses all of the following aspects of Marin's life EXCEPT his:

   A. political beliefs.

   B. physical appearance.

   C. artistic style.

   D. family life.

6. In saying that intellectuals "have in their makeup a form of Nazism," (line 46), Marin most probably means that:

   A. the academic establishment is clearly fascist in its structure.

   B. intellectuals often have leftist political and social leanings.

   C. critics often misread extremist political messages in the works of artists.

   D. the criticism and interpretation of art represents a sort of tyranny.

7. The author characterizes Marin's work as:

   A. fevered and energetic.

   B. simple and colorful.

   C. constrained and precise.

   D. tortured and impenetrable.

8. The author characterizes Marin's paintings as "studio works" in line 27 in order to make the point that:

   A. Marin's painting exhibit the influences of many studio artists.

   B. despite attempts at objectivity, Marin's works expressed the academic biases of his time.

   C. although Marin's work seemed spontaneous, it was the result of precise crafting.

   D. Marin's paintings never reflected his complexity and vivid imagination.

Did You Catch the Main Idea?

The author's intent was to contrast John Marin's flamboyant artistic style with his subdued personal life. We get the first hint of this theme in the second paragraph, where the author describes the ostensible mechanism by which Marin created his art ("mad wonder dancing"). The idea is further developed in the next paragraph, where we get the sense that the process through which Marin produced art was not as it seemed ("In truth, hardly anything Marin turned out was unrehearsed"). The fourth paragraph describes the subject's personal life, showing it to be as dull as his art was wild. The last paragraph begins with a clear statement of the passage's main idea; the rest of the paragraph solidifies the intent of the passage.

There's more to understanding the passage than just being able to figure out the main idea. You have to construct a mental outline of the structure of the passage so you'll be able to refer back to it while you answer the questions. The questions following a passage test your understanding of the passage, its structure, its implications, and its tone. It's important that you gather information about the passage as you read so you'll be able to answer the questions quickly and confidently.

Answer Review

1. **B**

    Choice (B) has the proper scope to reflect the main idea. Choice (A) makes reference to a minor point in the first paragraph, Choice (C) distorts an idea from the passage and magnifies a detail, and Choice (D) connects two ideas presented separately.

2. **B**

    The citation after the passage and the general tone of the writing suggest that "magazine art critic" is most fitting. Were the writer a painter, we would expect more information about the artwork. An investigative reporter would have a confrontational tone. Finally, we might expect that a museum curator would focus more on Marin's artwork and its effect on the public rather than on the relation between his art and his life.

3. **C**

    Go back to the passage to find the reference. We find it in conjunction with the writer's implication that the art world has a short attention span. This is most consistent with Choice (C). Choices (A) and (B) mistakenly connect Op Art to the work of Marin, a connection the author does not make in the passage. Choice (D) assumes a comparison also not drawn from the passage.

4. **D**

    Only Choice (D) matches the overall tone of the passage. Most tone questions have adjectives and nouns in the answer choices. Remember that both must match the passage for the choice to be correct.

5. **A**

    This type of question requires that you find an exception. Choice (A)—political beliefs—is the only aspect among the answer choices not discussed in the passage. If you misinterpreted Marin's "Nazi" quote as being political instead of philosophical, you might have had a hard time answering this question.

6. **D**

Here, you must show that you interpreted the quote correctly. Marin used the phrase *Nazism* to describe a repressive, tyrannical system of criticism—not a political attitude. Only Choice (D) resonates with the metaphorical interpretation of the phrase.

7. **A**

The answer can't be found in a particular line from the passage. You must conclude the best answer based on the attitude and tone of the passage. Choice (A) accurately reflects the writer's characterizations of Marin's work. Choice (B) might be tempting because the writer does describe Marin as simple, but in his personal life, not in reference to his art. Choice (C) describes Marin's life as depicted by the author but has no connection to his art. Finally, Choice (D) conveys too much negativity to match the tone of the passage.

8. **C**

Refer to the line referenced in the question stem to see how the sentence functions in the passage. We see that the author was trying to suggest that despite their seeming spontaneity, Marin's paintings were actually quite "crafted." Choice (C) is thus consistent with the intent of the passage. Choice (A) is a tricky interpretation of the sentence. Choice (B) sounds erudite, but it has no relation to the passage whatsoever. Lastly, Choice (D) makes an illogical leap to conclude that Marin's paintings showed no imagination, but the passage never suggests this is the case.

SIX QUESTION TYPES

There are six Verbal Reasoning question styles you'll find on the MCAT: Main Idea, Detail, Inference, Application, Tone, and Logic. Familiarity with the question types helps you anticipate the kinds of answers you should be choosing. The ability to anticipate correct answers will speed up your testing time, give you extra confidence, and ultimately boost your score!

1. Main Idea

Description: Main Idea questions ask for a restatement of the author's main point, the primary idea, or the overall gist of the passage. Question 1 in the preceding sample is a Main Idea question, because it's asking you for the point of the Marin excerpt.

Strategy: Look for the answer choice that best matches the scope of the main theme. Wrong answers will be either too narrow or too broad in their restatement of the author's main point, or will distort it in some way.

Strategy Applied: If you look for the "big idea" of the preceding sample passage as you read it, you see that your interpretation of the author's purpose matches only one answer choice, that there was a sharp contrast between Marin's artistic style and personal life.

2. Detail

Description: Detail questions require you to recall a specific point from the passage or to relocate it using information from the question stem. Correct answer choices will be those that approximate information directly from the passage. One type of Detail question—"Scattered Detail"—will ask you to consider many details from various places in the passage and may ask you to identify a detail as an exception among the answer choices. For example: "The author uses as evidence all the following EXCEPT . . . ." Question 5 in the preceding sample is a Scattered Detail question, because it requires that you recall or look back to the passage to determine a characteristic of Marin's life that is not mentioned.

Strategy: Refer to any notes you made in the margin or to notes in your mental outline to identify the detail under consideration. If the question is in the "all except" format, you should be looking for the exception, for the choice that fits the stimulus. By all means, look back to the passage. You're not supposed to memorize details!

Strategy Applied: In the case of the sample, you're looking for the exception, so you should ask yourself, "Does this fit the stimulus?" for each answer choice. The answer is "no" for only one—the passage does not discuss Marin's political beliefs.

3. Inference

Description: Inference questions ask you to make a small logical leap from the passage to another idea that would be consistent with the main idea. Correct answers to Inference questions will have the proper degree of "distance" from the passage itself—not so close as to be a detail but not so far as to be illogical.

Strategy: Choose an answer that is consistent with the passage but is not a simple restatement of information already presented.

Strategy Applied: There wasn't an Inference question in the sample, but let's say that you were asked how Marin's work was affected by critical interpretation. Since you're told that Marin did not like interpretation of his or anyone else's art, you can infer that he would not adjust his art to suit the critics, that his work would be unaffected.

4. Application

Description: Application questions ask you to take an essential idea from the passage and relate it to a different context. These questions may set up analogies or metaphors; you'll need to figure out how they relate to one another and determine which one presents an idea that parallels the passage. Question 2 in the sample is an Application question, because it asks you to use what you know about the passage to guess at the source of the passage.

Strategy: Pick an answer choice that effectively "translates" an idea from the passage into a new context or scenario.

Strategy Applied: Taking what you know about the sample passage (the author's point of view and tone) and applying this to a scenario outside the passage (the source of the piece), you can judge that the author was most likely a magazine art critic.

5. Tone

Description: Questions of Tone require you to identify the author's attitude or opinion about a passage's subject matter. Such questions may be focused on a detail or may refer to the tone of the whole passage. Question 4 from the sample passage is an example of a Tone question, because it asks you to determine the author's attitude.

Strategy: Go with the answer choice that is consistent with your "gut feel" from the passage—positive, neutral, or negative.

Strategy Applied: Based on the first paragraph in the sample passage, you know that the author holds Marin in high esteem, so the correct answer about the author's tone will have to reflect a completely positive attitude. Only one choice does so.

6. Logic

Description: Logic questions require that you analyze the function of certain portions of the passage. You may be asked how a particular detail serves the purpose of the passage, or you may be asked about overall passage structure. A Logic question is derived from the overall plan and layout of the passage—not from the specifics contained within the passage. Question 8 in the sample is a Logic question, because it asks you about the logical structure of the passage.

Strategy: Refer to your mental map and passage outline, the source of all logic questions. Choose an answer that maintains the integrity of your passage blueprint.

Strategy Applied: In the sample, you're asked to determine the meaning of the term *studio works*. To do so, you need to read a few sentences back from the term and figure out its context. You clearly see, then, that "studio works" refers to artistic pieces crafted out of a deliberate process.

KAPLAN TIPS

GETTING OFF ON THE RIGHT FOOT

- You don't have to do the passages in order. Do the easiest early on, leaving the intimidating or unfamiliar for last. Also, look for the passages with more questions, and do those first to maximize points.
- You usually won't save time by scanning the questions before reading the passage, since most of the questions are based on a holistic understanding of the passage. Besides, having the questions in mind can distract you from focusing on the passage.
- Read the opening lines of each paragraph slowly and carefully to "orient" yourself to the subject matter and its main point.
- Read for the Main Idea, often but not always expressed in the opening lines.

READING THE PASSAGES

- Read actively!
- Don't get emotional. Read with distance.
- Don't judge the passages. You'll need to overcome the hurdle of reading material that doesn't interest you.
- Create a mental map.
- Feel free to make notes in the margin.
- Don't try to memorize details. Know the purpose of the detail, not the detail itself.
- Look for structural keywords to help you anticipate new ideas in the passage.
- Check the citation at the end of the passage. It may give clues about tone or context.

FACING THE QUESTIONS

- When you're finished reading, don't rush to the questions. Take a moment to rephrase the main idea to yourself.
- Remember that wrong answer choices will distort or reverse the author's main point, blow a detail out of proportion, confuse or misplace details, or be totally irrational. Use a process of elimination to increase your chances of getting to the right answer.
- You should look back at the passage to find or clarify details while you're answering the questions.
- Answer questions based on the passage—not based on outside knowledge.
- If you don't know an answer, guess! Try to do so while you're still working on the passage, so you won't have to reread it later. There's no penalty for wrong answers.

USING THE GRID

- If time is running out and there are blank spaces on your grid, by all means, guess.
- Be careful marking your answer grid—especially if you're not answering the questions in numerical order.

Physical and Biological Sciences

3

- Find out why abstract thinking is much more important than memorization on the MCAT
- Review the content areas you can expect to find on the actual MCAT
- Learn key strategies to help you answer both passage-based questions and stand-alone questions

THE BIG PICTURE

The two science sections on the MCAT—Physical and Biological—are similar in their format, though their content obviously differs. In each 100-minute section you'll find about 10–11 passages, each followed by 4 to 8 multiple-choice questions (for a total of 62), and 15 stand-alone multiple-choice questions (also referred to as *discretes*)—not based on any passage. The Physical Sciences section is comprised of physics and general chemistry, approximately evenly divided in content though mixed throughout the section. The Biological Sciences section consists of biology and organic chemistry questions mixed throughout, with greater emphasis on biology (about 50–60 percent biology, 40–50 percent organic chemistry).

The passages, each 250–300 words in length, will describe experiments, situations, or ideas from which questions are drawn. The information may be presented in the guise of journal or textbook articles, experimental research, data analysis, or scientific-style editorials. When reading the science passages, you should think about extracting *information*—not meaning and structure as in Verbal Reasoning. Consider the passages to be data that you must interpret and understand so as to be able to apply it to the specific needs of the questions. The passage-and-question structure allows you to demonstrate many skills, among them:

- Understanding the science presented in the passage, no matter how obscure or foreign to you
- Confidently connecting elements of your scientific "repertoire" to new situations
- Quickly assessing the kinds of situations feasible given the information in the passage

The stand-alone questions will draw on your knowledge of particular concepts or themes in the respective sciences. They're "wild cards" in the sense that you cannot group them together in any formal way; in fact, they appear scattered throughout the sections. Ranging in scope from a quantitative problem to a conceptual thought experiment, they are the test maker's way of randomly tapping into your knowledge base.

THE MCAT ATTITUDE

It's important to approach both science sections with the same mindset: MCAT science is just a window into your mind. The test makers are trying to see how you reason, how you solve problems, and how well you command your knowledge. They are not after a data dump from your core memory. It's crucial that you demonstrate conceptual understanding of scientific material and show proficiency in applying scientific themes in new situations. This is the kind of mental flexibility that will get you a great MCAT score.

Abstract Thinking

Another way to describe flexibility is as a form of abstraction. To think abstractly is to lift ideas out of a specific context and place them in a new context. It's a skill that allows you passage into seemingly unfamiliar territory, and on the MCAT that could mean the question around the corner. In the science sections, this skill is tested repeatedly.

For example, passages may provide hypothetical scenarios or describe experiments you've never seen before. You'll need to take the unfamiliar and make it familiar, and that's where abstract thinking comes in. If you understand the basic framework of experimental design and scientific method, you won't be overwhelmed by a specific unfamiliar context. You'll be able to "rise above" the details rather than get tripped up by them.

What About Formulas and Math?

Contrary to what you may presume, the MCAT is not a math-intensive test. Despite the scientific language on the MCAT, there is nothing more mathematically complex than algebra, exponents, logs, and a little bit of trig. There is no calculus, differential equations, or matrix mechanics. You may need to recall sine and cosine for standard angles, though such values are provided if necessary. That's it! No higher math.

Similarly, many of the scientific formulas necessary to work through problems and answer questions will be provided on the test. This is just an indicator of how negligible is the value of "straight memorization." You gain little by having every nitty-gritty formula easily accessible unless you also have a broad understanding of what the formulas mean, what they imply, what their units indicate, how they relate to one another, and how to navigate among them.

In light of our discussion of concept-based testing, it makes sense that the MCAT will not reward you merely for the "brute force" of memorization. There will rarely be an opportunity on the MCAT to algebraically crunch away on a formula. The information you're given won't fit neatly into formulas. If it did, the MCAT would be nothing but a memory-and-algebra test. And, as we've discussed, it is much more. Again, you should not be concerned with memorizing formulas. You should be concerned with *understanding* formulas. The key point is that once you understand the scientific concepts behind a formula, you hardly need the formula itself anymore. Though this applies mostly to physics and chemistry, the underlying theme is relevant for both science sections: Think, don't compute!

A CLOSER LOOK

What follows is a review of the content areas you can expect to find in the science sections of the MCAT. This is not to suggest that your MCAT will actually cover all of these topics; instead, use this list as a guideline of the content that could possibly show up. All of these concepts are covered in detail in Kaplan's *MCAT Comprehensive Review* book.

PHYSICAL SCIENCES

Physics

- Basic Units/Kinematics
- Newtonian Mechanics
- Force and Inertia
- Thermodynamics
- Fluids/Solids
- Electrostatics
- Magnetism
- Circuits
- Periodic Motion, Waves, Sound
- Light and Optics
- Atomic Phenomena
- Nuclear Physics

General Chemistry

- Quantum Numbers
- Hund's Rule/Electron Configuration
- Periodic Table
- Reaction Types
- Balancing Equations
- Bonding
- Formal Charge/VSEPR Theory
- Intermolecular Forces
- Chemical Kinetics/Equilibrium
- Thermodynamics/Entropy
- Ideal Gas Law

- Phases of Matter
- Solutions
- Acids and Bases
- Electrochemistry

BIOLOGICAL SCIENCES

Biology

- Eukaryotic and Prokaryotic Cells
- Membrane Traffic
- Cell Division—Mitosis and Meiosis
- Embryogenesis
- Enzymatic Activity
- Cellular Metabolism
- Muscular and Skeletal Systems
- Digestive System
- Respiratory and Circulatory Systems
- Lymphatic System
- Immune System
- Homeostasis
- Endocrine System
- Nervous System
- Molecular Genetics/Inheritance
- Viruses
- Evolution

Organic Chemistry

- Nomenclature
- Stereochemistry
- Mechanisms
- Carboxylic Acids
- Amines
- Spectroscopy
- Carbohydrates and Lipids

- Hydrolysis and Dehydration
- Amino Acids and Proteins
- Oxygen-containing Compounds
- Hydrocarbons
- Laboratory Techniques
- IR and NMR Spectroscopy

SAMPLE PASSAGE AND QUESTIONS

This is probably your first chance to see what the passages, passage-based questions, and stand-alone questions will look like in the science sections. An answer key is provided, but try to work through these samples without consulting it. We'll use the following passage and questions to highlight general strategies. You'll find more MCAT-style practice questions in the practice tests found in section two of this workbook.

Passage

A physics class is attempting to measure the acceleration due to gravity, g, by throwing balls out of classroom windows. They performed the following two experiments:

Experiment 1

Two class members lean out of different windows at the same height, h = 5.2 m, above the ground and drop two different balls. One ball is made out of lead and has a mass of 5 kg. The other ball is made out of plastic and has a mass of 1 kg. The students measure the velocity of the lead ball just before impact with the ground and find it to be 10 m/s. They also find that when the plastic ball hits the ground it bounces, and its momentum changes by 18 kg × m/s.

Experiment 2

Instead of dropping the plastic ball, a student throws the ball out of a higher window and observes its projectile motion. The ball is thrown from a height of 10 m above the ground with a velocity of 4 m/s directed at an angle of 30° above the horizontal. (Note: Assume that the air resistance is negligible unless otherwise stated.)

Passage-Based Questions

1. The students did not account for air resistance in their measurement of g in Experiment 1. How does the value of g they obtained compare to the actual value of g?

    A. The value of g obtained in Experiment 1 is greater than the actual value of g because air resistance increases the time it takes the balls to fall from the windows to the ground.

    B. The value of g obtained in Experiment 1 is greater than the actual value of g because air resistance decreases the kinetic energy of the balls just before impact.

    C. The value of g obtained in Experiment 1 is less than the actual value of g because air resistance decreases the velocity of the balls just before impact.

    D. The value of g obtained in Experiment 1 is less than the actual value of g because air resistance decreases the time it takes the balls to fall from the windows to the ground.

2. Which of the following would change the measured value of g in Experiment 1?

    I.   Increasing the mass of the earth

    II. Using balls having a different mass but the same volume

    III. Throwing the balls horizontally instead of dropping them vertically

    A. I only

    B. III only

    C. I and II only

    D. II and III only

3. In Experiment 1, the change in momentum that the plastic ball experiences when it bounces off the ground does NOT depend on: (Note: Assume that the collision is perfectly elastic.)

    A. the velocity of the ball just before impact.

    B. the mass of the ball.

    C. the mass of Earth.

    D. the volume of the ball.

4. In Experiment 2, what was the maximum height above the window reached by the plastic ball? (Note: The acceleration due to gravity is $g = 9.8$ m/s^2, sin 30° = 0.50, and cos 30° = 0.866.)

    A. 10.2 cm

    B. 20.4 cm

    C. 30.6 cm

    D. 61.2 cm

5. In a third experiment, a student throws the lead ball out of the same window used in Experiment 1 with a velocity of 3 m/s in the horizontal direction. What is the ratio of the work done by gravity on the lead ball in the first experiment to the work done by gravity on the ball in the third experiment?

   A. 1:1

   B. 1:3

   C. 1:9

   D. 3:1

Stand-Alone Questions

6. In the figure below, the velocity vector of a particle is represented at successive times t. Which of the following best represents the acceleration vector?

   $$\xrightarrow{\hspace{2cm}} \xrightarrow{\hspace{1cm}} \rightarrow \leftarrow \xleftarrow{\hspace{1cm}} \xleftarrow{\hspace{2cm}}$$
   $$t = 0 \qquad t = 1 \quad t = 2 \quad t = 3 \quad t = 4 \qquad t = 5$$

   A. $\longrightarrow$

   B. $\longleftarrow$

   C.   The acceleration changes direction.

   D.   The acceleration is zero.

7. All of the following statements are true of most transition elements EXCEPT:

   A. they have partially filled d subshells.

   B. they have extremely high ionization energies.

   C. they exhibit metallic character.

   D. they have multiple oxidation states.

8. A patient is taking a drug that has the side effect of being a sympathetic nervous system inhibitor. Which of the following would most likely be seen as a result of this drug?

   A. Decreased bowel motility

   B. Decreased heart rate

   C. Increased pupil diameter

   D. Increased blood supply to skeletal muscles

Were You Able to Think Abstractly?

Did you get bogged down in details, or were you able to rise above them? Were you able to come up with your own answers before looking at the choices? As you review the following answer explanations you'll be able to assess your performance and pick up important strategies.

ANSWER REVIEW

Passage

The passage describes a series of experiments performed by some students. As you read, you should be making notes in the margins or underlining important information (i.e., the height = 5.2 meters, mass = 5 kg, etcetera). You might make a chart to list out the respective "given" data for each experiment:

Experiment 1	Experiment 2
2 balls	*height*
masses for each	*initial velocity*
height	*angle above horizon*
final velocity for lead ball	
plastic ball: change in momentum	

Passage-Based Questions

1. C

This is a question you could answer without reference to the passage. It's really asking about how a measurement of g would change depending on whether or not air resistance is considered (with all other variables presumed constant). Since air resistance is a force working in the opposite direction from gravity, it's a force of resistance, like friction. Therefore, it slows down the motion of the ball, making it take longer to fall the same distance. Thus the velocity just before impact decreases when air resistance is considered. We know that g is proportional to the square of the velocity (from solving for g in $v^2 = v_0^2 + 2ad$, where a would be g, and d would be the height). If the velocity is less (because the ball takes more time to travel the same distance if we consider air resistance), then g will also be less than the measured value. This line of reasoning rules out choices (A) and (B). choice (D) says that air resistance *decreases* the time it takes for the ball to fall. But we just discussed that resistance *adds* to the time for travel. So, choice (C) is correct.

Key Strategy: A chart helps you organize what you know from the passage, so you can access the information quickly while answering the questions. Remember, you're reading for data—not for meaning or structure. Be sure, however, that you understand the context of every piece of data you collect.

Key Strategy: Don't read more complexity into a question than is there. In some cases, passage-based questions will actually be testing in a stand-alone style, with little or no reference back to the passage.

2.   **A**

This Roman numeral–style question asks about what factors would change the measured value of g in the first experiment. Be careful to consider only the information from Experiment 1 when answering this question.

Let's consider the first statement. If it's wrong, then you can eliminate any answer choice that has it listed. If you decide it is true, then you must choose an answer that includes it in its list of numerals. In the first experiment, the students neglected air resistance, so we have only gravity to consider. The first statement requires that we think about how g is related to the mass of the earth. You should recall that the gravitational force between an object and the earth is $F = GmM/R^2$, where G is the universal gravitational constant, m is the mass of the object, M is the mass of the earth, and R is the distance between. But remember also that the weight of an object $= mg$. We can equate these two forces ($GmM/R^2 = mg$) to solve for $g = GM/R^2$. Therefore, changing the mass of the earth would indeed change the value of g. So, Statement I is true, and you can eliminate choices (B) and (D). Now we need only consider Statement II to decide between (A) and (C). Let's look at Statement II. It says that using balls with different mass but the same volume would change g. We know that in Experiment 1, the students ignored air resistance, so the volume of the balls is not relevant. What about the mass? Well, we saw above that g is independent of the object's mass. So, Statement II is not true and choice (A) is correct.

If you were unsure about Statement I, though, you'd have to work through Statement III to decide which answer choice is correct. The key to the third statement is realizing that vertical trajectory will be unchanged by any initial horizontal velocity. The same vertical force—gravity—will be at work. So, Statement III is untrue, confirming (A) as the correct answer choice.

Key Strategy: Use the structure of a Roman numeral question to your advantage! Eliminate choices as soon as you find them to be inconsistent with the truth or falsehood of a statement in the stimulus. Similarly, consider only those choices that include a statement that you've already determined to be true.

Key Strategy: You don't have to consider the statements in order. Knowing about any one of them will get you off to a great start answering the question, so if you're unsure about the first statement, go on to the second or third.

3.   **D**

This question asks which variable is *not* a factor in determining the change in momentum for the plastic ball in Experiment 1. You'll be looking for the answer choice that does not play a role in the momentum shift. One of the first things to note is that you're given a hint about the collision between the ball and the ground—it is elastic, implying that both kinetic energy and momentum are conserved during the collision. The question stimulus tells you, then, that at the time of impact, the two surfaces act like solid, hard surfaces (like billiard balls) with no energy lost to the collision.

Since the mass of the ball doesn't change, its change in momentum is dependent on its change in velocity. So change in momentum = $mv_{final} - mv_{initial}$. In considering the answer choices, however, there is no need to painstakingly step through calculations. There is one choice that jumps out as inconsistent. Choice (D) mentions a variable—the volume of the ball—which has no bearing on the ball's change in momentum. All the other choices mention variables which are relevant in considering the change in momentum of the ball as it hits the earth.

Key Strategy: Don't do more work than you have to on the test. Work smart. The MCAT rewards test takers who can save time by seeing a creative strategy (i.e., looking for a variable that's not relevant rather than plodding though every choice, solving equations, and wasting time).

4.   B

Be careful to read the question. It asks for the maximum height above the window reached by the plastic ball in Experiment 2. Thus, we're looking for the maximum height above the window. We know that at the instant the maximum height is attained, the vertical velocity will be 0 (that's when the ball stops and turns around to fall back to the ground). From the passage, we know that the ball's initial velocity is 4 meters per second at an angle of 30°. The initial vertical velocity component is $4 \times \sin 30°$, or $4 \times \frac{1}{2}$, which is 2 meters per second. Using kinematics, we know that $v_f^2 - v_0^2 = 2ay$, where v_f is the final velocity, v_0 is the initial velocity, a is the constant acceleration, and y is the distance. We know that $v_f = 0$ meters per second, $v_0 = 2$ meters per second, and we can estimate a which is the acceleration of gravity to be -10 meters per second squared. So $0^2 - 2^2 = 2(-10)y$, $-4 = -20y$, and y maximum $= \frac{1}{5} = 0.2$ meters or 20 centimeters. This is closest to choice (B), the correct answer. The height of the window doesn't even come into play. Notice that choice (D) derives from using the cosine rather than sine of 30° to find the vertical component of velocity. Choice (A) results from a simple calculation error. Choice (C) is incorrect as well.

Key Strategy: Estimate whenever you can to save time.

Key Strategy: Don't get flustered by unnecessary information. In this case, you had more information than you needed to solve the problem. Don't just plug in numbers and hope for a match. Think before you calculate!

5.   A

You're asked for a ratio. The implication is that some component of the problem is not solvable, so don't expect to work with actual numbers. In this case, you need to compare the work done in two different scenarios. We need to know that work is force through a distance, or $F \times d$. Since gravity works only along the vertical axis, we need to know the vertical distance traveled by both balls to compare the work done. In both cases, the ball drops 5.2 meters. The ball mentioned in the question has some horizontal velocity, but this has no bearing on the vertical dynamics. So, the distance traveled by the balls in the two different experiments is the same. Furthermore, because the mass is identical, the work done is the same. So, the ratio is 1:1, or choice (A).

Key Strategy: In many cases with ratio questions, you will not be able to solve for actual numbers. You may have to work with relationships, fractions, and formulas to arrive at the solution.

Key Strategy: We reviewed these questions in order, but you don't have to do the questions order. Start with the ones that seem most feasible and leave the ones that seem difficult or time intensive for last.

Stand-Alone Questions

6.   **B**

This question is a great example of how the MCAT rewards the careful thinker. You're told that the vectors represent successive measurements of velocity for a particle. You're then asked which answer choice best represents the acceleration vector. Without having actual numbers to work with, you have to be able to construct a relationship between velocity and acceleration and "visualize" that relationship using vectors. The way to approach this question is to ask yourself, "What is the connection between velocity and acceleration?" Once you answer that, you can begin to home in on an appropriate answer choice. So, what *is* the relationship? Recall that, dimensionally, acceleration is velocity per unit time or displacement per time squared. Theoretically speaking, acceleration is the *rate of change of velocity through a period of time.*

So, the answer choice will be a vector that matches the general rate of change amongst the given velocity vectors. At *t* = 0, the velocity is positive and at a maximum. At *t* = 1, it is still positive but the magnitude has decreased, indicating a *deceleration*. At *t* = 2, the velocity is still positive but is diminished in magnitude even more. What the vectors are describing is a particle, mass, car, thing, object, whatever, slowing down. At *t* = 3, something that looks a little tricky happens: The velocity becomes negative but with the same magnitude as *t* = 2. The object we're tracking has changed direction from "forward" to "reverse." The trend continues through *t* = 4 and *t* = 5; we see that the particle is going faster (greater magnitude) but in the opposite direction from its original orientation. Let's get a picture of what we've just figured out. A particle—suppose it's a car—is moving forward at some velocity. It slows down, stops at some point, and then reverses direction and speeds up.

OK, now that we understand the stimulus, we're ready to tackle the answer choices. Remember, we're looking for acceleration. We said earlier that acceleration is the rate of change in velocity. Even though the velocity vectors change direction, the acceleration vector maintains its negative direction throughout the time sampled. So, even though the car speeds up in the "negative" direction, its acceleration remains negative. It continually *decelerates* throughout its movement. The implication is that the force acting on the car is in a direction *opposing* the original direction of movement. Once this clicks, the correct answer choice—choice (B)—leaps out as correct.

Let's step through the others. Choice (A) suggests that the particle keeps accelerating, but the velocity vectors get *smaller* in magnitude at first, not larger. So, even if you forgot that the "negative acceleration" for time markers 3, 4, and 5 has a negative direction, there's no way choice (A) makes sense. Choice (C) replicates the behavior of the velocity vectors, and if you're not thinking careful-ly, you might fall for this choice because it *seems* to be consistent with the information you're given. Choice (D) presumes that you might visually "add up" all the vectors in the stimulus rather than apply them. If you do try to add them, you'll get a sum of 0. However, that sum is *not* the acceler-ation. In fact, it's the total *displacement*. The car essentially moves forward, slowing down to a stop, and then reverses, speeding up back to its original position.

Key Strategy: Understand the question clearly before you move to the answer choices. Otherwise, you'll be vulnerable to persuasive but incorrect choices.

Key Strategy: Use reason. Don't compute.

7. B

This question has the "all except" format, which means you're looking for the answer choice that is the *exception* (i.e., it's *not* true). The stimulus asks about transition elements. Before you rush to the answer choices, think about what you know of transition elements. They're in the middle of the periodic table and have partially filled *d* subshells. You might also recall that their electrons are loosely held by the nucleus and they are sometimes called *transition metals*.

Choice (B)—they have high ionization energies—is the correct choice because its statement about transition elements is false. Transition elements are easy to ionize because their electrons are not strongly bound. Choice (A) can't be the correct choice because it says something *true* about transi-tion elements. Choice (C) is also true—they do exhibit metallic properties because their electrons are mobile. Choice (D) is also true about transition elements; they can lose electrons from both *s* and *d* orbitals, resulting in multiple oxidation states.

Key Strategy: When answering a question in the "all except" format, remember that you're looking for the choice that is not true.

Key Strategy: When answer questions in the "all except" format, be sure to consider all the answer choic-es to be confident you've picked the most appropriate one.

8. B

This question is based on various functions of the different branches of the nervous system. Specifically, it requires knowledge of the pathways innervated by the sympathetic division of the autonomic nervous system. The autonomic nervous system is divided into two branches—the sympathetic and the parasym-pathetic. The sympathetic system mediates the "fight or flight" responses that ready the body for action. The parasympathetic system innervates those pathways that return the body to its normal state follow-ing fight or flight. The sympathetic system prepares the body by increasing heart rate, inhibiting diges-tion, causing vasoconstriction of blood vessels in the skin, causing vasodilation of blood vessels in skele-tal muscle, and promoting pupil dilation.

From this list of functions, you can eliminate choices (A), (C), and (D) since they're all functions of the sympathetic nervous system and would therefore not be likely responses to a drug that inhibits the activity of the sympathetic system. So by the process of elimination you see that choice (B) is the correct answer. Since sympathetic innervation normally increases heart rate, of the four choices, an inhibitor of the system would most likely result in a *decrease* in heart rate.

Key Strategy: If you approach a stand-alone question that tests specific knowledge you do not possess, skim the choices carefully to see if you can glean any clues or information from them. If not, guess quickly, don't look back, and move on. You don't have time to waste.

KAPLAN TIPS

READING THE PASSAGES

- Passages may sound difficult or unfamiliar. Don't be daunted!
- Feel free to skip around within each section. Tackle the easiest passages first, leaving the harder ones for later, and check for passages with the most questions. Maximize your opportunity for points.
- Make notes in the margin or draw diagrams to help you summarize the information presented.

FACING THE QUESTIONS

- Again, you can skip around. Tackle the easiest questions first, leaving the harder ones for later. The difficult questions are worth the same as the easy ones.
- Use numerical approximations when you can. Don't do any long calculations.
- Base your answers on the passage, not on your own knowledge.
- Use a process of elimination to get to the right answer, or to increase your chances of guessing the right answer.
- If you don't know an answer, guess! Try to do so while you're still working on the passage, so you won't have to reread it later. There's no penalty for wrong answers.

USING THE GRID

- If time is running out and there are blank spaces on your grid, guess.
- Be careful marking your answer grid—especially if you're not answering the questions in numerical order.

Writing Sample

4

- Familiarize yourself with the requirements of the three-task essay
- Learn Kaplan's Seven-Step Approach to the Writing Sample
- Find out exactly what the graders are looking for when they score your essays

THE BIG PICTURE

Medical schools want an assessment of your written communication skills, since this is a reflection of your ability to effectively convey information to your future patients, health-care colleagues, and the public. This is where the Writing Sample section of the MCAT comes in.

You'll be writing two essays during the MCAT, each in response to a stimulus and each within a half-hour allotment. The Writing Sample is the only section that is not comprised of multiple-choice questions. Like the Verbal Reasoning section, this one tends to be underestimated by MCAT test takers. Most think they can just apply their everyday writing skills to the MCAT and do OK on the essays. This is a dangerous presumption. In every facet, the MCAT is a test of analytical reasoning—even in the Writing Sample.

THE STIMULUS

The statement you're to respond to will be in a format along the lines of: *True leadership leads by example rather than by command.* It may be an opinion, a widely shared belief, a philosophical dictum, or an assertion regarding general policy concerns in such areas as history, political science, business, ethics, or art. You can be sure that the statement will not concern scientific or technical subjects, your reasons for entering the medical profession, emotionally charged religious or social issues, or obscure social or political issues that might require specialized knowledge. In fact, you will not need any specialized knowledge to do well on this part of the MCAT.

Most test takers make the mistake of using the essay stimulus as a platform from which to emote, lecture, convince, or just babble. Instead, your goal should be to analyze the statement, present it from two perspectives, and explain how and when you might apply the statement. Your essays need to be written with a critical mind, not an emotional one. This theme is in keeping with the overall goals and intentions of the MCAT—the test makers want to see how you think.

THE THREE-TASK ESSAY

Though worded slightly differently each time, the instructions that follow the statement will ask you to perform three tasks. When completed properly, the following tasks create a balanced essay.

Task One

Provide your interpretation or explanation of the statement. The degree to which you develop the statement in this first task dictates the depth and sophistication of your entire essay.

Task Two

Offer a concrete example that illustrates a point of view *directly opposite* to the one expressed in or implied by the statement. You must give an explicit counterexample; it can be factual or hypothetical.

Task Three

Explain how the conflict between the viewpoint expressed in the statement and the viewpoint you described in the second task might be resolved. You'll be coming up with a kind of "test" or rule that you could apply in situations to see whether or not the statement holds true.

A CLOSER LOOK

Here's an opportunity to begin familiarizing yourself with the essay subjects and an actual essay. You should try your hand at addressing the three tasks (observing the 30-minute time limit, of course), compare your essay with the sample that's provided below, and review the strategies that follow. You'll have the opportunity to boost your essay-writing skills in the practice tests in section two of this book.

The AAMC publishes an annual list of potential MCAT Writing Sample topics and tasks. This list is available online at www.aamc.org.

SAMPLE STIMULUS AND ESSAY

Stimulus

Consider this statement:

Heroes are people who place the needs of others above their own.

Write a unified essay in which you perform the following tasks:

- Explain what you think the above statement means.
- Describe a specific situation in which a person could be heroic while placing his or her own needs above the needs of others.
- Discuss what you think determines whether or not people who put their own needs above the needs of others can be heroes.

KAPLAN

Sample Essay

The statement suggests that being heroic means subjugating one's own needs to external forces of need, relinquishing one's inner compass to be directed by the power of others in need. The classic hero, of course, is the firefighter who runs back into a burning building to save a child. The urgency of momentary crisis can compel people to forget their own safety, their own need for security, in order to guarantee the safety or security of others. In that a hero, by definition, is someone who is emulated and respected, the statement above carries with it the assumption that we respect people who sacrifice themselves to the needs of others.

In a more sophisticated sense, however, many of our historical and fictional heroes have been men and women who stood strong against a tide of negative judgment—people who did not indulge the needs of others but rather played out their own needs. Shakespeare's famous line is often quoted: "This above all: To thine own self be true and good will follow thee as night the day." We make heroes out of individualists who implement unique and personal vision. Ayn Rand is famous and well-read in part because her characters—such as Howard Roark in *The Fountainhead*—refuse to place the needs of others above their own. Indeed, the more lyrical classic hero is the one who stands alone without the title of "hero" until long after the true heroism has passed—the heroism of maintaining a course consistent with one's principles regardless of outside pressure or persuasion. It is in the fuller circle of time that the person comes to be seen as heroic. These are the kinds of heroes who last through history—not just through tomorrow's news.

There are indeed times when sacrifice is heroic. No one would deny a soldier a Purple Heart earned in battle. However, we also see that there are circumstances in which self-actualization rather than self-denial is the heroic choice. Being a hero, then, seems to be more about courage and choice making than about any particular outcome or event. Heroes of all kind—those who put their own needs first (i.e., the "compassionate hero") and those who don't (i.e., the "principled hero")—are people who act according to a standard of "what is right." So, the thing that determines whether or not a sacrificial person can be a hero seems to be the gradient of courage he or she must climb on the way to action.

Did You Address All Three Tasks?

Don't be intimidated by this ideal essay. It's there for you to learn from, not for you to hold up as a standard that may be unrealistic considering the time limit. The sample completes all three tasks and does so with vivid examples and a strong organization. The statement is handled confidently, leading to an essay with interpretive depth, and the writing is crisp, focused, and easy to follow. On the whole the essay is well-balanced, with strong counter examples and a strong resolution.

It begins by immediately defining the "classic hero" and developing an understanding of what is meant by the word *hero*. This gives the reader a context for the essay. When we get to the next paragraph— where we see a discussion of heroes who don't place others' needs above their own—the polarity emerges immediately. Through a series of examples, the essay becomes balanced in its discussion of heroism in relation to self-sacrifice. The stage is set for the resolution in the last paragraph.

As you familiarize yourself with the following Seven-Step Approach to the Writing Sample, you'll see exactly how this particular essay follows each step.

SEVEN-STEP APPROACH TO THE WRITING SAMPLE

Your writing skills are directly linked to your ability to think analytically and logically. You might have a wonderful command of the English language, but if you can't get your thoughts organized and your ideas clear in your mind, your essay will be a jumbled mess.

Step 1: Read and Annotate

Purpose: Clarify for yourself what the statement says and what the instructions require.

Process: Read the statement and instructions carefully.

Annotate the statement, marking any words or phrases that are easy to miss but crucial to a good understanding, are ambiguous or confusing, or refer to vague or abstract concepts.

Annotate the instructions, numbering the tasks and marking any words that will help you remember exactly what it is you're supposed to do.

Application: Key words from the preceding sample statement, *heroes are people who place the needs of others above their own needs,* would be *hero, needs,* and *above*. These words form the seed of thought from which grows a personal interpretation of the statement.

Step 2: Prewrite the First Task

Purpose: Develop a clear interpretation of the statement.

Process: Think of one or more supporting examples.

Clarify/define/interpret abstract, ambiguous, or confusing words.

Ask yourself questions to get beyond the superficial meaning of the statement.

Application: For the preceding sample, you would want to expand the ideas in the statement by asking, "What is a hero? What are examples of self-sacrificial heroism, and what makes those situations heroic?" Try to distill the implications of the statement. This is where the idea of the classic hero comes in as a context for understanding the statement.

Step 3: Prewrite the Second Task

Purpose: Further explore the meaning of the statement by examining a situation that represents an opposing point of view.

Process: Think up one or more specific situations that demonstrate a way in which the statement is not true (even if you agree with the statement).

It's OK to discuss more than one example, but don't spread yourself too thin.

Application: Here's where, for the sample essay, you would consider opposing situations along the lines of, "When is a hero not sacrificial?" and "What are instances in which heroism has been defined by lack of self-sacrifice?" These extremes help balance and deepen the essay. Shakespeare's quote and Ayn Rand's characters help set up the duality of the essay by opposing the fireman example introduced earlier.

Step 4: Prewrite the Third Task

Purpose: Find a way to resolve the conflict between the statement given in the essay topic and the opposing situation(s) you conceived for the second task.

Process: Read the instructions for the third task carefully.

Look back at the ideas you generated for the first and second tasks.

Develop your response based on these ideas.

You don't have to resolve the conflict in support of, or in opposition to, the statement. It's your reasoning that counts, not your stance on the conflict.

Application: Once the seeming dichotomy is set up, as in the hero essay, you need to find a way to resolve it. Sometimes a hero must act to save another. Sometimes saving oneself from moral inconsistency is the heroic act. Both must exist in the context of heroism, so there must be some "deciding" factor. Perhaps it's the difficulty of the act—the amount of courage it requires—or the degree of risk taken in order to achieve one's goal, selfless or otherwise.

Step 5: Clarify the Main Idea and Plan

Purpose: Do final organization and clarification of ideas; take a mental "breath" before beginning to write.

Process: Take a quick moment to look back over your notes in light of the ideas you have reached in prewriting the third task.

Check to make sure your ideas are consistent with each other.

Decide in what order your essay will address the three tasks.

Application: Take note of how solid organization provides a sense of unity in the sample essay.

Step 6: Write

Purpose: Write a straightforward essay that thoroughly presents your response to each of the three tasks.

Process: Write on every other line so you have room for corrections.

Use your prewriting notes for guidance.

Stick to the tasks.

Think about the quality of the essay, not the length.

Try not to use clichés, slang expressions, redundant words or phrases (e.g., *refer back* instead of *refer*), and water-treading sentences (sentences that get you nowhere or serve only to restate the essay directions).

Vary sentence length and structure, to give your essay a rhythm.

Avoid making repeated references to yourself (e.g., *I feel*).

Application: You can see in the hero essay what a difference writing in a strong, confident voice makes.

Step 7: Proofread

Purpose: Quickly review your essay for blatant errors or significant omissions.

Process: You don't have time to revise your essay substantially.

Look for problems in meaning (missing words, sentence fragments, illegible words, confusing punctuation, etcetera) and problems in mechanics (misspelled words, capitalization, etcetera).

Learn the types of mistakes you tend to make and look for them.

Application: The sample essay would have made quite a different impression if words had been misspelled throughout. Reading through the essay carefully to see how it sounds is an important step.

YOUR ESSAY SCORE

Your essays will be graded on a six-tier scale, with Level 6 being the highest. Graders will be looking for an overall sense of your essay; they won't be assigning separate scores for specific elements like grammar or substance. They realize you're writing under time pressure and expect you to make a certain number of mistakes of this kind. However, a series of mistakes can mar your essay's overall impression, so work on any areas you're particularly weak in.

Two readers read each essay and score them independently. If the two graders differ by more than a point, a third grader is called in as a final judge. The four scores are added together, and this combined score will then be converted into an alphabetical rating (ranging from J to T). Statistically speaking, there will be few Level 6 essays. An essay of 4 or 5 would place you at the upper range of those taking the exam.

Here's a quick look at what determines your score:

Score Level 6
- Fulfills all three tasks
- Develops the statement in depth
- Demonstrates careful thought
- Presents an organized structure
- Uses language in a sophisticated manner

Score Level 5
- Fulfills all three tasks
- Interprets the statement in some depth
- Demonstrates some in-depth thought
- Presents a fairly organized essay
- Shows good command of word choice and structure

Score Level 4
- Addresses all three tasks
- Considers the statement somewhat but not in depth
- Shows logical thought but nothing very complex
- Shows overall organization but may have digressions
- Demonstrates strong skills in word use

Score Level 3
- Overlooks or misses one or more of the tasks
- Offers a barely adequate consideration of the statement
- Contains ideas that lack depth
- Shows basic control of word choice and essay structure
- May have problems with clarity of meaning

Score Level 2
- Glaringly omits or misinterprets one or more task
- Offers an unacceptable consideration of the statement
- Shows lack of unity or is incoherent
- Exhibits errors in basic grammar, punctuation, or word use
- May be hard to follow or understand

Score Level 1
- Shows significant problems in basic writing construction
- Presents confusing or disjointed ideas
- May disregard or ignore the given assignment

You can see by this scoring outline that in order to receive higher than a Level 3 score you must successfully address all three tasks. Also note that in order to receive a top-level score you need to develop the statement in depth and show sophisticated thought. Furthermore, for a great writing score, you must demonstrate a strong and logical style, a confident tone, and an eloquent use of language.

KAPLAN TIPS

GETTING OFF ON THE RIGHT FOOT

- Spend about five minutes prewriting, outlining your thoughts before you start writing.
- If you can't come up with real-life examples, use literary examples or your imagination.

WRITING THE ESSAY

- Write on every other line. This way it's easy to make corrections later.
- Write neatly. If you don't think your poor handwriting will work against you, guess again. Readers will be prejudiced against your Writing Sample if it's hard to decipher.
- Use a paragraph structure that matches the tasks, so your essay will be easy for readers to follow.
- Avoid clichés, slang expressions, junk phrases, redundant words or phrases, and water-treading sentences.
- Don't get emotional—graders don't care *what* you think, they care *how* you think.

REVIEWING YOUR ESSAY

- Be strict with yourself so you have at least a few minutes left at the end to read over what you've written. Don't let yourself get cut off.
- Go ahead and make corrections on your essay—these are timed first drafts, not polished term papers.
- Be sure you've addressed all three tasks. Your essay must be balanced.

Test Expertise

- Learn Kaplan's Five Basic Principles of Test Expertise
- Find out how to pace yourself during each individual section of the MCAT
- Make sure you know the smartest way to handle the answer grid

The first year of medical school is a frenzied experience for most students. In order to meet the requirements of a rigorous work schedule, they either learn to prioritize and budget their time or else fall hopelessly behind. It's no surprise, then, that the MCAT, the test specifically designed to predict success in the first year of medical school, is a high-speed, time-intensive test. It demands excellent time-management skills as well as that *sine qua non* of the successful physician: grace under pressure.

It's one thing to answer a Verbal Reasoning question correctly; it's quite another to answer 60 of them correctly in 85 minutes. And the same goes for Physical and Biological Sciences—it's a whole new ball game once you move from doing an individual passage at your leisure to handling a full section under actual timed conditions. You also need to budget your time for the Writing Sample, but this section isn't as time sensitive. But when it comes to the multiple-choice sections, time pressure is a factor that affects virtually every test taker.

So when you're comfortable with the content of the test, your next challenge will be to take it to the next level, test expertise, which will enable you to manage the all-important time element of the test.

THE FIVE BASIC PRINCIPLES OF TEST EXPERTISE

On some tests, if a question seems particularly difficult, you spend significantly more time on it, since you'll probably be given more points for correctly answering a hard question. Not so on the MCAT. Remember, every MCAT question, no matter how hard, is worth a single point. There's no partial credit or "A" for effort. And since there are so many questions to do in so little time, you'd be a fool to spend ten minutes getting a point for a hard question and then not have time to get a couple of quick points from three easy questions later in the section.

Given this combination—limited time, all questions equal in weight—you've got to develop a way of handling the test sections to make sure you get as many points as you can as quickly and easily as you can. Here are the principles that will help you do that:

1. FEEL FREE TO SKIP AROUND

One of the most valuable strategies to help you finish the sections in time is to learn to recognize and deal first with the questions and passages that are easier and more familiar to you. That means temporarily skipping those that promise to be difficult and time-consuming, if you feel comfortable doing so. You can always come back to these at the end, and if you run out of time, you're much better off not getting to questions you may have had difficulty with, rather than missing out on potentially feasible material. Of course, since there's no guessing penalty, always fill in an answer to every question on the test, whether you get to it or not. Remember, too, to work on those passages with the most questions, so you maximize your points.

This strategy is difficult for most test takers; we're conditioned to do things in order. But give it a try when you practice. Remember, if you do the test in the exact order given, you're letting the test makers control you. But *you* control how you take this test. On the other hand, if skipping around goes against your moral fiber and makes you a nervous wreck—don't do it. Just be mindful of the clock, and don't get bogged down with the tough questions.

2. LEARN TO RECOGNIZE AND SEEK OUT QUESTIONS YOU CAN DO

Another thing to remember about managing the test sections is that MCAT questions and passages, unlike items on the SAT and other standardized tests, are not presented in order of difficulty. There's no rule that says you have to work through the sections in any particular order; in fact, the test makers scatter the easy and difficult questions throughout the section, in effect rewarding those who actually get to the end. Don't lose sight of what you're being tested for along with your reading and thinking skills: efficiency and cleverness. If organic chemistry questions are your thing, head straight for them when you first turn to the Biological Sciences section.

Don't waste time on questions you can't do. We know that skipping a possibly tough question is easier said than done; we all have the natural instinct to plow through test sections in their given order. But it just doesn't pay off on the MCAT. The computer won't be impressed if you get the toughest question right. If you dig in your heels on a tough question, refusing to move on until you've cracked it, well, you're letting your ego get in the way of your test score. A test section (not to mention life itself) is too short to waste on lost causes.

3. USE A PROCESS OF ANSWER ELIMINATION

Using a process of elimination is another way to answer questions both quickly and effectively. There are two ways to get all the answers right on the MCAT. You either know all the right answers, or you know all the wrong answers. Since there are three times as many wrong answers, you should be able to eliminate some if not all of them. By doing so you either get to the correct response or increase your chances of guessing the correct response. You start out with a 25 percent chance of picking the right answer, and with each eliminated answer your odds go up. Eliminate one, and you'll have a 33 1/3 percent chance of picking the right one, eliminate two, and you'll have a 50 percent chance, and, of course, eliminate three, and you'll have a 100 percent chance. Increase your efficiency by actually crossing out the wrong choices in your test booklet. Remember to look for wrong-answer traps when you're eliminating. Some answers are designed to seduce you by distorting the correct answer.

4. REMAIN CALM

It's imperative that you remain calm and composed while working through a section. You can't allow yourself to become so rattled by one hard reading passage that it throws off your performance on the rest of the section. Expect to find at least one killer passage in every section, but remember, you won't be the only one to have trouble with it. The test is curved to take the tough material into account. Having trouble with a difficult question isn't going to ruin your score—but getting upset about it and letting it throw you off track will. When you understand that part of the test maker's goal is to reward those who keep their composure, you'll recognize the importance of not panicking when you run into challenging material.

5. KEEP TRACK OF TIME

Of course, the last thing you want to happen is to have time called on a particular section before you've gotten to half the questions. Therefore, it's essential that you pace yourself, keeping in mind the general guidelines for how long to spend on any individual question or passage. Have a sense of how long you have to do each question, so you know when you're exceeding the limit and should start to move faster.

So, when working on a section, always remember to keep track of time. Don't spend a wildly disproportionate amount of time on any one question or group of questions. Also, give yourself 30 seconds or so at the end of each section to fill in answers for any questions you haven't gotten to.

SECTION-SPECIFIC PACING

Let's now look at the section-specific timing requirements and some tips for meeting them. Keep in mind that the times per question or passage are only averages; there are bound to be some that take less time and some that take more. Try to stay balanced. Remember, too, that every question is of equal worth, so don't get hung up on any one. Think about it—if a question is so hard that it takes you a long time to answer it, chances are you may get it wrong anyway. In that case, you'd have nothing to show for your extra time but a lower score.

PHYSICAL AND BIOLOGICAL SCIENCES

Averaging over each section, you'll have about one minute and 20 seconds per question. Some questions, of course, will take more time, some less. A science passage plus accompanying questions should take about eight to nine minutes, depending on how many questions there are. Stand-alone questions can take anywhere from a few seconds to a minute or more. Again, the rule is to do your best work first.

VERBAL REASONING

Allow yourself approximately eight or ten minutes per passage and respective questions. It may sound like a lot of time, but it goes quickly. Do the easiest passages first. Within a section, if you're deciding which passage to do based on time alone, do the one with the most questions. That way you maximize your reading efficiency. However, keep in mind that some passages are longer than others. On average, give yourself about three or four minutes to read and then four to six minutes for the questions.

Also, don't feel that you have to understand everything in a passage before you go on to the questions. You may not need that deep an understanding to answer questions, since a lot of information may be extraneous. You should overcome your perfectionism and use your time wisely.

WRITING SAMPLE

You have exactly 30 minutes for each essay. As mentioned in discussion of the seven-step approach to this section, you should allow approximately five minutes to prewrite the essay, 23 minutes to write the essay, and two minutes to proofread. It's important that you budget your time, so you don't get cut off.

ANSWER GRID EXPERTISE

An important part of MCAT test expertise is knowing how to handle the answer grid. After all, you not only have to get right answers; you also have to transfer those right answers onto the answer grid in an efficient and accurate way. It sounds simple but it's extremely important: **Don't make mistakes filling out your answer grid!** When time is short, it's easy to get confused going back and forth between your test book and your grid. If you know the answer, but misgrid, you won't get the point. Here are a few methods of avoiding mistakes on the answer grid.

ALWAYS CIRCLE THE QUESTIONS YOU SKIP

Put a big circle in your test book around the number of any question you skip (you may even want to circle the whole question itself). When you go back, such questions will then be easy to locate. Also, if you accidentally skip an oval on the grid, you can easily check your grid against your book to see where you went wrong.

ALWAYS CIRCLE THE ANSWERS YOU CHOOSE

Circle the correct answers in your test booklet, but don't transfer the answer to the grid right away. Circling your answers in the test book will also make it easier to check your grid against your book.

GRID FIVE OR MORE ANSWERS AT ONCE

As we said, don't transfer your answers to the grid after every question. Transfer your answers after every five questions, or at the end of each passage (find the method that works best for you). That way, you won't keep breaking your concentration to mark the grid. You'll save time and improve accuracy. Just make sure you're not left at the end of the section with ungridded answers!

SAVE TIME AT THE END FOR A FINAL GRID CHECK

Make sure you have enough time at the end of every section to make a quick check of your grid, to make sure you've got an oval filled in for each question in the section. Remember, a blank grid has no chance of earning a point, but a guess does.

<table>
<tr><td>Test Mentality</td><td>6</td></tr>
</table>

HIGHLIGHTS

- Learn Kaplan's Four Basic Principles of Good Test Mentality
- Find out how to handle stress leading up to and during the exam
- Review Kaplan's Top Ten MCAT Tips

In this section, we first glanced at the content that makes up each specific section of the MCAT, focusing on the strategies and techniques you'll need to tackle individual questions and passages. Then we discussed the test expertise involved in moving from individual items to working through full-length sections. Now we're ready to turn our attention to the often overlooked attitudinal aspects of the test, to put the finishing touches on your comprehensive MCAT approach.

THE FOUR BASIC PRINCIPLES OF GOOD TEST MENTALITY

Knowing the test content arms you with the weapons you need to do well on the MCAT. But you must wield those weapons with the right frame of mind and in the right spirit. Otherwise, you could end up shooting yourself in the foot. This involves taking a certain stance toward the entire test. Here's what's involved:

1. TEST AWARENESS

To do your best on the MCAT, you must always keep in mind that the test is like no other test you've taken before, both in terms of content and in terms of the scoring system. If you took a test in high school or college and got a number of the questions wrong, you wouldn't receive a perfect grade. But on the MCAT, you can get a handful of questions wrong and still get a "perfect" score. The test is geared so that only the very best test takers are able to finish every section. But even these people rarely get every question right.

What does this mean for you? Well, just as you shouldn't let one bad passage ruin an entire section, you shouldn't let what you consider to be a subpar performance on one section ruin your performance on the entire test. If you allow that subpar performance to rattle you, it can have a cumulative negative effect, setting in motion a downward spiral. It's that kind of thing that could potentially do serious damage to your score. Losing a few extra points won't do you in, but losing your cool will.

Remember, if you feel you've done poorly on a section, don't sweat it. Chances are it's just a difficult section, and that factor will already be figured into the scoring curve. The point is, remain calm and collected. Simply do your best on each section, and once a section is over, forget about it and move on.

2. STAMINA

You must work on your test-taking stamina. Overall, the MCAT is a fairly grueling experience, and some test takers simply run out of gas on the last section. To avoid this, you must prepare by taking a few full-length practice tests in the weeks before the test, so that on test day, three sections plus a writing sample will seem like a breeze. (Well, maybe not a breeze, but at least not a hurricane.)

Take the full-length practice test included in this book. You'll be able to review answer explanations and assess your performance. For additional practice material, visit the Association of American Medical Colleges website (www.aamc.org) to order the MCAT Practice Tests it publishes. The AAMC also publishes MCAT Practice Items, which are booklets of MCAT-style passages and sample essay topics. You should, of course, keep in mind that every MCAT administration differs; you can't be assured that your actual score will be predicted by your score on a practice test. The score you'll get on any practice test is less important than the practice itself.

For those students who want more intensive preparation, Kaplan offers a wide range of MCAT prep options, including classroom-based courses, private tutoring, and online courses. **MCAT STAT: Science Basics** is an online course featuring a thorough review of key concepts in organic chemistry, physics, general chemistry, and biology. Another online course, **MCAT STAT: Plus**, includes the Science Basics course described above, along with exclusive strategies and practice quizzes for Verbal Reasoning and the Writing Sample. Visit kaptest.com for more information or to enroll in these courses.

Your best option, if you have time, would be to take the live Kaplan course. We'll give you access to all the released material plus loads of additional material (more than 500 MCAT-style passages in total), so you can really build up your MCAT stamina. You'll also have the benefit of our expert live instruction on every aspect of the MCAT. To go this route, call 1-800-KAP-TEST or visit kaptest.com for a Kaplan center location near you.

Reading this chapter is a great start in your preparation for the test, but it won't get you your best score. That can happen only after lots of practice and skill building. You've got to train your brain to be test smart! Kaplan has been helping people do that for over 60 years, so giving us a call would be a great way to move your test prep into high gear!

3. CONFIDENCE

Confidence feeds on itself, and unfortunately, so does the opposite of confidence—self-doubt. Confidence in your ability leads to quick, sure answers and a sense of well-being that translates into more points. If you lack confidence, you end up reading the sentences and answer choices two, three, or four times, until you confuse yourself and get off track. This leads to timing difficulties, which only perpetuate the downward spiral, causing anxiety and a tendency to rush in order to finish sections.

If you subscribe to the MCAT Mindset we've described, however, you'll gear all of your practice toward the major goal of taking control of the test. When you've achieved that goal—armed with the principles, techniques, strategies, and approaches set forth in this book—you'll be ready to face the MCAT with supreme confidence. And that's the one sure way to score your best on test day.

4. THE RIGHT ATTITUDE

Those who approach the MCAT as an obstacle, who rail against the necessity of taking it, who make light of its importance, who spend more time making fun of the AAMC than studying for the test, usually don't fare as well as those who see the MCAT as an opportunity to show off the reading and reasoning skills that the medical schools are looking for. Don't waste time making value judgments about the MCAT. It is not going to go away, so deal with it. Those who look forward to doing battle with the MCAT—or, at least, who enjoy the opportunity to distinguish themselves from the rest of the applicant pack—tend to score better than do those who resent or dread it.

It may sound a little dubious, but take our word for it: Attitude adjustment is a proven test-taking technique. Here are a few steps you can take to make sure you develop the right MCAT attitude:

- Look at the MCAT as a challenge, but try not to obsess over it; you certainly don't want to psyche yourself out of the game.

- Remember that, yes, the MCAT is obviously important, but, contrary to what some premeds think, this one test will not single-handedly determine the outcome of your life.

- Try to have fun with the test. Learning how to match your wits against the test makers can be a very satisfying experience, and the reading and thinking skills you'll acquire will benefit you in medical school as well as in your future medical career.

- Remember that you're more prepared than most people. You've trained with Kaplan. You have the tools you need, plus the know-how to use those tools.

QUICK TIPS FOR THE DAYS JUST BEFORE THE EXAM

- The best test takers do less and less as the test approaches. Taper off your study schedule and take it easy on yourself. Give yourself time off, especially the evening before the exam. By that time, if you've studied well, everything you need to know is firmly stored in your memory bank.

- Positive self-talk can be extremely liberating and invigorating, especially as the test looms closer. Tell yourself things such as "I will do well," rather than "I hope things go well"; "I can," rather than "I cannot." Replace any negative thoughts with affirming statements that boost your self-esteem.

- Get your act together sooner rather than later. Have everything (including choice of clothing) laid out in advance. Most important, make sure you know where the test will be held and the easiest, quickest way to get there. You'll have great peace of mind by knowing that all the little details— gas in the car, directions, etcetera—are set before the day of the test.

- Go to the test site a few days in advance, particularly if you are especially anxious. Better yet, bring some practice material and do at least a section or two.

- Forego any practice on the day before the test. It's in your best interest to marshal your physical and psychological resources for 24 hours or so. Even race horses are kept in the paddock and treated like princes the day before a race. Keep the upcoming test out of your consciousness; go to a movie, take a pleasant hike, or just relax. Don't eat junk food or tons of sugar. And, of course, get plenty of rest the night before—just don't go to bed too early. It's hard to fall asleep earlier than you're used to, and you don't want to lie there worrying about the test.

HANDLING STRESS DURING THE TEST

The biggest stress monster will be the test itself. Fear not; there are methods of quelling your stress during the test.

- Keep moving forward instead of getting bogged down in a difficult question. You don't have to get everything right to achieve a fine score. So, don't linger out of desperation on a question that is going nowhere even after you've spent considerable time on it. The best test takers skip difficult material temporarily in search of the easier stuff. They mark the ones that require extra time and thought.

- Don't be thrown if other test takers seem to be working more busily and furiously than you are. Don't mistake the other people's sheer activity as signs of progress and higher scores.

- Keep breathing! Weak test takers tend to share one major trait: They don't breathe properly as the test proceeds. They might hold their breath without realizing it, or breathe erratically or arrhythmically. Improper breathing hurts confidence and accuracy. Just as important, it interferes with clear thinking.

- Some quick isometrics during the test—especially if concentration is wandering or energy is waning—can help. Try this: Put your palms together and press intensely for a few seconds. Concentrate on the tension you feel through your palms, wrists, forearms, and up into your biceps and shoulders. Then, quickly release the pressure. Feel the difference as you let go. Focus on the warm relaxation that floods through the muscles. Now you're ready to return to the task.

- Here's another isometric that will relieve tension in both your neck and eye muscles: Slowly rotate your head from side to side, turning your head and eyes to look as far back over each shoulder as you can. Feel the muscles stretch on one side of your neck as they contract on the other. Repeat five times in each direction.

With what you've just learned here, you're armed and ready to do battle with the test. This book and your studies have given you the information you'll need to answer the questions. It's all firmly planted in your mind. You also know how to deal with any excess tension that might come along, both when you're studying for and taking the exam. You've experienced everything you need to tame your test anxiety and stress. You're going to get a great score.

KAPLAN'S TOP TEN MCAT TIPS

1. **Relax!**

2. **Remember: It's primarily a thinking test.** Never forget the purpose of the MCAT: It's designed to test your powers of analytical reasoning. You need to know the content, as each section has its own particular "language," but the underlying MCAT intention is consistent throughout the test.

3. **Feel free to skip around within each section.** Attack each section confidently. You're in charge. Move around if you feel comfortable doing so. Work your best areas first to maximize your opportunity for MCAT points. Choose the order in which to complete passages. Don't be a passive victim of the test structure!

4. **For passage-based questions, choose an answer based on the information given.** Be careful not to be "too smart for your own good." Passages—especially those that describe experimental findings (an MCAT favorite, by the way)—often generate their own data. Your answer choices must be consistent with the information in the passage, even if that means an answer choice is inconsistent with the science of ideal theoretical situations.

5. **Avoid wrong-answer traps.** Try to anticipate answers before you read the answer choices. This helps boost your confidence and protects you from persuasive or tricky incorrect choices. Most wrong answer choices are logical twists on the correct choice.

6. **Think, think, think!** We said it before, but it's important enough to say again: Think. Don't compute.

7. **Don't look back.** Don't spend time worrying about questions you had to guess on. Keep moving forward. Don't let your spirit start to flag, or your attitude will slow you down. You can recheck answers within a section if you have time left, but don't worry about a section after time has been called.

8. **Be careful transferring answers to your grid.** Be sure that you are very careful transcribing answers to your grid, especially if you do skip around within the test sections.

9. **Don't leave any blanks on your answer grid.** There are no points taken off for wrong answers, so if you're not sure of an answer, guess. And guess quickly, so you'll have more time to work through other questions.

10. **Call us! We're here to help!** 1-800-KAP-TEST. Or visit us on the Web at **kaptest.com.**

Section Two

Practice Tests

Full-Length Practice Test I

MCAT Overview

PHYSICAL SCIENCES

Time	100 minutes
Format	77 multiple-choice questions:
	approximately 10–11 passages with 4–8 questions each;
	12–17 stand-alone questions (not passage-based)

VERBAL REASONING

Time	85 minutes
Format	60 multiple-choice questions:
	approximately 9–10 passages with 6–9 questions each

WRITING SAMPLE

Time	60 minutes
Format	2 essay questions (3 tasks per essay)

BIOLOGICAL SCIENCES

Time	100 minutes
Format	77 multiple-choice questions:
	approximately 10–11 passages with 4–8 questions each;
	12–17 stand-alone questions (not passage-based)

INSTRUCTIONS FOR TAKING THE FULL-LENGTH PRACTICE TEST

Before taking this Full-Length Practice Test, find a quiet place where you can work uninterrupted. Make sure you have a comfortable desk and several No. 2 pencils.

Use the answer grid on the following page to record your answers. Time yourself according to the time limits shown at the beginning of each section.

You'll find the answer key, the score converter, and detailed answer explanations following the test.

Good luck.

MARK ONE AND ONLY ONE ANSWER TO EACH QUESTION. BE SURE TO FILL IN COMPLETELY THE SPACE FOR YOUR INTENDED ANSWER CHOICE. IF YOU ERASE, DO SO COMPLETELY. MAKE NO STRAY MARKS.

RIGHT MARK: ● WRONG MARKS: ✓ ✗ ◉

#	A B C D		#	A B C D		#	A B C D		#	A B C D
1	Ⓐ Ⓑ Ⓒ Ⓓ		41	Ⓐ Ⓑ Ⓒ Ⓓ		81	Ⓐ Ⓑ Ⓒ Ⓓ		121	Ⓐ Ⓑ Ⓒ Ⓓ
2	Ⓐ Ⓑ Ⓒ Ⓓ		42	Ⓐ Ⓑ Ⓒ Ⓓ		82	Ⓐ Ⓑ Ⓒ Ⓓ		122	Ⓐ Ⓑ Ⓒ Ⓓ
3	Ⓐ Ⓑ Ⓒ Ⓓ		43	Ⓐ Ⓑ Ⓒ Ⓓ		83	Ⓐ Ⓑ Ⓒ Ⓓ		123	Ⓐ Ⓑ Ⓒ Ⓓ
4	Ⓐ Ⓑ Ⓒ Ⓓ		44	Ⓐ Ⓑ Ⓒ Ⓓ		84	Ⓐ Ⓑ Ⓒ Ⓓ		124	Ⓐ Ⓑ Ⓒ Ⓓ
5	Ⓐ Ⓑ Ⓒ Ⓓ		45	Ⓐ Ⓑ Ⓒ Ⓓ		85	Ⓐ Ⓑ Ⓒ Ⓓ		125	Ⓐ Ⓑ Ⓒ Ⓓ
6	Ⓐ Ⓑ Ⓒ Ⓓ		46	Ⓐ Ⓑ Ⓒ Ⓓ		86	Ⓐ Ⓑ Ⓒ Ⓓ		126	Ⓐ Ⓑ Ⓒ Ⓓ
7	Ⓐ Ⓑ Ⓒ Ⓓ		47	Ⓐ Ⓑ Ⓒ Ⓓ		87	Ⓐ Ⓑ Ⓒ Ⓓ		127	Ⓐ Ⓑ Ⓒ Ⓓ
8	Ⓐ Ⓑ Ⓒ Ⓓ		48	Ⓐ Ⓑ Ⓒ Ⓓ		88	Ⓐ Ⓑ Ⓒ Ⓓ		128	Ⓐ Ⓑ Ⓒ Ⓓ
9	Ⓐ Ⓑ Ⓒ Ⓓ		49	Ⓐ Ⓑ Ⓒ Ⓓ		89	Ⓐ Ⓑ Ⓒ Ⓓ		129	Ⓐ Ⓑ Ⓒ Ⓓ
10	Ⓐ Ⓑ Ⓒ Ⓓ		50	Ⓐ Ⓑ Ⓒ Ⓓ		90	Ⓐ Ⓑ Ⓒ Ⓓ		130	Ⓐ Ⓑ Ⓒ Ⓓ
11	Ⓐ Ⓑ Ⓒ Ⓓ		51	Ⓐ Ⓑ Ⓒ Ⓓ		91	Ⓐ Ⓑ Ⓒ Ⓓ		131	Ⓐ Ⓑ Ⓒ Ⓓ
12	Ⓐ Ⓑ Ⓒ Ⓓ		52	Ⓐ Ⓑ Ⓒ Ⓓ		92	Ⓐ Ⓑ Ⓒ Ⓓ		132	Ⓐ Ⓑ Ⓒ Ⓓ
13	Ⓐ Ⓑ Ⓒ Ⓓ		53	Ⓐ Ⓑ Ⓒ Ⓓ		93	Ⓐ Ⓑ Ⓒ Ⓓ		133	Ⓐ Ⓑ Ⓒ Ⓓ
14	Ⓐ Ⓑ Ⓒ Ⓓ		54	Ⓐ Ⓑ Ⓒ Ⓓ		94	Ⓐ Ⓑ Ⓒ Ⓓ		134	Ⓐ Ⓑ Ⓒ Ⓓ
15	Ⓐ Ⓑ Ⓒ Ⓓ		55	Ⓐ Ⓑ Ⓒ Ⓓ		95	Ⓐ Ⓑ Ⓒ Ⓓ		135	Ⓐ Ⓑ Ⓒ Ⓓ
16	Ⓐ Ⓑ Ⓒ Ⓓ		56	Ⓐ Ⓑ Ⓒ Ⓓ		96	Ⓐ Ⓑ Ⓒ Ⓓ		136	Ⓐ Ⓑ Ⓒ Ⓓ
17	Ⓐ Ⓑ Ⓒ Ⓓ		57	Ⓐ Ⓑ Ⓒ Ⓓ		97	Ⓐ Ⓑ Ⓒ Ⓓ		137	Ⓐ Ⓑ Ⓒ Ⓓ
18	Ⓐ Ⓑ Ⓒ Ⓓ		58	Ⓐ Ⓑ Ⓒ Ⓓ		98	Ⓐ Ⓑ Ⓒ Ⓓ		138	Ⓐ Ⓑ Ⓒ Ⓓ
19	Ⓐ Ⓑ Ⓒ Ⓓ		59	Ⓐ Ⓑ Ⓒ Ⓓ		99	Ⓐ Ⓑ Ⓒ Ⓓ		139	Ⓐ Ⓑ Ⓒ Ⓓ
20	Ⓐ Ⓑ Ⓒ Ⓓ		60	Ⓐ Ⓑ Ⓒ Ⓓ		100	Ⓐ Ⓑ Ⓒ Ⓓ		140	Ⓐ Ⓑ Ⓒ Ⓓ
21	Ⓐ Ⓑ Ⓒ Ⓓ		61	Ⓐ Ⓑ Ⓒ Ⓓ		101	Ⓐ Ⓑ Ⓒ Ⓓ		141	Ⓐ Ⓑ Ⓒ Ⓓ
22	Ⓐ Ⓑ Ⓒ Ⓓ		62	Ⓐ Ⓑ Ⓒ Ⓓ		102	Ⓐ Ⓑ Ⓒ Ⓓ		142	Ⓐ Ⓑ Ⓒ Ⓓ
23	Ⓐ Ⓑ Ⓒ Ⓓ		63	Ⓐ Ⓑ Ⓒ Ⓓ		103	Ⓐ Ⓑ Ⓒ Ⓓ		143	Ⓐ Ⓑ Ⓒ Ⓓ
24	Ⓐ Ⓑ Ⓒ Ⓓ		64	Ⓐ Ⓑ Ⓒ Ⓓ		104	Ⓐ Ⓑ Ⓒ Ⓓ		144	Ⓐ Ⓑ Ⓒ Ⓓ
25	Ⓐ Ⓑ Ⓒ Ⓓ		65	Ⓐ Ⓑ Ⓒ Ⓓ		105	Ⓐ Ⓑ Ⓒ Ⓓ		145	Ⓐ Ⓑ Ⓒ Ⓓ
26	Ⓐ Ⓑ Ⓒ Ⓓ		66	Ⓐ Ⓑ Ⓒ Ⓓ		106	Ⓐ Ⓑ Ⓒ Ⓓ		146	Ⓐ Ⓑ Ⓒ Ⓓ
27	Ⓐ Ⓑ Ⓒ Ⓓ		67	Ⓐ Ⓑ Ⓒ Ⓓ		107	Ⓐ Ⓑ Ⓒ Ⓓ		147	Ⓐ Ⓑ Ⓒ Ⓓ
28	Ⓐ Ⓑ Ⓒ Ⓓ		68	Ⓐ Ⓑ Ⓒ Ⓓ		108	Ⓐ Ⓑ Ⓒ Ⓓ		148	Ⓐ Ⓑ Ⓒ Ⓓ
29	Ⓐ Ⓑ Ⓒ Ⓓ		69	Ⓐ Ⓑ Ⓒ Ⓓ		109	Ⓐ Ⓑ Ⓒ Ⓓ		149	Ⓐ Ⓑ Ⓒ Ⓓ
30	Ⓐ Ⓑ Ⓒ Ⓓ		70	Ⓐ Ⓑ Ⓒ Ⓓ		110	Ⓐ Ⓑ Ⓒ Ⓓ		150	Ⓐ Ⓑ Ⓒ Ⓓ
31	Ⓐ Ⓑ Ⓒ Ⓓ		71	Ⓐ Ⓑ Ⓒ Ⓓ		111	Ⓐ Ⓑ Ⓒ Ⓓ		151	Ⓐ Ⓑ Ⓒ Ⓓ
32	Ⓐ Ⓑ Ⓒ Ⓓ		72	Ⓐ Ⓑ Ⓒ Ⓓ		112	Ⓐ Ⓑ Ⓒ Ⓓ		152	Ⓐ Ⓑ Ⓒ Ⓓ
33	Ⓐ Ⓑ Ⓒ Ⓓ		73	Ⓐ Ⓑ Ⓒ Ⓓ		113	Ⓐ Ⓑ Ⓒ Ⓓ		153	Ⓐ Ⓑ Ⓒ Ⓓ
34	Ⓐ Ⓑ Ⓒ Ⓓ		74	Ⓐ Ⓑ Ⓒ Ⓓ		114	Ⓐ Ⓑ Ⓒ Ⓓ		154	Ⓐ Ⓑ Ⓒ Ⓓ
35	Ⓐ Ⓑ Ⓒ Ⓓ		75	Ⓐ Ⓑ Ⓒ Ⓓ		115	Ⓐ Ⓑ Ⓒ Ⓓ		155	Ⓐ Ⓑ Ⓒ Ⓓ
36	Ⓐ Ⓑ Ⓒ Ⓓ		76	Ⓐ Ⓑ Ⓒ Ⓓ		116	Ⓐ Ⓑ Ⓒ Ⓓ		156	Ⓐ Ⓑ Ⓒ Ⓓ
37	Ⓐ Ⓑ Ⓒ Ⓓ		77	Ⓐ Ⓑ Ⓒ Ⓓ		117	Ⓐ Ⓑ Ⓒ Ⓓ		157	Ⓐ Ⓑ Ⓒ Ⓓ
38	Ⓐ Ⓑ Ⓒ Ⓓ		78	Ⓐ Ⓑ Ⓒ Ⓓ		118	Ⓐ Ⓑ Ⓒ Ⓓ		158	Ⓐ Ⓑ Ⓒ Ⓓ
39	Ⓐ Ⓑ Ⓒ Ⓓ		79	Ⓐ Ⓑ Ⓒ Ⓓ		119	Ⓐ Ⓑ Ⓒ Ⓓ		159	Ⓐ Ⓑ Ⓒ Ⓓ
40	Ⓐ Ⓑ Ⓒ Ⓓ		80	Ⓐ Ⓑ Ⓒ Ⓓ		120	Ⓐ Ⓑ Ⓒ Ⓓ		160	Ⓐ Ⓑ Ⓒ Ⓓ

#	A B C D
161	Ⓐ Ⓑ Ⓒ Ⓓ
162	Ⓐ Ⓑ Ⓒ Ⓓ
163	Ⓐ Ⓑ Ⓒ Ⓓ
164	Ⓐ Ⓑ Ⓒ Ⓓ
165	Ⓐ Ⓑ Ⓒ Ⓓ
166	Ⓐ Ⓑ Ⓒ Ⓓ
167	Ⓐ Ⓑ Ⓒ Ⓓ
168	Ⓐ Ⓑ Ⓒ Ⓓ
169	Ⓐ Ⓑ Ⓒ Ⓓ
170	Ⓐ Ⓑ Ⓒ Ⓓ
171	Ⓐ Ⓑ Ⓒ Ⓓ
172	Ⓐ Ⓑ Ⓒ Ⓓ
173	Ⓐ Ⓑ Ⓒ Ⓓ
174	Ⓐ Ⓑ Ⓒ Ⓓ
175	Ⓐ Ⓑ Ⓒ Ⓓ
176	Ⓐ Ⓑ Ⓒ Ⓓ
177	Ⓐ Ⓑ Ⓒ Ⓓ
178	Ⓐ Ⓑ Ⓒ Ⓓ
179	Ⓐ Ⓑ Ⓒ Ⓓ
180	Ⓐ Ⓑ Ⓒ Ⓓ
181	Ⓐ Ⓑ Ⓒ Ⓓ
182	Ⓐ Ⓑ Ⓒ Ⓓ
183	Ⓐ Ⓑ Ⓒ Ⓓ
184	Ⓐ Ⓑ Ⓒ Ⓓ
185	Ⓐ Ⓑ Ⓒ Ⓓ
186	Ⓐ Ⓑ Ⓒ Ⓓ
187	Ⓐ Ⓑ Ⓒ Ⓓ
188	Ⓐ Ⓑ Ⓒ Ⓓ
189	Ⓐ Ⓑ Ⓒ Ⓓ
190	Ⓐ Ⓑ Ⓒ Ⓓ
191	Ⓐ Ⓑ Ⓒ Ⓓ
192	Ⓐ Ⓑ Ⓒ Ⓓ
193	Ⓐ Ⓑ Ⓒ Ⓓ
194	Ⓐ Ⓑ Ⓒ Ⓓ
195	Ⓐ Ⓑ Ⓒ Ⓓ
196	Ⓐ Ⓑ Ⓒ Ⓓ
197	Ⓐ Ⓑ Ⓒ Ⓓ
198	Ⓐ Ⓑ Ⓒ Ⓓ
199	Ⓐ Ⓑ Ⓒ Ⓓ
200	Ⓐ Ⓑ Ⓒ Ⓓ

#	A B C D
201	Ⓐ Ⓑ Ⓒ Ⓓ
202	Ⓐ Ⓑ Ⓒ Ⓓ
203	Ⓐ Ⓑ Ⓒ Ⓓ
204	Ⓐ Ⓑ Ⓒ Ⓓ
205	Ⓐ Ⓑ Ⓒ Ⓓ
206	Ⓐ Ⓑ Ⓒ Ⓓ
207	Ⓐ Ⓑ Ⓒ Ⓓ
208	Ⓐ Ⓑ Ⓒ Ⓓ
209	Ⓐ Ⓑ Ⓒ Ⓓ
210	Ⓐ Ⓑ Ⓒ Ⓓ
211	Ⓐ Ⓑ Ⓒ Ⓓ
212	Ⓐ Ⓑ Ⓒ Ⓓ
213	Ⓐ Ⓑ Ⓒ Ⓓ
214	Ⓐ Ⓑ Ⓒ Ⓓ

Physical Sciences Test

Time: 100 minutes—Questions 1–77

DIRECTIONS: Most of the questions in the following Physical Sciences test are organized into groups, with a descriptive passage preceding each group of questions. Study the passage, then select the single best answer to each question in the group. Some of the questions are not based on a descriptive passage; you must also select the best answer to these questions. If you are unsure of the best answer, eliminate the choices that you know are incorrect, then select an answer from the choices that remain. A periodic table is provided below for your use with the questions.

Periodic Table of the Elements

1 H 1.0																	2 He 4.0
3 Li 6.9	4 Be 9.0											5 B 10.8	6 C 12.0	7 N 14.0	8 O 16.0	9 F 19.0	10 Ne 20.2
11 Na 23.0	12 Mg 24.3											13 Al 27.0	14 Si 28.1	15 P 31.0	16 S 32.1	17 Cl 35.5	18 Ar 39.9
19 K 39.1	20 Ca 40.1	21 Sc 45.0	22 Ti 47.9	23 V 50.9	24 Cr 52.0	25 Mn 54.9	26 Fe 55.8	27 Co 58.9	28 Ni 58.7	29 Cu 63.5	30 Zn 65.4	31 Ga 69.7	32 Ge 72.6	33 As 74.9	34 Se 79.0	35 Br 79.9	36 Kr 83.8
37 Rb 85.5	38 Sr 87.6	39 Y 88.9	40 Zr 91.2	41 Nb 92.9	42 Mo 95.9	43 Tc (98)	44 Ru 101.1	45 Rh 102.9	46 Pd 106.4	47 Ag 107.9	48 Cd 112.4	49 In 114.8	50 Sn 118.7	51 Sb 121.8	52 Te 127.6	53 I 126.9	54 Xe 131.3
55 Cs 132.9	56 Ba 137.3	57 La* 138.9	72 Hf 178.5	73 Ta 180.9	74 W 183.9	75 Re 186.2	76 Os 190.2	77 Ir 192.2	78 Pt 195.1	79 Au 197.0	80 Hg 200.6	81 Tl 204.4	82 Pb 207.2	83 Bi 209.0	84 Po (209)	85 At (210)	86 Rn (222)
87 Fr (223)	88 Ra 226.0	89 Ac† 227.0	104 Unq (261)	105 Unp (262)	106 Unh (263)	107 Uns (262)	108 Uno (265)	109 Une (267)									

*	58 Ce 140.1	59 Pr 140.9	60 Nd 144.2	61 Pm (145)	62 Sm 150.4	63 Eu 152.0	64 Gd 157.3	65 Tb 158.9	66 Dy 162.5	67 Ho 164.9	68 Er 167.3	69 Tm 168.9	70 Yb 173.0	71 Lu 175.0
†	90 Th 232.0	91 Pa (231)	92 U 238.0	93 Np (237)	94 Pu (244)	95 Am (243)	96 Cm (247)	97 Bk (247)	98 Cf (251)	99 Es (252)	100 Fm (257)	101 Md (258)	102 No (259)	103 Lr (260)

GO ON TO THE NEXT PAGE.

Passage I (Questions 1-5)

When light enters the eye, it forms an image on the retina. First, light from the object passes through the cornea, a converging lens within the eye, and then through a liquid known as the aqueous humor. After this it passes through a second crystalline converging lens into the eyeball, which is filled with a fluid known as the vitreous humor. The light is refracted by the cornea and by the crystalline lens, and is focused on the retina, which transmits electrical impulses along the optic nerve to the brain.

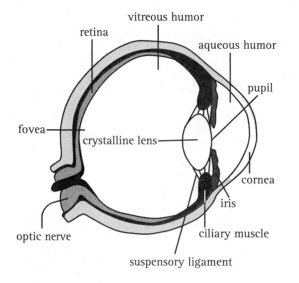

The cornea has a constant focal length, and is responsible for most of the refraction of the light from the object. The crystalline lens has a variable focal length, which enables the eye to focus the image on the retina, even though the object distance varies. The focal length of the crystalline lens is varied by tensing and relaxing the ciliary muscle that surrounds the lens. It is relaxed when focusing on a distant object, and tensed when focusing on a near object. It is important to note that when the ciliary muscle is tensed, the lens assumes a more spherical shape, thus decreasing the focal length.

The cornea and the crystalline lens may be considered two thin lenses in contact, and therefore thought of as a single converging lens at a distance of 2.0 centimeters from the retina. When an object is at an infinite distance away, the focal length of the lens is equal to the distance between the lens and the retina When the distance to the object is appreciably smaller, the focal length of the lens changes so that the image is still focused on the retina.

There are several defects of vision. The two most common are myopia and hyperopia. Myopia, or nearsightedness, is caused when the image of an object at infinity is focused in front of the retina. Hyperopia, or farsightedness, is caused when an object at infinity is focused behind the retina. (Note: In the following questions, assume that the distance from the lens to the retina is 2 cm.)

1. The index of refraction of the vitreous humor is greater than the index of refraction of the aqueous humor which is greater than the index of refraction of air. What is the relationship of the speed of light in each of these media?

    A. Fastest in air, slower in aqueous humor, slowest in vitreous humor
    B. Fastest in vitreous humor, slower in aqueous humor, slowest in air
    C. Equal in all three
    D. Depends on the index of refraction of the lenses which separate the media

2. In order for a normal eye to focus on an object 20 cm away, what is the required focal length of the eye's lens?

    A. 0.05 cm
    B. 1.8 cm
    C. 2.0 cm
    D. 2.2 cm

GO ON TO THE NEXT PAGE.

3. Two converging lenses are in contact. If the focal lengths are each 5 cm, what is the equivalent focal length of the combination?

   A. 0.1 cm
   B. 2.5 cm
   C. 5.0 cm
   D. 10.0 cm

4. A myopic person's eye has a relaxed focal length of 1.9 cm. What is the maximum distance from the eye at which she can see an object clearly, and what is the magnification of the lens for an object at this point?

   A. $O = 1$ cm, $m = -\frac{1}{2}$
   B. $O = 38$ cm, $m = -\frac{1}{38}$
   C. $O = 38$ cm, $m = -\frac{1}{19}$
   D. $O = 50$ cm, $m = -\frac{1}{50}$

5. Which of the following is true of the image formed on the retina?

   I. It is real.

   II. It is inverted.

   III. It is reduced.

   A. I only
   B. I and II only
   C. II and III only
   D. I, II, and III

GO ON TO THE NEXT PAGE.

Passage II (Question 6–11)

A mixture of two volatile solvents that exhibits ideal behavior will boil when the total vapor pressure is equal to the atmospheric pressure. The concentration of the more volatile component will always be greater in the vapor than in the solution. If the vapor above the boiling mixture is condensed and boiled again, it will be even richer in the more volatile component. With successive condensations and boilings, it is possible to separate the individual components. This process is known as fractional distillation.

There are, however, a number of solvent systems that do not behave ideally, and consequently cannot be separated. Figure 1 shows a boiling-point diagram for a system that is called a *minimum-boiling azeotrope*. In a system such as this, the attraction between unlike molecules is weaker than the attraction between like molecules; as a result, the solution boils at a lower temperature than the pure components. Systems that have a maximum on the boiling-point diagram are called *maximum-boiling azeotropes*. Fractional distillation of these nonideal systems will, at best, give one pure component and the azeotrope.

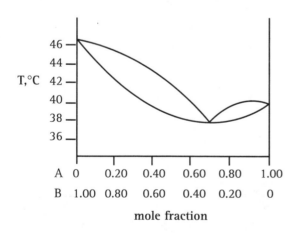

mole fraction

6. Which of the following best describes the mechanism by which two substances form a maximum-boiling azeotrope?

A. Each substance increases the specific heat of the other.

B. Each substance decreases the specific heat of the other.

C. Each substance increases the vapor pressure of the other.

D. Each substance decreases the vapor pressure of the other.

7. Which of the following combinations would be likely to form a minimum-boiling azeotrope?

A. Water and chlorobenzene

B. Water and nitric acid

C. Water and hydrogen peroxide

D. Water and acetone

8. Which of the following shows the boiling point of an aqueous sodium chloride solution as a function of the percent sodium chloride in the solution by weight?

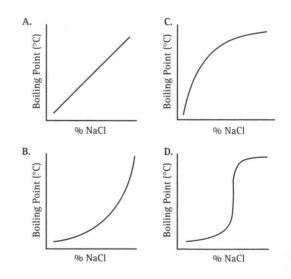

GO ON TO THE NEXT PAGE.

9. Based on Figure 1, if a mixture of Solution A and Solution B boils at 40°C, what is the mole fraction of B in the vapor?

   A. 0.04 or 0.70
   B. 0.20 or 0.40
   C. 0.30 or 0.96
   D. 0.60 or 0.80

10. An ethanol and water solution can be distilled to, at best, a 95 percent ethanol solution, which boils at 78°C. What can be said about this mixture?

    A. It is a minimum-boiling azeotrope with water as the most volatile component.
    B. It is a minimum-boiling azeotrope with ethanol as the most volatile component.
    C. It is a maximum-boiling azeotrope with water as the most volatile component.
    D. It is a maximum-boiling azeotrope with ethanol as the most volatile component.

11. Which of the following describes the effect on boiling point when a nonvolatile solute is added to a liquid?

    A. $\Delta T_b = K_b M$
    B. $\Delta T_b = K_b / M$
    C. $\Delta T_b = K_b m$
    D. $\Delta T_b = K_b / m$

GO ON TO THE NEXT PAGE.

Passage III (Questions 12–17)

Robert Millikan is credited with showing experimentally that the electron has a definite, finite charge. His experiment, in a somewhat simplified form, is described below. The setup is shown in Figure 1.

Two horizontal parallel plates, A and B, are placed 1 cm apart, and are insulated from one another. A potential difference V_{AB} is applied across the plates, producing an electric field between them.

Drops of oil between 10^{-6} and 10^{-5} cm in diameter are sprayed through a hole in the top plate into the electric field. The drops accumulate electric charge, and are therefore affected by the electric field. In the case of a negatively charged drop, the potential difference across the plates is adjusted until the drop is motionless, the gravitational force being exactly balanced by the upward electrostatic force. The mass of the droplet and the potential difference across the plates is measured, and from this the electric charge on the drop can be determined. This procedure is then repeated with another drop.

Millikan found, when he calculated the electric charge required from the balanced forces, that the measured charges were integer multiples of a specific electric charge. This "unit" charge was assumed to be the charge of a single electron. (Note: Acceleration due to gravity = 9.8 m/s²; density of oil = 800 kg/m³.)

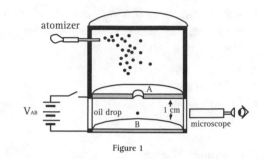

Figure 1

12. What is the electric field between the plates in Figure 1 if the voltage V_{AB} is 20 volts?

    A. 0.02 V/m
    B. 0.2 V/m
    C. 20 V/m
    D. 2×10^3 V/m

13. What is the direction of an electric field between the plates that holds a negatively charged droplet motionless?

    A. Upwards
    B. Downwards
    C. To the left
    D. To the right

14. If the separation of the plates is reduced, but the potential difference across them remains constant, which of the following statements must be true?

    I.   The electric field increases.
    II. The magnetic field increases.
    III. The capacitance increases.

    A. I only
    B. I and II only
    C. I and III only
    D. II ant III only

GO ON TO THE NEXT PAGE.

68

15. An oil drop is stationary within an electric field of 490 V/m that is set up between two parallel plates. If the volume of the oil drop is 4×10^{-19} m³, how many excess electrons does it carry? (Note: The fundamental unit of charge e = 1.6×10^{-19} C.)

    A. 1
    B. 4
    C. 10
    D. 40

16. A negatively charged droplet has a mass of 5×10^{-16} kg and carries a charge of 8×10^{-18} C. The droplet falls through the hole in the upper plate when the electric field is 0 V/m. How does the drop move within the plates as the electric field is increased slowly from 0 V/m to 800 V/m? (Note: Assume that the drop remains between the plates at all times.)

    A. It moves downwards, stops, then moves upwards.
    B. It moves downwards, accelerating all the time.
    C. It moves downwards, stops, then moves downwards again.
    D. It moves downwards, stops, and remains stationary.

17. A drop of oil of mass 5×10^{-16} kg is at rest on the bottom plate of a parallel plate combination when the electric field is zero. An electric field of 4×10^3 V/m is then applied between the plates, accelerating the drop towards the top plate. What will be the resultant acceleration of the drop if it carries a negative charge of 3×10^{-18} C? (Note: Neglect the effects of air resistance.)

    A. 9.8 m/s²
    B. 14.2 m/s²
    C. 24.0 m/s²
    D. 28.4 m/s²

Questions 18 through 22 are NOT based on a descriptive passage.

18. What is the calcium concentration of a solution formed by adding 1 mol of $CaCl_2$ to 1 L of distilled water at 298K?

    A. $1M$
    B. $1m$
    C. $2M$
    D. $2m$

19. Two blocks of the same density are completely submerged in water. One block has a mass equal to m and volume equal to V. The other has a mass equal to $2m$. What is the ratio of the first block's apparent weight to the second block's apparent weight?

    A. 1:1
    B. 1:2
    C. 2:1
    D. 4:1

20. In which atomic orbital(s) to the alkaline earth elements contain valence electrons?

    A. s
    B. d
    C. s and d
    D. s, d, and p

GO ON TO THE NEXT PAGE.

21. In the arrangement shown below, a current flows from P to Q and the ammeter A_1 reads 3.0 A. If each ammeter has negligible resistance, what is the reading on ammeter A_2?

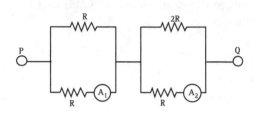

A. 1.0 A
B. 1.5 A
C. 2.0 A
D. 4.0 A

22. What is the ratio of the maximum possible number of f electrons to the maximum possible number of p electrons?

A. 2:1
B. 4:1
C. 7:3
D. 15:6

GO ON TO THE NEXT PAGE.

Passage IV (Questions 23–27)

A chemistry teacher wishes to set up a demonstration of a redox reaction for her class. Students are provided with the materials necessary to set up the apparatus shown below.

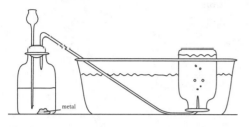

Experiment 1:
Students were provided with 1 *M* hydrochloric acid and offered a choice of various metals. The metals offered to the students, along with their reduction potentials, are listed below.

Metal	E°(V)
Silver	0.80
Copper	0.34
Tin	−0.14
Nickel	−0.25
Iron	−0.44

Each student group tested a different metal for reactivity by placing it in a beaker and observing the gas produced (if any) from the reaction. Each metal's reaction was timed and the rate at which gas was produced was recorded.

Experiment 2:
Students were given the supplies necessary to set up a galvanic cell for the purpose of determining the reduction potential of zinc, also using hydrochloric acid. The reduction potential was determined to be −0.76V.

Both experiments were carried out at 25°C and 1 atm.

23. When hydrochloric acid is added to each of the metals listed in Table 1, which metals will produce a reaction?
    A. Ag, Cu
    B. Sn, Ni, Fe
    C. All of the metals
    D. None of the metals

24. Of the metals listed, which will produce the most vigorous reaction?
    A. Silver
    B. Copper
    C. Tin
    D. Iron

25. In Experiment 2, which of the following galvanic cell setups would be most useful for determining the reduction potential of zinc?
    A. Zinc electrode as anode in a 1 *M* Zn^{2+} solution; hydrogen electrode as cathode in a 1 *M* H^+ solution
    B. Zinc electrode as cathode in a 1 *M* Zn^{2+} solution; hydrogen electrode as anode in a 1 *M* H^+ solution
    C. Zinc electrode as anode in a 1 *M* Zn^{2+} solution; copper electrode as cathode in a 1 *M* Cu^{2+} solution
    D. Zinc electrode as cathode in a 1 *M* Zn^{2+} solution; copper electrode as anode in a 1 *M* Cu^{2+} solution

GO ON TO THE NEXT PAGE.

26. What is the role of HCl in Experiment 2?

    A. It is a reducing agent.
    B. It is an oxidizing agent.
    C. It is a catalyst.
    D. It is a solvent.

27. If Experiment 1 were carried out using zinc, what would be the maximum weight of the sample that could be used to ensure that all the gas produced could be collected in a 1 L bottle?

    A. 1.3g
    B. 1.4g
    C. 2.6g
    D. 2.9g

GO ON TO THE NEXT PAGE.

Passage V (Questions 28–32)

The most commonly used electric lights in homes today are incandescent. Incandescent light is created by applying a potential difference to a filament of thin, high-resistance wire. Electrons moving in the current collide with atoms in the wire, transferring energy to these atoms. This energy is dissipated in the form of radiation, almost all of which is in the infrared range. When the wire becomes hot enough, the spectrum produced begins to enter the red end of the visible range. As the temperature of the resistor increases, the visible spectrum produced becomes closer to the spectrum of white light. However, a high temperature decreases the life of the light bulb by increasing the rate of vaporization of the filament. Early incandescent lamps used vacuum bulbs; later on, filling the bulb with an inert gas became common. The gas distributes the light more evenly over the visible spectrum, and also increases the life of the filament.

Fluorescent lights work by an entirely different method. An electric arc is created between two electrodes in a tube in which a small amount of mercury has been vaporized. The mercury produces ultraviolet light, and this light is then intercepted by a phosphor that coats the inside of the glass tube. The phosphor absorbs the ultraviolet and emits visible radiation of a longer wavelength. The wavelength produced can be controlled by varying the phosphor composition. A "warm white" lamp produces more light on the red end of the spectrum than does a "cool white" lamp.

With the recent interest in the effect of light on mood, a market has developed for lamps that simulate the spectrum of outdoor light. The natural light spectrum on a sunny day is of more or less equal intensity over the range from 540 to 700 nanometers, although the intensity is lower at shorter wavelengths, particularly from about 400 to 460 nanometers. On a cloudy day, the greatest natural light intensity occurs on the blue end of the spectrum, with the red end somewhat less intense. Of course, the greatest difference between the artificial light generally used in homes and natural light is the intensity.

28. Why does an incandescent light have a longer life when an inert gas is used rather than a vacuum?

    A. The filament vaporizes more slowly.
    B. Heat is removed from the filament.
    C. The bulb is less likely to implode when subjected to vibration.
    D. The gas directly absorbs energy from the electrons in the filament.

29. An advertiser argues that incandescent lights are not adequate for improving mood on a cloudy day because they do not provide enough light of short wavelength. What argument could be made against this position?

    A. Incandescent lights provide mostly light of short wavelength.
    B. Outdoor light is more intense at longer wavelengths on a sunny day than on a cloudy day.
    C. Outdoor light is more intense at shorter wavelengths on a sunny day than on a cloudy day.
    D. The spectrum produced by electric lights is irrelevant since their intensity is so low.

GO ON TO THE NEXT PAGE.

30. Which of the lamps described in the passage can produce excess exposure to ultraviolet radiation when operating normally?

   A. Incandescent lamps only
   B. Fluorescent lamps only
   C. Both incandescent and fluorescent lamps
   D. Neither kind of lamp

31. Which kind of lamp, incandescent or fluorescent, is more efficient?

   A. Incandescent lamps, because they release all of the radiation they originally produce
   B. Fluorescent lamps, because they produce only radiation in the visible range
   C. Incandescent lamps, because no energy is lost in the conversion of energy from one wavelength to another
   D. Fluorescent lamps, because they multiply the intensity of radiation as it is converted from ultraviolet to visible light

32. What would a manufacturer of fluorescent lamps have to do in order to change his "warm white" lamps to "cool white" lamps?

   A. Change the amount of mercury vapor in the lamp to produce less ultraviolet light.
   B. Change the thickness of the glass tube to get a greater index of refraction.
   C. Change the composition of the electrodes to produce a weaker electric arc.
   D. Change the composition of the phosphor to emit more light at the blue-violet end of the spectrum.

GO ON TO THE NEXT PAGE.

Passage VI (Questions 33–39)

One equation that physicists use to describe fluid dynamics is Bernoulli's equation:

$$P + \rho v^2/2 + \rho g y = \text{constant}$$

where P is the absolute pressure, ρ is the density of the fluid, v is the speed of the fluid, g is the acceleration due to gravity, and y is the height of the fluid. A second more familiar equation is the continuity equation

$$vA = \text{constant}$$

where A is the cross-sectional area of the fluid flow.

A domestic water heating system is a good example of a dynamical fluid system. Figure 1 shows a water heating system used to provide hot water in British homes. An open water storage tank located in the attic is fed with cold water by the street water mains. The water level of the storage tank is kept constant at all times.

Water from the storage tank in the attic fills a hot water cylinder which holds 60 kg of water. The hot water cylinder is a storage tank that is thermally insulated from the outside environment. The water in the cylinder is heated by an immersion heater, which is a wire coil encased in a metal jacket. Current passes through the coil and dissipates energy. This heats up the metal jacket which then heats the surrounding water. The resistance of the wire coil is 20 Ω, and the voltage across it is 240 V. When the hot water faucet is turned on, the water that leaves the hot water cylinder is immediately replaced with cold water from the storage tank. Thus, the hot water cylinder always remains full, and the entire hot water system can be considered a single pipe.

Water leaving the hot water cylinder is directed through pipes to various rooms in the house. These pipes supply hot water to the bathroom shower and sink on the second floor, the kitchen

and bathroom sinks on the first floor, and the washing machine in the basement. Cold water is supplied in separate pipes which are shaded in Figure 1. (Note: Assume the cross-sectional area of the pipes is constant everywhere unless otherwise stated. The density of water is 1,000 kg/m³, and its specific heat is 4,200 J/kg • °C. The acceleration of gravity is $g = 10$ m/s².)

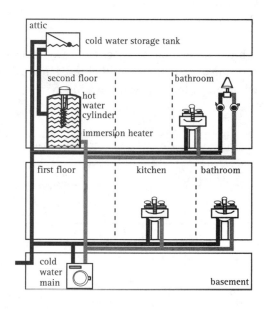

Figure 1

33. If the flow in the pipes is laminar, what can be said about the streamlines of the water's flow?

    A. The streamlines of the flow are uniform and regular.

    B. The streamlines of the flow are complex.

    C. The streamlines are far apart.

    D. Nothing can be deduced about the streamlines with the information given.

GO ON TO THE NEXT PAGE.

34. When all the taps are shut, the hot water cylinder is full of water at 10°C. If the taps remain shut, approximately how long does it take the heater to raise the temperature of the water to 50°C? (Note: Assume that the metal casing of the immersion heater is a perfect thermal conductor.)

    A. 20 minutes
    B. 1 hour
    C. 2 hours
    D. 3 hours

35. Which of the following circuits would have a resistance equivalent to the resistance of the wire coil in the hot-water heating system?

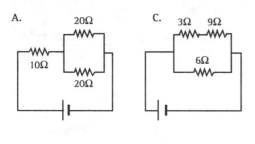

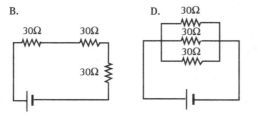

36. Some space heating systems use the heat released when steam condenses into water. The existence of this heat of vaporization can be explained by the fact that:

    A. water at 100°C has the same internal energy as steam at 100°C.
    B. water at 100°C has a larger internal energy than steam at 100°C.
    C. water at 100°C has a smaller internal energy than steam at 100°C.
    D. the temperature at which the water boils depends on the pressure in the pipes.

37. Suppose that the hot water is running in the shower on the second floor. If the fill level in the open storage tank is allowed to decrease, then the water at the shower opening will:

    I. increase in pressure.
    II. decrease in pressure.
    III. decrease in velocity.

    A. II only
    B. III only
    C. I and III only
    D. II and III only

38. Assuming that all of the faucets are shut, where in Figure 1 will the water have the greatest pressure?

    A. At the shower faucet on the second floor
    B. At the kitchen and bathroom faucets on the first floor
    C. At the bathroom sink faucet on the second floor
    D. At the intake valve of the washing machine in the basement

39. The height of the water in the open storage tank is 1.25 m. If someone working in the attic accidentally punctures a very small hole in the bottom of the tank, what will the approximate speed of the water be as it exits the hole?

    A. 1 m/s
    B. 5 m/s
    C. 12 m/s
    D. 25 m/s

GO ON TO THE NEXT PAGE.

Questions 40 through 44 are NOT based on a descriptive passage.

40. When an electron falls from n = 3 to n = 2 in a hydrogen atom, what is the value of the energy released, given that A is the energy needed to remove an electron from the ground state of a hydrogen atom to an infinite distance from the atom?

    A. 0.14A
    B. 0.17A
    C. 1.00A
    D. 5.00A

41. A Boeing 737 aircraft has a mass of 150,000 kg, and a cruising velocity of 720 km/hr. Its engines can create a total thrust of 200,000 N. If air resistance, change in altitude, and fuel consumption can be ignored, how long does it take for the plane to reach its cruising velocity starting from rest?

    A.   100 s
    B.   150 s
    C.   540 s
    D.   1944 s

42. If the pK_a of a weak acid is 5, the pH will be 6:

    A. when the concentration of dissociated acid is one-tenth the concentration of undissociated acid.
    B. when half the acid is dissociated.
    C. when the concentration of dissociated acid is ten times the concentration of undissociated acid.
    D. only after a base has been added.

43. A certain metal plate is completely illuminated by a monochromatic light source. Which of the following would increase the number of electrons ejected from the surface of the metal?

    I.   Increasing the intensity of the light source
    II. Increasing the frequency of the light source
    III. Increasing the surface area of the metal plate

    A. I only
    B. I and II only
    C. I and III only
    D. II and III only

44. An apparatus is set up to measure the standard potential of a chemical reaction. When the apparatus is in operation, which of the following correctly describes of the movement of electrons?

    A. Through the ammeter to the anode
    B. Through the ammeter to the cathode
    C. Through the voltmeter to the anode
    D. Through the voltmeter to the cathode

GO ON TO THE NEXT PAGE.

Passage VII (Questions 45–49)

Thin films are layers of material between 2 nm and 1 μm thick, which correspond to a range of a few to several hundred atomic layers. Since these thin films are so fragile, they are often formed on, and continuously supported by, a rigid base known as a substrate. This substrate is very often simply a glass microscope slide. To create a thin film sample the substrate is first covered with a thin metal coating, known as an electrode. The thin film is built on top of this to the desired thickness, and then covered with a second metal electrode. This effectively forms a parallel-plate capacitor with the thin film acting as the dielectric and the electrodes acting as the parallel plates. Figure 1 below shows the structure of such a thin film device.

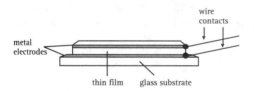

Figure 1

Some thin films are pyroelectric. These are materials that respond to a change in temperature by generating a small current across the opposite faces of the thin film. The magnitude of the current generated by a pyroelectric material is determined by the equation:

$$i = pA\frac{\Delta T}{t}$$

where i is the current, p is the pyroelectric coefficient, A is the area of the electrodes, ΔT is the change in temperature, and t is the time. The pyroelectric coefficient is a measure of the performance of a pyroelectric material; the higher the pyroelectric coefficient, the more efficient the pyroelectric material is.

The pyroelectric thin film used here has a thickness of 1 μm, and a pyroelectric coefficient of 20 $\times$ 10^{-6} C/m² • °C. The area of the metal electrodes is 3 $\times$ 10^{-4} m². (Note: The condition for maximum intensity of light reflected off of a thin film is $2dn = (m +1/2)\lambda$, m is an integer equal to or greater than 0, where n is the index of refraction of the film, d is the thickness of the film, and λ is the wavelength of light.)

45. Which of the following would increase the magnitude of the current generated by the pyroelectric thin film?

    I.   Increasing the rate of change in temperature

    II. Increasing the area of the electrodes

    III. Increasing the thickness of the film

  A. I only
  B. I and II only
  C. II and III only
  D. I, II, and

46. The current, i, generated by the pyroelectric is equal to Q/t, where $+Q$ and $-Q$ are equal to the charge deposited on the positive and negative electrodes, respectively. If a pyroelectric is charged up and then connected in parallel to a resistor, what will be the maximum voltage across the resistor? (Note: The capacitance of the pyroelectric is C, and the resistance of the resistor is R.)

  A. $pA(\Delta T)/RC$
  B. $pA(\Delta T)/C$
  C. $pA(\Delta T)/R$
  D. $pA(\Delta T)RC$

GO ON TO THE NEXT PAGE.

47. Which of the following graphs best illustrates the relationship between the thickness and the capacitance of the thin film?

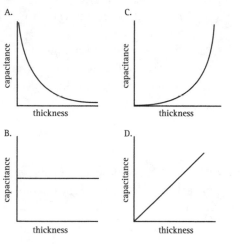

A.

B.

C.

D.

48. If the area of the electrodes and the thin film are doubled, the dielectric constant of the film will then:

A. be cut in half.
B. remain unchanged.
C. double.
D. quadruple.

49. A thin film of unknown thickness and index of refraction $n = 1.5$ is not in contact with any electrodes or substrate. Monochromatic light of variable wavelength is incident on the film. If the reflected light is maximum for a wavelength of 480 nm, what is the minimum thickness of the film?

A. 80 nm
B. 160 nm
C. 240 nm
D. 480 nm

GO ON TO THE NEXT PAGE.

Passage VIII (Questions 50–57)

Aggregated gas molecules, known as clusters, are found in abundance in the upper atmosphere. Atmospheric scientists have devised several ways of artificially synthesizing clusters, which are bound together by weak intermolecular forces. The most common method of producing bimolecular clusters in the laboratory is via a supersonic nozzle. Such a nozzle consists of a tiny pinhole, a few microns in diameter, through which a gas under high pressure (up to 100 atm) expands into a vacuum chamber. During expansion the molecules collide with one another, and many "stick together" as clusters. Conditions such as pressure and nozzle diameter can be adjusted to favor clusters containing different numbers of molecules.

The strength of the forces holding these aggregations together can be determined by irradiating samples with a laser. The threshold frequency of light needed to break the clusters down into their constituent molecules is used to derive the energy of the clusters. The table below shows several types of intermolecular attractive forces and examples of clusters for which each type of force predominates. In contrast to the strengths of these intermolecular forces, the strength of a chemical bond is typically tens of thousands of wavenumbers.

Table 1

FORCE	STRENGTH (cm^{-1})	EXAMPLES
H-bonding	~1,200 – 2,000	F–H • • • F–H
Dipole-Dipole	~30 – 1,000	HCl • • • SO$_2$
Dipole-Induced Dipole	~20 – 500	H$_2$O • • • Ar
Dispersion	~3 – 150	Ar • • • Ar

50. What is meant by the "energy of the clusters" mentioned in the second paragraph of the passage?

    A. The energy released when a cluster is formed
    B. The energy shared among the molecules of the cluster
    C. The bond energy of the molecules in the cluster
    D. The energy released when a cluster breaks up

51. Which of the following clusters would you expect to be most strongly bound?

    A. NO • • • Ar
    B. Ar • • • Ar
    C. CCl$_4$ • • • Ar
    D. HCl • • • Ar

52. If clusters are broken up using lasers in the near-infrared to the radio-frequency range of the spectrum, what frequencies could be used to break a chemical bond?

    A. Far infrared
    B. Microwave
    C. Ultraviolet
    D. Red light

53. What is the strongest intermolecular interaction between H$_2$O and CH$_3$OH molecules?

    A. Dipole-dipole
    B. Dipole-induced dipole
    C. H-bonding
    D. Dispersion

GO ON TO THE NEXT PAGE.

54. What type of intermolecular force(s) can exist between two neon atoms?

    I.   Dispersion forces
    II. Dipole-induced dipole
    III. Dipole-dipole

    A. I only
    B. II only
    C. I and II only
    D. I and III only

55. Why do dipole-dipole interactions occur between molecules of CO and molecules of NO?

    A. They both contain at least one electronegative element.
    B. They both have dipole moments.
    C. One is more polar than the other.
    D. They both contain oxygen.

56. The example given in Table 1 of a system exhibiting dipole-dipole interactions shows the molecule SO_2. What is the shape of this molecule?

    A. Linear
    B. Bent
    C. T-shaped
    D. Trigonal planar

57. If a cluster can be broken up by a photon with a wave number of 1000 cm^{-1}, what is the cluster's energy? (Note: Planck's constant = 6.6×10^{-34} J • s.)

    A. 6.6×10^{-31} J
    B. 6.6×10^{-29} J
    C. 2.0×10^{-26} J
    D. 2.0×10^{-20} J

GO ON TO THE NEXT PAGE.

Passage IX (Questions 58–64)

A bomb calorimeter measures the heat of combustion of unknown materials. Inside a pressurized heavy-duty steel canister (the "bomb") filled with pure oxygen gas, is placed a compressed disc of the unknown sample, through which a fine wire runs. The wire is connected to electrodes on the canister, and is ignited with a jolt of electricity. Both sample and wire burn rapidly in the oxygen, raising the calorimeter's temperature.

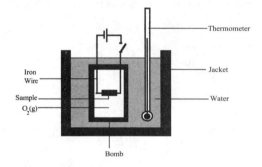

Figure 1 Bomb Calorimeter

The energy of combustion ΔE_{comb} of the sample may be determined from the sample's heat capacity C_v at constant volume, the rise in temperature of the calorimeter ΔT, and the heat capacity of the iron wire C_{Fe}. We assume that sufficient oxygen is available in the bomb to allow the combustion reaction to go to completion.

$$\Delta E_{comb} = (C_v\Delta T - C_{Fe}m_{Fe})/m_{sample} \text{ [Equation I]}$$

$$C_{calorimeter} = -\Delta E/\Delta T \text{ [Equation II]}$$

The following experimental data were taken by a student.

Property	Value
m_{sample}	1.3916 g
m_{wire}	0.0068 g
C_{Fe}	1400 cal/g
$C_{calorimeter}$	2417 cal/°C
T_i	25.01 °C
T_f	29.93 °C
C_v	8541.9 cal/g

Table 1 Bomb Calorimetry of Sample

From the data listed in Table 1, the student determined that the sample was benzophenone, $(C_6H_5)_2CO$.

58. Which expression gives the correct energy of combustion for benzophenone?

   A. $\Delta E_{comb} = 13\Delta E_{f,CO_2} + 5\Delta E_{f,H_2O} - \Delta E_{f,benzophenone}$
   B. $\Delta E_{comb} = \Delta E_{f,benzophenone} + \Delta E_{f,O_2} - \Delta E_{f,CO_2} - \Delta E_{f,H_2O}$
   C. $\Delta E_{comb} = \Delta E_{f,benzophenone} + 15\Delta E_{f,O_2} + 13\Delta E_{f,CO_2} + 5\Delta E_{f,H_2O}$
   D. $\Delta E_{comb} = 13\Delta E_{f,CO_2} + 5\Delta E_{f,H_2O} - \Delta E_{f,benzophenone} - \Delta E_{f,CO_2}$

59. When performing bomb calorimetry, which of the following conditions best applies to the combustion of a sample?

   A. constant P
   B. constant T
   C. constant V
   D. constant n

GO ON TO THE NEXT PAGE

60. Below is a plot of the temperature of the calorimeter versus time:

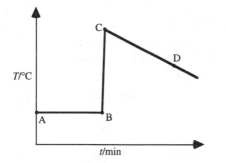

Which point on the graph represents T_f?

A. A
B. B
C. C
D. D

61. About how many moles of oxygen were consumed in the calorimeter?

A. 0.001 mol
B. 0.01 mol
C. 0.1 mol
D. 1 mol

62. About how much energy was required to raise the calorimeter's temperature by 4.92 °C?

A. 2.4 kJ
B. 12 kJ
C. 30 kJ
D. 490 J

63. Which of the following two assumptions is (are) invoked when using a bomb calorimeter to measure energy of combustion?

I. The system is adiabatic with respect to the environment.
II. The system maintains an approximately constant pressure throughout the process.

A. I only
B. II only
C. I and II
D. neither I nor II

64. What is the molar heat capacity of the iron wire?

A. 1.4 kcal/mol
B. 9.5 cal/mol
C. 25 cal/mol
D. 78 kcal/mol

GO ON TO THE NEXT PAGE

Passage X (Questions 65–71)

Among the many atmospheric industrial pollutants are the various oxides of nitrogen, often denoted NO_x. A major source of NO_x pollution is automobile exhaust. A chain of reactions involving NO_x may start with $NO(g)$, which is formed from burning $N2(g)$ in the automobile engine:

$$N_2(g) + O_2(g) \leftrightarrow 2NO(g) \text{ [Equation I]}$$

The K_{eq} at 25 °C for Equation I is about 10–15, which increases to about 0.05 at 2100 °C, the temperature inside a engine cylinder undergoing compression. The enthalpy of formation of NO is 181 kJ/mol. Upon entering the atmosphere, NO is oxidized to form $NO_2(g)$. $NO_2(g)$ exists in equilibrium with a dimeric form:

$$N_2O_4(g) \leftrightarrow 2NO_2(g) \text{ [Equation II]}$$
colorless   brown

The K_{eq} at 25 °C for Equation II is 0.115. Above 140 °C, dissociation is complete. The dissociation energy of N_2O_4 is 57 kJ/mol. Both species in Equation II are highly toxic. The reddish-brown NO_2 is a major component of the famous brownish haze that often covers the Los Angeles area of California, as well as other major metropolitan centers. The NO_2 gas attacks metals rapidly, and reacts with water:

$$2NO_2 + H_2O \leftrightarrow HNO_3 + HNO_2 \text{ [Equation III]}$$

Equation III shows how atmospheric NO_2 contributes to so-called "acid rain," which is a suspected cause of the lowering of soil and freshwater pH in industrialized areas.

Note that $h = 6.63 \times 10^{-34}$ J s, $R = 0.08206$ L·atm/mol·K, and $c = 3.00 \times 10^8$ m/s.

65. In the presence of the nitrogen oxides shown in Equations II and III, atmospheric acidity is more likely to form under conditions of

   A. heat and dry weather
   B. cold and dry weather
   C. heat and humidity
   D. cold and humidity

66. Suppose, in a darkened room, we place a piece of iron in a glass vessel containing the equilibrium mixture of gases in Equation II. We could most easily promote corrosion of the iron if we irradiate the vessel with a(n)

   A. radio-frequency generator
   B. microwave oven
   C. CO_2 laser which emits at 10µm
   D. ultraviolet quartz lamp

67. Using Lewis structures, which molecule would be described as a radical?

   A. H_2O
   B. NO_2
   C. N_2O_4
   D. HNO_3

68. All of the following experimental methods might be used to detect the presence of NO2 in a glass vessel initially charged with pure N_2O_4, EXCEPT

   A. UV-visible spectroscopy
   B. manometer
   C. wet litmus paper
   D. gravimetric analysis

GO ON TO THE NEXT PAGE

69. What is the correct sequence of oxidation states through which nitrogen goes from N_2 to NO to NO_2 to HNO_3?

   A. 0, +2, +4, +5
   B. 0, −2, −4, −5
   C. +5, 0, −2, −3
   D. +5, −2, −4, −5

70. An equilibrium mixture of gases in Equation II is compressed. What would be the effect of compression on the mixture?

   A. The mixture would become more intensely colored
   B. The mixture would become less intensely colored
   C. The color of the mixture would remain about the same
   D. The passage does not provide enough information to determine what happens to the color.

71. A car emits $NO(g)$ at a rate of 0.30 g/km through its exhaust pipe. How many liters of $NO(g)$ is this at standard temperature and pressure?

   A. 0.021 L/km
   B. 0.22 L/km
   C. 2.0 L/km
   D. 200 L/km

Questions 72 through 77 are NOT based on a descriptive passage.

72. Which form of energy transfer occurs most readily in a vacuum?

   A. Convection
   B. Conduction
   C. Radiation
   D. Two of the above

73. $^{204}_{84}Po$ undergoes radioactive decay with a half-life of 3.8 hours by emitting alpha particles. Two moles of pure $^{204}_{84}Po$ are isolated and put on a scale. After 7.6 hours a reading of the sample's mass is made. Its mass is found to be

   A. 201 grams.
   B. 203 grams.
   C. 400 grams.
   D. 402 grams.

74. A sound wave that has a velocity of 10,000 ft/s and a frequency of 1000 Hz is emitted by a source at rest. When the source is moving at a constant velocity of 2,000 ft/s, what is the ratio of the wavelength that would be heard by a stationary observer behind the moving source to an observer in front of the moving source?

   A. 1:1
   B. 2:3
   C. 3:2
   D. 9:11

GO ON TO THE NEXT PAGE

75. Gas A is at 30 °C and gas B is at 20° C. Both gases are at 1 atmosphere. What is the ratio of the volume of 1 mole of gas A to 1 mole of gas B?

  A. 1:1
  B. 2:3
  C. 3:2
  D. 303:293

76. Which of the following elements has an ionic radius that is larger than its atomic radius?

  A. Na
  B. K
  C. Mg
  D. Cl

77. When there are 2 electrons in the $3s$ subshell

  A. They must be occupying different orbitals.
  B. The Heisenberg uncertainty principle predicts that they must periodically jump to the $3p$ subshell.
  C. The oxidation state of the atom must be +2.
  D. They must have opposite spins.

STOP.

IF YOU FINISH BEFORE TIME HAS EXPIRED, CHECK YOUR WORK.
YOU MAY GO BACK TO ANY QUESTION IN THIS PART ONLY.

Verbal Reasoning Test

Time: 65 minutes—Questions 78–137

DIRECTIONS: There are nine passages in this Verbal Reasoning test. Each passage is followed by several questions. After reading a passage, select the one best answer to each question. If you are not certain of an answer, eliminate the alternatives that you know to be incorrect and then select an answer from the remaining alternatives.

Passage I (Questions 78–84)

Although many may argue with my stress on the continuity of the essential traits of American character and religion, few would question the
Line thesis that our business institutions have reflect-
5 ed the constant emphasis in the American value system on individual achievement. From the earliest comments of foreign travelers down to the present, individuals have identified a strong materialistic bent as being a characteristic
10 American trait. The worship of the dollar, the desire to make a profit, the effort to get ahead through the accumulation of possessions, all have been credited to the egalitarian character of the society, that is, to the absence of aristocracy. As
15 Tocqueville noted in his discussion of the consequences of a democracy's destruction of aristocracy: "They have swept away the privileges of some of their fellow creatures which stood in their way, but they have opened the door to uni-
20 versal competition." And a study of the comments on American workers of various nineteenth-century foreign travelers reveals that most of these European writers, among whom were a number of socialists, concluded that "social and economic
25 democracy in America, far from mitigating compensation for social status, intensified it. . . ."

American secular and religious values both have facilitated the "triumph of American capitalism," and fostered status striving. The focus on
30 equalitarianism and individual opportunity has also prevented the emergence of class consciousness among the lower classes. The absence of a socialist or labor party, and the historic weakness of American trade-unionism, appear to attest to
35 the strength of values which depreciated a concern with class. The growth of a large trade-union movement during the 1930s, together with the greater political involvement of labor organizations in the Democratic party, suggested to some
40 that the day—long predicted by Marxists—was arriving in which the American working class would finally follow in the footsteps of its European brethren. Such changes in the structure of class relations seemed to these observers to
45 reflect the decline of opportunity and the hardening of class lines. To them, such changes could not occur without modification in the traditional value system. . . .

A close examination of the character of the
50 American labor movement, however, suggests that it, like American religious institutions, may be perceived as reflecting the basic values of the larger society. Although unions, like all other American institutions, have changed in various
55 ways consistent with the growth of an urban industrial civilization, the essential traits of American trade unions, as of business corporations, may still be derived from key elements in the American value system. . . .
60

Although the American labor movement is similar to others in many respects, it differs from those of other stable democracies in ideology, class solidarity, tactics, organizational structure, and patterns of leadership behavior. American

GO ON TO THE NEXT PAGE.

65 unions are more conservative; they are more narrowly self-interested; their tactics are more militant; they are more decentralized in their collective bargaining; and they have more full-time
salaried officials, who are on the whole much
70 more highly paid. . . . American unions have also
organized a smaller proportion of the labor force
than have unions in these other nations.

78. If the claims made in the passage about
American and foreign labor unions are correct,
how would they be expected to react during a
strike against a corporation?

A. American labor unions would be less likely
than foreign unions to use violence against
a corporation.

B. American labor unions would be more
likely than foreign unions to use violence
against a corporation.

C. American labor unions would be less likely
than foreign unions to bargain with a
corporation.

D. American labor unions would be more
likely than foreign unions to bargain with
a corporation.

79. The existence of which of the following phenomena would most strongly challenge the
information in the passage?

A. American union leaders who are highly
paid to negotiate on behalf of workers

B. American labor organizations that avoid
involvement in non-labor issues

C. American workers with a weak sense of
group solidarity

D. American corporations that are more
interested in helping people than in
making a profit

80. Based on the passage, which of the following
is/are NOT true?

I. American society emphasizes class solidarity over individual achievement.

II. American unions are less interested in
non-labor issues than unions in other
democracies.

III. American labor organizations and
American religious institutions share
some of the same values.

A. I only

B. II only

C. II and III

D. I, II, and III

81. Suppose that an American union decides that its
members should take an active part in national
politics. What effect would this information
have on the author's view of American unions?

A. It would support that view.

B. It would contradict that view.

C. It would neither support nor contradict
that view.

D. It would support that view only if it could
be shown that getting involved in politics
was for society's good.

82. In the context of the passage, the phrase *strong
materialistic bent* (lines 8–9) refers to:

A. European socialists' view of aristocrats.

B. European travelers' concern with
democracy.

C. American society's emphasis on acquiring
wealth.

D. American religion's criticism of secular
values.

GO ON TO THE NEXT PAGE.

83. According to the passage, all of the following have influenced the outlook of the American labor movement EXCEPT:

    A. secular values.

    B. religious values.

    C. urban industrial civilization.

    D. foreign labor movements.

84. According to the passage, which of the following is a part of the "traditional value system"?

    A. Class solidarity

    B. Individual achievement

    C. Urban industrialization

    D. Marxist ideology

GO ON TO THE NEXT PAGE.

Passage II (Questions 85–91)

There are a great many points about coral reefs that remain subjects of scientific puzzlement. One mystery concerns the relationship between *Scleractinia*, the coral type whose colonization produces reefs, and their symbiotic partners the *zooxanthellae,* the unicellular algae present in the corals' endodermic tissues. It is known that each symbiont plays an integral part in the formation of a reef's protective limestone foundation. The coral polyps secrete calceous exoskeletons which cement themselves into an underlayer of rock, while the algae deposit still more calcium carbonate, which reacts with sea salt to create an even tougher limestone layer. It is also known that, due to the algal photosynthesis, the reef environment is highly oxygen-saturated, while the similarly high amounts of carbon dioxide are carried off rapidly. All this accounts for the amazing renewability of coral reefs despite the endless erosion caused by wave activity. However, the precise manner in which one symbiont stimulates the secretion of calcium carbonate by the other remains unclear.

Scientists have also proposed various theories to explain the transformation of "fringing reefs," those connected above sea level to land masses, into "barrier reefs" that are separated from shorelines by wide lagoons, and then into free-floating atolls. Though the theory postulated by Charles Darwin is considered at least partially correct, some scientists today argue that the creation of the reef forms has more to do with the rise of sea level that accompanied the end of the Ice Age than with the gradual submergence of the volcanic islands to which the fringing reefs were originally attached. However, recent drillings at Enewetak atoll have uncovered a large underlay of volcanic rock, which suggests that Darwin's explanation may have been more valid after all.

Even the name give to the reefs is something of a misnomer. The *Scleractinia* themselves generally comprise no more than 10 percent of the biota of the average reef community: *zooxanthellae* can account for up to 90 percent of the reef mass, along with *foraminifera,* annelid worms, and assorted mollusks. Moreover, the conditions under which reef growth occurs are determined by the needs of the algae, not the corals. Reefs can flourish only in shallow, highly saline waters above 70° F, because the algae require such circumstances; yet non-reef-building corals—corals which lack the algal presence—occur worldwide under various environmental conditions, from the Arctic to the Mediterranean, home of the red coral prized for jewelry. The most likely reason that the term "coral reefs" persists is that the brilliant variety of coral shapes and colors makes aesthetic considerations more vivid than biological ones.

85. All of the following are puzzling to reef scientists EXCEPT:

    A. how the *zooxanthellae* stimulate *Scleractinia* to secrete calcium carbonate.
    B. how barrier reefs become separated from land masses by vast expanses of water.
    C. how the reef environment reaches such high levels of oxygen saturation.
    D. how fringing reefs develop into barrier reefs and then into atolls.

GO ON TO THE NEXT PAGE.

86. Some scientists consider the term *coral reef* a misnomer because:

    A. the beautiful shapes and colors of reefs are produced by the *Scleractinia* rather than the *zooxanthellae*.
    B. the coral portion of a reef has little to do with the reef's survival.
    C. "non-reef-building" corals are found throughout the world.
    D. the majority of a reef's substance comprises *zooxanthellae, foraminifera,* annelid worms, and assorted molluscs while a small portion comprises the *Scleractinia*.

87. Opponents of Darwin's theory regarding coral reef transformation would disagree with which of the following statements?

    A. Coral reefs change from fringing reefs to barrier reefs, and then into free-floating atolls.
    B. Atolls are farther from land masses than are barrier reefs.
    C. Fringing reefs inevitably developed into barrier reefs because volcanic islands gradually sank into the ocean.
    D. As a result of the end of the Ice Age, increased expanses of water aided in the transformation of fringing reefs into barrier reefs.

88. Based on the passage, which of the following is probably an assumption of scientists studying coral reefs?

    A. The theories of reef evolution through glacial melting and through volcanic subsidence are mutually exclusive.
    B. The three main types of coral reefs did not develop independently of one another.
    C. *Zooxanthellae* are always found with coral.
    D. Intense calcification single-handedly protects reefs from destruction by waves and other natural causes.

89. In the passage, the mention of the recent drillings at the Enewetak atoll serves to:

    A. stengthen the claims made by scientists today concerning reef transformation.
    B. weaken the claims made by scientists today concerning reef transformation.
    C. strengthen the claims made by Darwin concerning reef transformation.
    D. weaken the claims made by Darwin concerning reef transformation.

90. According to the author, the theory proposed by Charles Darwin:

    A. is less persuasive on the topic of reef formation in light of recent discoveries.
    B. shows that each type of coral reef developed by separate, distinct processes.
    C. accurately described the transformation of fringing reefs into atolls.
    D. focused on the idea of submerging volcanic islands.

91. Suppose that marine biologists discovered that the calceous exoskeletons produced by coral polyps stimulate the *zooxanthellae* to deposit calcium carbonate via a chemical stimulus. How would this finding be relevant to the study of reefs?

    A. It would explain how reefs maintain a high level of oxygen saturation.
    B. It would clarify the symbiotic relationship between *Scleractinia* and *zooxanthellae* during their formation of the protective limestone foundation.
    C. It would identify the chemical components of the reef's protective layer.
    D. It would explain the intense colors and formations often seen in coral reefs.

GO ON TO THE NEXT PAGE.

Passage III (Questions 92–98)

Archaeopteryx lithographica lived during the latter part of the Jurassic period, approximately 150 million years ago, just south of what today is
Line central Germany. This ancient creature, which
5 combined a reptilian body and tail with birdlike wings and feathers, has provided a wealth of information about the evolution of flight in birds. However, fossil and skeletal studies indicate that it was not capable of flight. . . .

10 None of the *Archaeopteryx* fossils discovered to date, including the most mature specimens, exhibits an ossified or bony sternum, the wide bone that extends from the chest to the pelvic area in most modern birds. The main purposes of this
15 structure are to protect internal organs during flight and to act as a sturdy anchoring point for the enormous pectoral muscles necessary for flight. There is no indication that *Archaeopteryx* ever developed strong pectoral muscles, and per-
20 haps this is one reason why it never developed a sternum. Instead, it retained reptilian gastral ribs, thin braces in the abdominal region, which were not attached to the skeleton and which served only to support and protect internal organs. These
25 fishbonelike structures appear too fragile to have supported pectoral muscles. Researchers believe that flight would have been highly unlikely in an animal with such skeletal characteristics.

Furthermore, the bones in the manus of
30 *Archaeopteryx* do not seem to have been fused. In modern birds, these bones are fused in order to support the wing. In addition, the ulna of modern birds is marked with small knobs where feathers are anchored firmly to the bone by ligaments. The
35 ulna in *Archaeopteryx*, however, is smooth, indi- cating that its feathers were not firmly anchored into the skeleton.

Finally, the skeletal characteristics of *Archaeopteryx* seem to indicate that this animal

40 was most adapted to terrestrial movement. Its hind legs and pelvis closely resemble those of bipedal theropods and dinosaurs, suggesting that, like these other bipeds, it was adept at running along the ground. In contrast to the posture of
45 modern birds, whose bodies are suspended at the pelvis like a seesaw with the thighbones horizon- tal, it stood up on its hind legs with its long rep- tilian tail serving to balance it as well as enhance its ability to coordinate abrupt changes of direc-
50 tion while running. In modern birds all that remains of the tail is a shrunken, fused structure called a pygostyle. Although the foot of *Archaeopteryx* was birdlike, with fused metatarsals, it was also adapted to running and
55 serves as further evidence that this ancient animal had probably not developed the faculty of flight. . . .

Despite the fact that *Archaeopteryx litho- graphica* possessed many birdlike features,
60 including wings and advanced feathers, most of the fossil evidence of its existence overwhelm- ingly indicates that this animal was not capable of flight. By way of its peculiar mix of features, it seems to represent a kind of transitionary
65 phase, illustrating an evolutionary leap from rep- tile to bird and providing insight into the devel- opment of flight. . . .

92. For which of the following claims does the pas- sage provide some supporting evidence or explanation?

   A. Many scientists believe that *Archaeopteryx lithographica* could fly.

   B. Most ancient birds had some reptilelike characteristics.

   C. *Archaeopteryx lithographica* cannot be classified as either a reptile or a bird.

   D. Very few ancient reptiles could move around on dry land.

GO ON TO THE NEXT PAGE.

93. Suppose that scientists have recently found the skeleton of a bird capable of flight embedded in pre-Jurassic period rock. What effect would this discovery most likely have on their thinking about *Archaeopteryx lithographica*?

   A. It would support the view that *Archaeopteryx lithographica* represented a transitionary species between reptiles and birds.
   B. It would undermine the view that *Archaeopteryx lithographica* represented a transitionary species between reptiles and birds.
   C. It would neither support nor undermine the view that *Archaeopteryx lithographica* represented a transitionary species between reptiles and birds.
   D. It would support the view that *Archaeopteryx lithographica* failed to develop the pectoral muscles necessary for flight.

94. Based on information in the passage, which of the following statements is NOT true?

   A. *Archaeopteryx lithographica's* skeleton is similar to the skeleton of a modern bird.
   B. *Archaeopteryx lithographica's* tail played a larger role in its daily life than the tail of a modern bird plays in its daily life.
   C. Scientists have studied *Archaeopteryx lithographica* in order to learn about the development of flight.
   D. *Archaeopteryx lithographica* shared some characteristics in common with dinosaurs.

95. In the context of the passage, the phrase *wealth of information* (lines 6–7) refers to:

   A. knowledge of recent research projects on the evolution of flight.
   B. knowledge about *Archaeopteryx lithographica's* skeletal structure.
   C. knowledge acquired by scientists studying the development of birds.
   D. knowledge of fossil discoveries in what is now central Germany.

96. The author suggests which of the following about *Archaeopteryx lithographica*?

   A. It did not have as well-developed a tail as a modern bird.
   B. Its wings had a different function than the wings of a modern bird.
   C. It was less intelligent than a modern bird.
   D. Its skeletal structure made it much larger than a modern bird.

97. Suppose scientists were to find a skeleton of *Archaeopteryx lithographica* that has a sternum similar to the sternum of a modern bird. According to the passage, which of the following beliefs would this finding most strongly challenge?

   A. The belief that *Archaeopteryx lithographica* lived in what is today Europe
   B. The belief that *Archaeopteryx lithographica* lived in the Jurassic period
   C. The belief that *Archaeopteryx lithographica* lacked birdlike feathers
   D. The belief that *Archaeopteryx lithographica* lacked the ability to fly

98. Researchers believe that *Archaeopteryx* differs from modern birds for all of the following reasons EXCEPT:

   A. a lack of feathers.
   B. pectoral muscle development.
   C. ossification of the sternum.
   D. knobs found on the ulna.

GO ON TO THE NEXT PAGE.

 93

Passage IV (Questions 99–106)

Now that the sheep has faltered, Australians ride more and more upon the marsupial's back. . . . To a large extent, but more difficult to quantify, Australia's fauna and flora are being used as a unique resource. In scientific disciplines from reproductive physiology and evolutionary biology to medicine, Australia's native species are hailed as a unique and priceless heritage. They are providing insights into the way the world, and humans themselves, work. . . .

Australia's rainforests—those "unimportant appendages"—are now widely acknowledged as being the most ancient of humanity's land-based ecosystems, which gave rise to most others. It is also becoming increasingly accepted that rainforests arose on the southern continents and that Australia has some of the most ancient rainforests on Earth. Australian rainforests are thus filled with primitive plants. Botanical discoveries of world importance are being made in them every year. Australian botanists have recently completed a catalogue of Australian plants, in which they list 18,000 species. Their taxonomic work over recent years has resulted in a 50 percent increase in the number of species in the groups examined. Yet they estimate that about 7,000 undiscovered plant species still exist in Australia. Many surely inhabit Australian rainforests and are members of ancient and bizarre families, like the southern pine (*Podocarpus* species) recently found growing in a steep valley in Arnhem Land, thousands of kilometers distant from its nearest relatives.

Research on newly discovered Australian dinosaur faunas is challenging previous conceptions of what dinosaurs were like. So important are these discoveries that an Australian dinosaur recently made it onto the cover of a major international magazine. It was discovered in one of only two deposits in the world which was laid down near the South Pole during the age of dinosaurs. The chicken-sized species survived three months of darkness each year in a refrigerated world. Study of these fossils is teaching us much about the greenhouse effect as well as the lives of the dinosaurs themselves.

Far from being fixed on Earth, scientists now know that Australia has wandered over the face of the planet for billions of years, sometimes lying in the northern hemisphere, sometimes in the south. For 40 million years, after finally cutting the umbilicus with Antarctica, it slowly drifted northwards, in isolation, at about half the rate at which a human hair grows.

For scientists are finally understanding that evolution in Australia, in contrast to evolution on some other continents, is not driven solely by nature "red in tooth and claw." Here, a more gentle force—that of coadaptation—is important. This is because harsh conditions force individuals to cooperate to minimize the loss of nutrients, and to keep them cycling through the ecosystem as rapidly as possible. Thus, entire ecosytems have evolved in Australia that, when untampered with, recycle energy and nutrients in the most extraordinarily efficient ways. . . .

99. For which of the following claims does the passage provide some supporting evidence or explanation?
    I. Scientists have catalogued thousands of Australian plant species.
    II. Australia has shifted its position on the Earth's surface over millions of years.
    III. Australia has more plant species than any other continent.

    A. I only
    B. II only
    C. I and II
    D. I and III

GO ON TO THE NEXT PAGE.

100. The author of this passage would probably give his greatest support to which of the following actions by the Australian government?

A. Funding further research on plant species in Australia's rainforests

B. Cutting down some of Australia's rainforests to make more room for agriculture

C. Making sure that Australia's flora and fauna get international press coverage

D. Convincing other governments to fight the greenhouse effect

101. According to the passage, the author suggests which of the following about the process of evolution in Australia?

A. The plant species that this process has produced in Australia are also found on other continents.

B. It has not received the attention that it deserves from the international scientific community.

C. It has been a less violent process in Australia than it has been in other parts of the world.

D. This process has only taken place over the last 40 million years.

102. The author would most likely agree with which of the following statements about dinosaurs?

A. Australian dinosaurs were generally small in size.

B. Modern marsupials are descended from dinosaurs.

C. Dinosaurs became extinct before rainforests appeared.

D. Not all dinosaur species lived in warm environments.

103. Based on information in the passage, which of the following is NOT true?

A. Australia has moved from one hemisphere to the other over time.

B. Most Australian plant species remain undiscovered.

C. Important information is being gathered by studying Australian plants.

D. Australian rainforests are different from other rainforests.

104. In the context of the passage, the phrase *unimportant appendages* (lines 11–12) refers to:

A. the author's view of Australia's rainforests.

B. a characteristic of Australia's plant species.

C. the discovery of the southern pine species.

D. a view of Australia's rainforests that the author dismisses.

105. Suppose that a previously unknown species of plant that is capable of producing medicine is found in an Australian rainforest. How would this information affect the author's opinion of Australian rainforests?

A. It would support the author's opinion.

B. It would contradict the author's opinion.

C. It would neither support nor contradict the author's opinion.

D. It would contradict the author's opinion only if this species of plant cannot be found anywhere else.

106. According to the passage, all of the following are considered benefits of studying Australian ecosystems EXCEPT:

A. to increase knowledge of reproductive physiology and medicine.

B. to gain information concerning evolutionary trends.

C. to better understand the uses of hydroelectric power and solar energy.

D. to provide insight into ancient ecosystems.

GO ON TO THE NEXT PAGE.

 95

Passage V (Questions 107–113)

The latest prominent principle of criminal sentencing is that of "selective incapacitation." Selective incapacitation, like general incapacitation, involves
Line sentencing with the goal of protecting the communi-
5 ty from the crimes that an offender would commit if he were on the street. It differs from general incapacitation in its attempt to replace bluntness with selectivity. Under a strategy of selective incapacitation, probation and short terms of incarceration are
10 given to convicted offenders who are identified as being less likely to commit frequent and serious crimes, and longer terms of incarceration are given to those identified as more crime prone.

An attractive aspect of the selective incapacita-
15 tion concept is its potential for bringing about a reduction in crime without an increase in prison populations. This reduction could be substantial. . . .

Is selective incapacitation truly an effective and appropriate proposal, an "idea whose time has
20 come," or is it . . . a proposal that carries with it a potential for injustice? . . .

Reserving prison and jail space for the most criminally active offenders may in some instances conflict not only with other norms of legal justice,
25 but with norms of social justice as well. Repeat offenders fall basically into two categories: those who are prone to violence and those who are not. If we reserve the sanction of incarceration only for the dangerous repeat offender, excluding the
30 white-collar offender and certain other criminals who pose no serious threat of physical injury to others, we may end up permitting harmful people from the middle class to evade a sanction that less privileged offenders cannot. Some white-collar
35 offenders, after all, impose greater costs on society than many dangerous street offenders, and it is clearly unjust to allow the former to pay a smaller price for their crimes than the latter must pay. . . .

One of the most pervasive criticisms of selec-
40 tive incapacitation is that it is based on the statistical prediction of dangerousness; because such predictions are often erroneous, according to this point of view, they should not be used by the court. This criticism is related to both the nature of the errors
45 and to the use of certain information for predicting a defendant's dangerousness.

Let's first consider the nature of errors in prediction. Prediction usually results in some successes
50 and in two kinds of errors: predicting that a phenomenon such as recidivism will occur when in fact it does not ("false positives") and predicting that it will not occur when in fact it does ("false negatives"). The problem of false positives in sentencing is costly
55 primarily to incarcerated defendants who are not really so dangerous, while false negative predictions impose costs primarily on the victims of subsequent crimes committed by released defendants. In predicting whether a defendant will recidivate or "go
60 straight," the problem of false positives is widely regarded as especially serious, for many of the same reasons that it has been regarded in our society as better to release nine offenders than to convict one innocent person. . . .
65

A tempting alternative is to reject prediction altogether; obviously, if we do not predict, then no errors of prediction are possible. A flaw in this logic is that, whether we like it or not, criminal justice decisions are now, and surely always will be, based
70 on predictions, and imperfect ones, at that. Attempts to discourage prediction in sentencing may in fact produce the worst of both worlds: the deceit of predictive sentencing disguised as something more tasteful, and inferior prediction as well.
75

If we are to reserve at least some prison and jail space for the most criminally active offenders, then the prediction of criminal activity is an inescapable task . . . .

GO ON TO THE NEXT PAGE.

107. Suppose the number of dangerous criminals that would be imprisoned under selective incapacitation but otherwise set free is greater than the number of harmless criminals who would be set free under selective incapacitation but otherwise imprisoned. How would this information be relevant to the passage?

    A. It weakens the claim that the goal of selective incapacitation is to protect the community.
    B. It strengthens the claim that there are more violent than nonviolent criminals.
    C. It weakens the claim that selective incapacitation would not increase prison populations.
    D. It strengthens the claim that white-collar criminals unfairly receive shorter sentences.

108. Implicit in the author's discussion of the idea of rejecting statistical prediction is the idea that:

    A. statistical prediction will always be imperfect.
    B. a judge may well make more errors than a flawed statistical formula would.
    C. prediction will never attain widespread accceptance in the criminal justice system.
    D. sentencing should not take into account a criminal's future behavior.

109. Which of the following would the author advocate LEAST as a defense of the idea that we should employ statistical prediction in sentencing?

    A. Prediction always has been used in sentencing.
    B. Prediction will reduce the overcrowding in prisons.
    C. Rejecting statistical prediction leaves us with no predictive basis for sentencing.
    D. Making some predictive errors is better than not predicting at all.

110. The author's statement that selective incapacitation may "end up permitting harmful people from the middle class to evade a sanction that less privileged offenders cannot" (lines 32–34) assumes that:

    A. there are more offenders in the lower class than in the middle class.
    B. the dangerous repeat offenders are lower class and not middle class.
    C. harmful middle class people can use their money to avoid prison.
    D. lower class offenders do not deserve to suffer incarceration.

111. Based on the information in the passage, if one's goal is to protect the community, one would employ a predictive formula that:

    A. maximized the number of "false positives" and "false negatives."
    B. minimized the number of "false negatives."
    C. minimized the number of "false positives."
    D. minimized the number of "false positives" and maximized the number of "false negatives."

112. Based on the passage, which of the following would most likely be cited by an opponent of statistical prediction of dangerousness as the reason that prediction should be abandoned?

    A. The possibility of letting a dangerous criminal loose is too great.
    B. The possibility of imprisoning a man who should be allowed to go free is too great.
    C. The court makes more accurate decisions when statistics is employed.
    D. Dangerousness has yet to be adequately defined as a legal concept.

GO ON TO THE NEXT PAGE.

97

113. Which of the following is a claim made by the author but NOT supported in the passage by evidence, explanation, or example?

   A. Selective incapacitation may conflict with norms of social justice.
   B. The criticism of statistical dangerousness is related to the nature of predictive errors.
   C. Under selective incapacitation, first-time offenders would get short terms of incarceration.
   D. Some white-collar offenders impose greater costs on society than many dangerous street offenders.

GO ON TO THE NEXT PAGE.

Passage VI (Questions 114–120)

It is becoming increasingly clear that the comfort of a good fit between man and machine is largely absent from the technology of the
Line information age. Consider the humble wristwatch,
5 which has been transformed into a kind of wrist-mounted personal computer, with a digital display and a calculator pad whose buttons are too small to be pressed by a human fingertip . . . By replacing the watch's conventional stem-winding mechanism
10 with a mystifying arrangement of tiny buttons, the manufacturers created a watch that was hard to reset. One leading manufacturer was distressed to discover that a line of its particularly advanced digitals was being returned as defective by the
15 thousands, even though the watches actually worked perfectly well. Further investigation revealed that they were coming back soon after purchase and thereafter in two large batches—in the spring and the fall, when the time changed.

20 Charles Mauro, a consultant in New York City, is a prominent member of a branch of engineering generally known as ergonomics, or human-factors—the only field specifically addressing the question of product usability. Mauro . . . was
25 brought in to provide some help to the watch manufacturer, which was experiencing what Mauro calls the "complexity problem." With "complexity" defined as "a fundamental mismatch between the demands of a technology and the capabilities of its
30 user," the term nicely captures the essence of our current technological predicament . . . .

When confronted by some mystifying piece of high-tech gadgetry, consumers naturally feel that there is something wrong with them if they can't
35 figure it out. In truth it is usually not their fault. Mauro attributes the confusion to the fact that most products are "technology-driven," their nature determined not by consumers and their needs and desires but by engineers who are too often
40 entranced with the myriad capabilities of the microprocessors that lie at the devices' hearts . . . .

The engineers' blindness to consumers' needs may be at the root of a deeper problem—how so much baffling technology enters the market. The
45 problem has been blamed on the "waterfall method": new technological equipment tumbles out of a corporation, never encountering a typical user until it is bought.

A growing number of technologists think that
50 the development process should be reversed, and they speak of user-centered design as a means of scrupulously maintaining the user's perspective from start to finish, adding technology only where necessary to accomplish a particular task . . . .

55 Much of the work is a matter of finding the "mental models" . . . by which users instinctively interpret a technology. Especially when the workings of a device are invisible, these models may very well be erroneous. For instance, many
60 people set an electric burner on high thinking that it will heat up faster that way: they have the mental model of a gas stove, whose knobs actually do increase the heat's intensity. On an electric stove, however, the knob is merely a
65 switch that turns on the burner and then turns it off when a certain temperature is reached.

A cause of fatal mining accidents was once the peculiar configuration of the controls on the trams shuttling along mineshafts. Each tram had a
70 steering wheel that rose straight up from the floor, with a brake pedal on one side and an accelerator pedal on the other. There was no room to turn the tram around, so to reverse direction the driver simply took a seat on the other side of the steer-
75 ing wheel, whereupon what had been the brake became the accelerator, and vice versa. While this may sound ingenious, it proved disastrous . . . .

No single approach will eliminate all the complexity problems posed by current technolo-
80 gy. But user-centered design can certainly help solve these problems, if only by encouraging manufacturers to consider the needs and abilities

GO ON TO THE NEXT PAGE.

of the average user early on in the product-development process . . . .

114. Based on the passage, an ergonomics expert would be likely to place high value on a product that:

A. required no instruction at all to use.
B. did not incorporate modern technology.
C. could be easily manipulated by hand.
D. solved complex problems for its user.

115. Suppose a watch manufacturer were to market a watch with a conventional winding mechanism and the watch was returned as defective by the thousands. How would this information affect the argument made in the first paragraph?

A. It would weaken the argument.
B. It would support the argument.
C. It would weaken the argument if the watches were coming back because they didn't run correctly.
D. It would weaken the argument if the watches were coming back right after the time changed.

116. The claim that "no single approach will eliminate all the complexity problems posed by current technology" (lines 78–80) is:

A. necessarily true, given the information presented in the passage.
B. perhaps true, and supported by the information presented in the passage.
C. perhaps true, but not supported by any information in the passage.
D. necessarily false, given the information presented in the passage.

117. The author claims that poor design of tram controls was to blame for fatal mining accidents. The designer of the tram controls might best counter this by arguing that:

A. it should not have been that difficult to adjust to the change in direction.
B. the driver should not have switched the pedals.
C. the tram was never intended to move in the reverse direction.
D. the driver's erroneous "mental model" was to blame for the accidents.

118. When consumers feel that there is something wrong with them if they can't figure a high-tech gadget out, which of the following assumptions are they making?

A. The gadget was designed for ready use by the average consumer.
B. Technology can only be understood by engineer types.
C. The gadget designers were blind to the consumers' needs.
D. Everyone is equally capable of understanding new technology.

119. Which of the following would most weaken the contention that the nature of technological products is not determined by consumers and their needs and desires?

A. Many of a product's features are added because they are eye-catching in the showroom.
B. Consumers are buying more technological products now than ever.
C. Computers are upgraded so rapidly that new models are obsolete in a year.
D. The answering machine has come to be regarded as a necessity rather than a luxury.

GO ON TO THE NEXT PAGE.

120. According to one consumer survey, a third of all VCR owners have given up trying to program their machines for time-delayed viewing. How would the author probably explain this fact?

    A. VCR owners have not yet found the correct mental model by which to interpret the VCR.
    B. Those owners have concluded that the VCR was not well designed.
    C. Those trying to program the machine are not as technologically savvy as they should be.
    D. The VCR is the result of technology-driven rather than user-centered design.

GO ON TO THE NEXT PAGE.

Passage VII (Questions 121–126)

Because self-deception and secrecy from self
point to self-inflicted and often harmful ignorance, they invite moral concern: judgments
about responsibility, efforts to weigh the degree of
5   harm imposed by such ignorance, and questions
of how to help reverse it. If the false belief is
judged harmless and even pleasurable, as may be
the case with the benevolent light in which most
of us see our minor foibles, few would consider
10 interfering. But clearly there are times when people are dangerously wrong about themselves. The
anorexic girl close to starving to death who thinks
that she looks fat in the mirror, and the alcoholic
who denies having a drinking problem, are both
15 in need of help; yet the help cannot consist merely in interference, but must somehow bring about
a recognition on their part of their need and the
role they play in not perceiving it accurately.

Judgments about when and how to try to
20 help people one takes to be in self-inflicted danger depend on the nature and the seriousness of
the danger, as well as on how rational one thinks
they are. To attribute self-deception to people is to
regard them as less than rational concerning the
25 danger one takes them to be in, and makes intervention, by contrast, seem more legitimate. But
this is itself dangerous because of the difficulties
of establishing that there is self-deception in the
first place. Some feel as certain that anyone who
30 does not believe in their deity, their version of the
inevitable march of history, or their views of the
human psyche deceives himself as they might feel
about the self-deception of the anorexic and the
alcoholic. Frequently, the more improbable their
35 own views, the stronger is their need to see the
world as divided up into those who perceive the
self-evident and those who persist in deluding
themselves.

Aiding the victims of such imputed self-
40 deception can be hard to resist for true believers
and enthusiasts of every persuasion. If they come
to believe that all who do not share their own
views are not only wrong but actually know they
are wrong in one part of their selves that keeps the
45 other in the dark, they can assume that it is an act
of altruism to help the victimized, deceived part
see through the secrecy and the self-deception . . .

Zealots can draw on their imputing self-
deception to nonbelievers in yet another way, to
50 nourish any tendency they might have to a conspiracy theory. If they see the self—their own and
that of others—as a battleground for a conspiracy,
they may then argue that anyone who disagrees
with them thereby offers proof that his mind has
55 been taken over by the forces they are striving to
combat. It is not long before they come to see the
most disparate events not only as connected but as
intended to connect. There are no accidents, they
persuade themselves . . . .
60

Indeed, calling something trivial or far-
fetched counts, for holders of such theories, as further evidence of its significance. And denying what
they see as self-evident is still more conclusive
proof. How well we recognize the tone in which the
65 eminent sixteenth-century philosopher and jurist
Jean Bodin denounced those who scoffed at the
belief in the existence of witches. Their protesta-
tions of disbelief, he declared, showed that they
were most likely witches themselves. He wrote of
70 the pact that "confessed" witches . . . said they had
signed with Satan. It obliged them to ridicule all
talk of witchcraft as superstitious invention and
contrary to reason. They persuaded many naive
persons, Bodin insisted, whose arrogance and self-
75 deception was such that they would dismiss as
impossible even the actions of witches that were
right before their eyes . . . .

GO ON TO THE NEXT PAGE.

121. Which of the following general theories would be most in agreement with the theme of the passage?

    A. One's own beliefs shape one's judgment of the beliefs of others.
    B. One should strive to rid oneself of all self-deception.
    C. One is always aware at least to some degree of one's self-delusions.
    D. One can never conclusively show that another person is deceiving himself.

122. Suppose one knows that a friend is not nearly as physically fit as the friend believes himself to be. According to the passage, one should:

    A. attempt to persuade the friend that he is deceiving himself.
    B. prevent the friend from engaging in strenuous physical activity.
    C. disabuse the friend of his belief if his lack of fitness endangers him.
    D. realize that one may be wrong about the friend's level of physical fitness.

123. Given the information in the passage, if someone who believed there was a government conspiracy to cover up visits by extraterrestrials were to watch a TV program that debunks the idea of extraterrestrials, that person would most likely:

    A. conclude that the program's producers were part of the conspiracy.
    B. begin to suspect that she was suffering from self-delusion.
    C. claim that the idea behind the program was trivial or far-fetched.
    D. argue that the narrator of the program was himself an extraterrestrial.

124. Based on the information in the passage, the author believes that someone with very unorthodox views of the human psyche is:

    A. probably suffering from harmless self-deception.
    B. acting as irrationally as an alcoholic or an anorexic.
    C. likely to perceive differing views as self-delusional.
    D. unable to establish the presence of self-delusion in others.

125. Based on the passage, the author would probably agree that people who believe in a conspiracy theory:

    A. believe themselves to be protected from harm.
    B. know that in one part of themselves they are wrong.
    C. should not be allowed to voice their radical opinions.
    D. will not be dissuaded from their belief by even strong evidence.

126. Which of the following, if true, would most weaken the author's argument in the final paragraph?

    A. The "confessed" witches were burned at the stake by townspeople.
    B. A significant percentage of the modern American population believes in witches.
    C. The supposed sixteenth-century witches never confessed or signed a pact.
    D. Those whom Bodin accused of witchcraft were really witches.

GO ON TO THE NEXT PAGE.

 103

Passage VIII (Questions 127–132)

. . . Evidence of the earliest known Maya, who
cleared and farmed land bordering swamps as
early as 2,500 B.C., has emerged from a site in
Line northern Belize, researchers recently reported at
5 the annual meeting of the Society for American
Archaeology . . . .

. . . Until now, the oldest Maya settlements dated
to about 1,000 B.C. These sites yielded extensive
pottery remains and led many investigators to
10 assume that any prior farmers of the Yucatan
Peninsula also fashioned ceramic vessels . . . . Yet
current evidence suggests that the first agricultur-
ists in this region did not use pottery. Beginning
around 2500 B.C., they introduced crops from
15 Mexico, or perhaps beyond, and left behind distinctive stone tools . . . .

. . . Later Maya occupations of the same site, called
Colha, have undergone excavation since 1979 . . . .
But in 1993, researchers made the first systematic
20 effort to document a pre-ceramic presence at the
tropical, forested location. Early Colha farmers
inhabited the area in two phases. There are stone
tools in deeper soil layers dating from 2500 B.C. to
1700 B.C., based on radiocarbon age estimates of
25 accompanying charcoal bits. Comparable dates
come from an adjacent swamp, where pollen
analysis documents forest clearance by 2500 B.C . .
. . The pollen provides evidence for the existence of
several cultivated crops soon thereafter, mainly
30 corn and manioc, a starchy plant . . . . From about
1400 B.C. to 1000 B.C., Colha residents made foot-
shaped stone tools that were chipped and
sharpened on one side. Preliminary scanning
electron microscope analysis of polish on these
35 tools . . . . suggests that inhabitants used them to
cut away vegetation after controlled burning of
trees, and, perhaps, also to dig . . . .

. . . An example of the same tool, known as a constricted uniface, also emerged last year at

40 Pulltrouser Swamp, a Maya site 20 miles north-
west of Colha . . . . with a preliminary radiocarbon date of 1300 B.C. to 1000 B.C. for the artifact .
. . . Its unusual design led researchers to suspect
that Colha might have harbored an extremely
45 early Maya population. Another sharpened stone
point retrieved at Pulltrouser Swamp dates to
between 2500 B.C. and 2000 B.C. Several other sites
in Belize have yielded constricted unifaces, but
archaeologists have been unsure of their ages and
50 origins . . . .

. . . Techniques used to manufacture constricted
unifaces show gradual refinement and modification in stone tools of Colha residents living after
1000 B.C.. Continuity in stone tool design and
55 manufacture suggests that pre-ceramic Maya
inhabited Colha, rather than non-Maya peoples
who migrated to the area and later left or were
incorporated into Maya villages. "None of us had
any reason to suppose that Colha would produce
60 a pre-ceramic Maya occcupation," remarks the
director of excavations at Cuello, a Maya site that
dates to about 1000 B.C. . . . . "This is a bit of
archaeological serendipity." The earliest Central
American farmers probably settled at the edges of
65 swampland that they had cleared and cultivated .
. . . Excavations of pre-ceramic Colha so far have
focused on quarry and field areas. However, some
pottery may still show up in early residential
structures . . . .

127. The recent findings reported at the Society for
American Archaeology provide new insight into
Mayan civilization because:

  A. Mayans may have settled extensively
     throughout the Yucatan penninsula.
  B. ceramic pottery may have been used by the
     Mayans.
  C. Mayans may have settled in regions much
     earlier than previously thought.
  D. stone tools were never used by the
     Mayans.

GO ON TO THE NEXT PAGE.

128. The passage implies that archaeologists previously believed which of the following theories concerning ceramic use and Mayan civilization?

  A. Stone tools were used by the Mayans to create elaborate clay pottery.
  B. The cultivation of crops and the development of pottery occurred simultaneously.
  C. Mayan settlements could be identified by the existence of ceramic pottery remains.
  D. Mayans did not use ceramics unless they inhabited an area near a swamp.

129. Which of the following statements clarifies the significance of Pulltrouser Swamp and Colha?

  A. Pottery retrieved at Colha and stone tools discovered at Pulltrouser Swamp show that non-Mayans and Mayans co-existed in the Yucatan.
  B. Stone tools retrieved from excavation sites at Pulltrouser Swamp lead scientists to believe that non-Mayan peoples inhabited this area.
  C. The discovery of a uniquely-designed stone tool in a known Maya site indicates that Mayans may have inhabited the sight before 1000 B.C.
  D. The findings at Pulltrouser Swamp and Colha offer scientists no conclusive evidence.

130. According to the passage, early Colha farmers were probably:

  A. Mayans who used stone tools.
  B. Mayans who did not use stone tools.
  C. non-Mayans who used stone tools.
  D. non-Mayans who made ceramics.

131. In the context of the passage, the term "archaeological serendipity" (line 63) refers to:

  A. the discovery of stone tools.
  B. the unexpected findings that gave researchers a new understanding of ancient settlements.
  C. the method used by archaeologists to excavate ancient civilizations.
  D. the Mayans' ability to work with their environment.

132. Which of the following discoveries would lead archaeologists to change their recently formed opinions on pre-ceramic Mayan populations?

  A. Careful study of a "constricted uniface" shows that this tool was used to clear away vegetation.
  B. After extensive excavation of the Colha dwellings, researchers discovered ceramic pottery remains dating back to 2500 B.C.
  C. Continued excavation at Colha has produced stone tools dating back to 2500 B.C.
  D. At a known Maya settlement, archaeologists recently uncovered pottery dating back to 1000 B.C.

GO ON TO THE NEXT PAGE.

Passage IX (Questions 133–137)

The tsetse fly, belonging to any of approximately twenty species composing the genus *Glossina,* is indigenous to Africa and is found
Line primarily in forests and savannas south of the
5 Tropic of Cancer. Dependent on vertebrate blood for nourishment, the tsetse fly is equipped with a long proboscis which is sharp enough to penetrate most animal skins and powerful enough to enable the tsetse to drink quantities of blood up to three times
10 its own body weight. Measuring less than half an inch in length, this tiny pest has emerged at the center of health and environmental controversies.

At the same time that the tsetse drains blood, it can also transmit a variety of dangerous
15 diseases. A bite from a tsetse fly can induce African sleeping sickness in human beings and nagana, a similar ailment, in domestic livestock. The agent of these diseases is the *trypanosome,* a unicellular, flagellated parasite which feeds
20 primarily on the blood of vertebrates and is generally transmitted by an intermediary leech or insect host, such as the tsetse fly. In humans the *trypanosome* causes damage to the brain and spinal cord, leading to extreme lethargy and,
25 ultimately, death; in livestock, *trypanosomes* destroy red blood cells, causing fatal anemia.

The immune system is ill-equipped to counter *trypanosomes.* As the immune system attempts to counter disease, antibodies are produced to attack
30 microbes whose antigens, surface proteins, are foreign to the body. Various antibodies are specific for particular antigens. However, the *trypanosome* is capable of disguising itself by altering its genetic code, thereby changing its antigen coating in
35 resistance to each new antibody that evolves. This "quick change" has confounded pathologists and made the development of effective vaccines elusive.

Since the protozoan cannot be conquered through antibodies or vaccines, scientists have
40 begun efforts to prevent the transmission of the *trypanosome* parasite by eliminating the tsetse. Attempts to eradicate the tsetse fly, however, have met with little success. Rhodesia used to combat tsetse by extensive brush cleaning, game shooting,
45 and chemical attack, yet the fly persisted. Aerial pesticide treatments have produced inconclusive results. The reproductive cycle of the tsetse fly is such that a larva pupates underground for several weeks before it emerges as an adult fly. This makes
50 repetitive chemical sweeping at intermittent periods an inconvenient necessity. A third method, called the "soft approach," makes use of the tsetse's attraction to the odors of carbon dioxide, acetone, and octenol. Open bottles of these compounds are hung behind
55 black screens and nets permeated with insecticides. Massive numbers of flies, attracted to the chemicals from great distances, are lured into the nets where they are poisoned and die. All of these methods, however, share the weakness of dependence on
60 harmful chemicals, such as DDT, which threaten both the health of the humans who handle them and the environment in which their toxic residues amass.

Thus, a controversy has been sparked between proponents of the elimination of the tsetse fly and
65 African environmentalists. Those in favor of eradication feel that in addition to reducing disease, the removal of the tsetse fly will open immense tracts of land to cattle breeding. This, however, is precisely what the opposition fears. Environmentalists and
70 conservationists dread the day when cattle and livestock, permitted to roam and graze freely, will uncontrollably devour plush African grasslands, converting them into barren desert. They argue that the tsetse fly must remain for the sake of the land.
75

With efforts to eradicate the tsetse fly largely unsuccessful, a compromise between tsetse control and tsetse elimination need not be forced. As elimination of the tsetse seems unlikely and may be impossible, control of the tsetse population
80 offers the only available option for the interests of both health and environment.

GO ON TO THE NEXT PAGE.

133. All of the following statements correctly describe the relationship between the tsetse fly, the *trypanosome,* and vertebrates EXCEPT:

    A. Vertebrate blood provides the nourishment for the transport of *trypanosomes.*
    B. The "bite" of a tsetse fly can kill vertebrates since it often injects a deadly chemical.
    C. Both the tsetse fly and the *trypanosome* utilize vertebrate blood for nourishment.
    D. Vertebrates may die after *trypanosome* contamination via a tsetse proboscis.

134. Which of the following is NOT identified in the passage as a characteristic of the tsetse fly?

    A. Dependence upon vertebrate blood
    B. Ability to transmit a fatal parasite to livestock and humans
    C. Ability to alter its genetic code
    D. Ability to influence the African cattle population

135. The passage implies that the tsetse fly must be controlled for all of the following reasons EXCEPT:

    A. to prevent the spread of disease throughout the African continent.
    B. because many human and animal lives are threatened by *trypanosomes.*
    C. because cattle in Africa are reproducing at an alarming rate.
    D. because *trypanosomes* cannot be overcome by vaccine.

136. In many warm climates, locusts feed on agricultural crops and lizards feed on locusts. Which of the following is most analogous to the effect that eradicating the tsetse fly would have on African grasslands?

    A. Locusts transmit a deadly parasite from the agricultural crops to the lizards.
    B. Lizards are dependent upon both the locusts and the grasslands for nourishment.
    C. Elimination of the locusts results in bumper wheat crops.
    D. Elimination of lizards results in locust infestation and devastation of agricultural crops.

137. Which of the following would the author most likely consider the best solution to the tsetse problem?

    A. Using repeated insecticide treatment during the fly's pupal period
    B. Clearing away large tracts of tsetse infested brush
    C. Strictly-regulated use of the "soft approach" in predetermined areas
    D. Continued research toward the development of a *trypanosome* vaccine

STOP.

IF YOU FINISH BEFORE TIME HAS EXPIRED, CHECK YOUR WORK.
YOU MAY GO BACK TO ANY QUESTION IN THIS PART ONLY.

Writing Sample

Time: 60 minutes
2 Prompts, Separately Timed—30 Minutes Each

DIRECTIONS: You are allotted 60 minutes to work on this part of the exam. You may work on only the Writing Sample part during that time. Should you finish early, you are permitted to check your work in this part of the exam only.

The Writing Sample test examines your writing skills. The test contains two assignments, Part 1 and Part 2, and you will have 30 minutes to complete each assignment.

You are permitted to work only on Part 1 during the first 30 minutes of the test and only on Part 2 during the second 30 minutes of the test. Should you finish writing on Part I before the time is up, you may review your work on Part 1, but do not begin writing on Part 2. Similarly, should you finish writing on Part 2 before the time is up, you are permitted to review your work on Part 2 only.

Use your time efficiently. Read the assignment carefully before you begin writing a response. Please ensure thorough comprehension of the assignment. Use the space located below each writing assignment for notation in planning your responses.

Your response to each part should be an essay composed of complete sentences and paragraphs, as this is a test of your writing skills. Your responses should be as well organized and clearly written as possible, given your time restrictions. Corrections or additions should be placed neatly between the lines of your responses.

Please note that illegible essays cannot be scored.

TURN THE PAGE AND BEGIN.

Part I

Consider the following statement:

The pursuit of knowledge is always justified.

Write a unified essay in which you perform the following tasks. Explain what you think the above statement means. Describe a specific situation in which the pursuit of knowledge is *not* justified. Discuss what you think determines when the pursuit of knowledge is justified and when it is not.

Part 2

Consider the following statement:

Testing is the most accurate predictor of intelligence.

Write a unified essay in which you perform the following tasks. Explain what you think the above statement means. Describe a specific situation in which testing is *not* the most accurate predictor of intelligence. Discuss what you think determines when testing is the most accurate predictor of intelligence.

STOP.

IF YOU FINISH BEFORE TIME HAS EXPIRED, CHECK YOUR WORK.
YOU MAY GO BACK TO ANY QUESTION IN THIS PART ONLY.

Biological Sciences Test

Time: 100 minutes—Questions 138–214

DIRECTIONS: Most of the questions in the following Biological Sciences test are organized into groups, with a descriptive passage preceding each group of questions. Study the passage, then select the single best answer to each question in the group. Some of the questions are not based on a descriptive passage; you must also select the best answer to these questions. If you are unsure of the best answer, eliminate the choices that you know are incorrect, then select an answer from the choices that remain. A periodic table is provided below for your use with the questions.

Periodic Table of the Elements

1 H 1.0																	2 He 4.0
3 Li 6.9	4 Be 9.0											5 B 10.8	6 C 12.0	7 N 14.0	8 O 16.0	9 F 19.0	10 Ne 20.2
11 Na 23.0	12 Mg 24.3											13 Al 27.0	14 Si 28.1	15 P 31.0	16 S 32.1	17 Cl 35.5	18 Ar 39.9
19 K 39.1	20 Ca 40.1	21 Sc 45.0	22 Ti 47.9	23 V 50.9	24 Cr 52.0	25 Mn 54.9	26 Fe 55.8	27 Co 58.9	28 Ni 58.7	29 Cu 63.5	30 Zn 65.4	31 Ga 69.7	32 Ge 72.6	33 As 74.9	34 Se 79.0	35 Br 79.9	36 Kr 83.8
37 Rb 85.5	38 Sr 87.6	39 Y 88.9	40 Zr 91.2	41 Nb 92.9	42 Mo 95.9	43 Tc (98)	44 Ru 101.1	45 Rh 102.9	46 Pd 106.4	47 Ag 107.9	48 Cd 112.4	49 In 114.8	50 Sn 118.7	51 Sb 121.8	52 Te 127.6	53 I 126.9	54 Xe 131.3
55 Cs 132.9	56 Ba 137.3	57 La* 138.9	72 Hf 178.5	73 Ta 180.9	74 W 183.9	75 Re 186.2	76 Os 190.2	77 Ir 192.2	78 Pt 195.1	79 Au 197.0	80 Hg 200.6	81 Tl 204.4	82 Pb 207.2	83 Bi 209.0	84 Po (209)	85 At (210)	86 Rn (222)
87 Fr (223)	88 Ra 226.0	89 Ac† 227.0	104 Unq (261)	105 Unp (262)	106 Unh (263)	107 Uns (262)	108 Uno (265)	109 Une (267)									

	58 Ce 140.1	59 Pr 140.9	60 Nd 144.2	61 Pm (145)	62 Sm 150.4	63 Eu 152.0	64 Gd 157.3	65 Tb 158.9	66 Dy 162.5	67 Ho 164.9	68 Er 167.3	69 Tm 168.9	70 Yb 173.0	71 Lu 175.0
†	90 Th 232.0	91 Pa (231)	92 U 238.0	93 Np (237)	94 Pu (244)	95 Am (243)	96 Cm (247)	97 Bk (247)	98 Cf (251)	99 Es (252)	100 Fm (257)	101 Md (258)	102 No (259)	103 Lr (260)

GO ON TO THE NEXT PAGE.

Passage I (Questions 138–144)

A common disease that afflicts the digestive system is *peptic ulcer disease*. In humans, this condition occurs when the concentration of gastric juice overwhelms the protection provided by the mucous lining of the stomach and the neutralizing secretions of the pancreas. This acidity damages the stomach walls, causing pain, bleeding, or laceration of the digestive tract. The most frequent site of peptic ulcers is the first few centimeters of the duodenum.

Parietal cells in the stomach secrete HCl. HCl secretion is stimulated by gastrin, acetylcholine (ACh), and histamine. There are two negative feedback mechanisms that regulate acid secretion. First, excess HCl in the duodenum stimulates the secretion of the hormone secretin, which increases the rate and volume at which pancreatic juice containing bicarbonate ion is secreted. Second, gastrin inhibits HCl secretion when the stomach pH reaches a certain minimum.

138. All of the following structures secrete digestive juices EXCEPT the:

   A. oral cavity.
   B. esophagus.
   C. stomach.
   D. small intestine.

139. It has recently been hypothesized that the triggering event for some ulcers is bacterial infection. If this is true, which of the following would be the most effective method to eliminate the ulcer?

   A. Stimulate ACh release.
   B. Inhibit the formation of formylmethionyl-tRNA, which is the initiator aminoacyl-tRNA found in prokaryotes only.
   C. Administer puromycin, which is an aminoacyl-tRNA analog in both prokaryotes and eukaryotes.
   D. Inject excess clotting factors to reduce bleeding.

140. Based on information in the passage, which of the following is NOT a plausible cause of peptic ulcer disease?

   A. Excessive gastrin production
   B. Weakness in mucosal barriers
   C. Decrease in parietal cell sensitivity to histamine
   D. Abnormally high density of parietal cells in the stomach

141. Which of the following treatments would most likely NOT alleviate peptic ulcer disease?

   A. Surgical removal of part of the stomach
   B. Administration of a drug that neutralizes stomach acid
   C. Coating the stomach lining with an exogenous substance
   D. Increasing stomach acidity to stimulate the negative feedback mechanism

GO ON TO THE NEXT PAGE.

142. Which of the following organs is involved in neutralizing gastric acidity?

   A. Pancreas
   B. Large intestine
   C. Stomach
   D. Liver

143. Which of the following best explains why gastric pH must be precisely controlled?

   A. Gastric enzymes are most active at a low pH.
   B. High gastric pH stimulates the release of pancreatic secretions.
   C. Low intracellular pH is necessary for proper parietal cell function.
   D. Gastric juices create the optimal environment for nutrient absorption in the large intestine.

144. Which of the following is implied by the term *negative feedback mechanism* as used in the passage?

   A. An increase in acid secretion decreases the rate at which bicarbonate ion is secreted into the duodenum.
   B. A decrease in acid secretion increases the rate at which bicarbonate ion is secreted into the duodenum.
   C. An increase in gastric pH increases acid secretion.
   D. A decrease in gastric pH increases acid secretion.

GO ON TO THE NEXT PAGE.

 115

Passage II (Questions 145–150)

The pseudomonad bacteria are a diverse group of microorganisms that are able to use many exotic compounds as food sources. In particular, certain pseudomonad strains can metabolize aromatic compounds such as toluene, xylenes, phenols, benzoic acids, and an assortment of toxic man-made organic pollutants. This degradation begins with oxidative cleavage of the aromatic ring. The resulting compounds are then broken down into an assortment of respiratory-chain intermediates, from which the bacteria can easily extract energy. Although it is not clear whether this occurs in nature, many of these strains can be grown successfully in the laboratory using aromatic compounds as their only source of energy.

Certain strains of *Pseudomonas putida,* isolated from mud on the bottom of the Hudson River, have been shown to have not one but two separate metabolic pathways that they can use to degrade aromatic compounds. The two pathways are known as the *meta* and *ortho* pathways. The genes for the *ortho* pathway are carried on the bacterial chromosome, while the genes for the *meta* pathway are borne on plasmids, small circular pieces of DNA that are independent of the bacterial chromosome and may be transmitted from one bacterium to another. Figure 1 shows the sequence of steps for the two pathways; the substrate is benzoate, the negatively charged ion of benzoic acid.

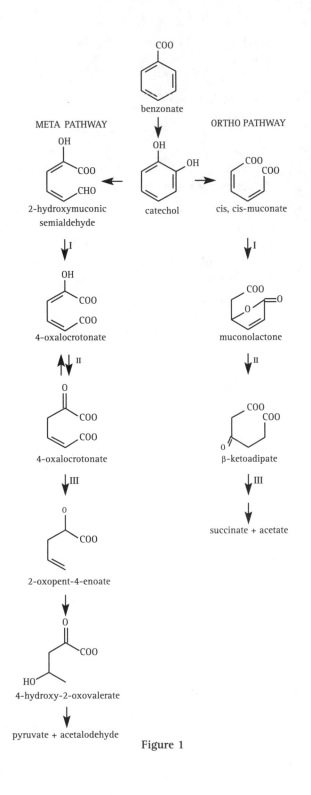

Figure 1

GO ON TO THE NEXT PAGE.

145. The *ortho* and *meta* designations of the two pathways refer to:

A. the two carbon atoms between which the ring is cleaved, with respect to the carboxylate group of benzoate.

B. the farther of the two carbon atoms between which the ring is cleaved, with respect to the carboxylate group of benzoate.

C. the carbon atom that is oxidized to an aldehyde group during the cleavage step.

D. the carbon atom that is oxidized to a carboxyl group during the cleavage step.

146. Most enzymes are named according to their chemical function. What is the most likely name for the enzyme that catalyzes Step II in the *meta* pathway?

A. 4-oxalocrotonate isomerase

B. 4-oxalocrotonate dehydrogenase

C. 4-oxalocrotonate tautomerase

D. 4-oxalocrotonate hydrolase

147. Based on its structure, which of the following compounds could NOT possibly be degraded via the *meta* pathway?

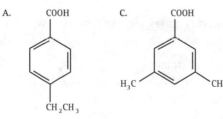
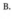
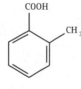
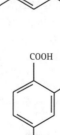

148. Which of the following could be used to synthesize β-ketoadipate from muconolactone by purely chemical means?

A. Treatment with aqueous base followed by addition of potassium dichromate

B. Treatment with hydrogen over platinum followed by addition of aqueous sulfuric acid

C. Treatment with hydrogen over platinum followed by addition of aqueous potassium hydroxide

D. Treatment with hydrogen over platinum followed by addition of aqueous potassium hydroxide and then potassium dichromate

149. The enzyme-catalyzed conversion of 4-hydroxy-2-oxovalerate to pyruvate, CH_3COCOO^-, and acetaldehyde, CH_3CHO, represents cleavage of the carbon skeleton between carbons 3 and 4, along with:

A. oxidation.

B. reduction.

C. isomerization.

D. enolization.

150. If a researcher needed to distinguish between catechol and 2-hydroxymuconic semialdehyde, which of the following types of spectroscopy would be useful?

   I. Mass spectroscopy

   II. NMR spectroscopy

   III. Infrared spectroscopy

A. I only

B. I and II only

C. II and III only

D. I, II, and III

GO ON TO THE NEXT PAGE.

Passage III (Questions 151–158)

Capillaries are very narrow blood vessels that link the arterial circulation to the venous circulation, and are the site of nutrient and gas exchange between the tissues and blood. However, nutrients and gases do not travel directly from capillaries into cells. Rather, they must first travel through the interstitial fluid. The capillary can be thought of as a selective filter for transport between blood and interstitial fluid.

There are three basic ways by which nutrients and gases enter and leave capillaries. First, lipid-soluble molecules diffuse through the capillary membrane. The capillary membrane is composed of a lipid bilayer that allows nonpolar molecules to travel through it; however, very small polar molecules can also cross the membrane. Second, nutrients diffuse through the pores in capillary walls. This diffusion is limited by the size of the pores. For example, albumin, a plasma protein, cannot filter into the nephron through the glomerulus. Third, substances cross the capillary wall via endocytosis.

The interactions between the hydrostatic pressure differential (the net hydrostatic pressure of the blood and the tissue) and the osmotic pressure differential (the net osmotic pressure of the blood and the tissue) determine whether nutrients, fluid, gases, and wastes will move into or out of the capillaries. The values of these pressures (in mmHg), and how they affect the movement of particles across the capillary membrane, are shown in Figure 1. The hydrostatic pressure differential tends to force fluid out of the capillary, the osmotic pressure differential tends to force fluid into the capillary, because of the blood's relatively high solute concentration in comparison to that of the tissue.

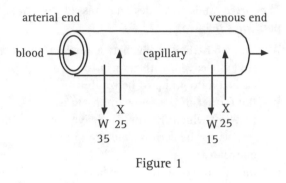

Figure 1

151. According to Figure 1, what is the net pressure at the arterial end of the capillary?

A. 35 mm Hg out
B. 25 mm Hg in
C. 10 mm Hg out
D. 10 mm Hg in

152. In Figure 1, what do the arrows labeled "W" represent?

A. Hydrostatic pressure differential
B. Osmotic pressure differential
C. The net flow of fluid out of the capillary at the arterial end
D. The net flow of fluid out of the capillary at the venous end

153. Respiratory gases are exchanged between blood and interstitial fluid via:

A. active transport.
B. passive diffusion.
C. facilitated diffusion.
D. exocytosis.

GO ON TO THE NEXT PAGE.

154. If the protein C1INH cannot pass through a specific segment of capillary walls, which of the following conclusions CANNOT be drawn?

    A. C1INH is too large to pass through its pores.
    B. C1INH is a large polar molecule.
    C. C1INH is a lipid-soluble molecule.
    D. The concentration of C1INH is the same on both sides of the capillary walls.

155. Which of the following is NOT a property of capillary walls?

    A. They are muscular.
    B. They are semipermeable.
    C. They are composed of endothelial cells.
    D. They are porous.

156. According to Figure 1, the hydrostatic pressure differential and the osmotic pressure differential:

    A. both decrease along the length of the capillary.
    B. both increase along the length of the capillary.
    C. are inversely proportional to each other at both ends of the capillary.
    D. oppose each other at both ends of the capillary.

157. Which of the following would most likely cause an increase in blood pressure within the capillaries?

    A. Closure of precapillary sphincters
    B. Decreased venous resistance
    C. Decreased arteriolar pressure
    D. Increased arteriolar pressure

158. The *oncotic pressure* of the blood is the fraction of the total osmotic pressure exerted by plasma proteins. Although it represents only 2.4 percent of the total osmotic pressure, the oncotic pressure plays a key role in fluid exchange across the capillary wall because:

    A. plasma proteins diffuse into the interstitial fluid.
    B. most plasma proteins are too large to cross the capillary wall.
    C. plasma proteins enhance the dissociation of oxyhemoglobin.
    D. plasma proteins facilitate fluid exchange by binding to fluid molecules.

GO ON TO THE NEXT PAGE.

Questions 159 through 163 are NOT based on a descriptive passage.

159. Differentiation of the ectoderm in a developing mammalian embryo eventually gives the animal the ability to:

   A. produce urine.
   B. digest food.
   C. respond to stimuli.
   D. breathe.

160. If an endothelial cell were placed in distilled water, the cell would most likely:

   A. shrivel.
   B. divide.
   C. remain the same size.
   D. lyse.

161. Which of the following compounds has the most stable structure?

   A. Cyclopropane
   B. Cyclohexane
   C. Cyclononane
   D. Cyclodecane

162. Why is carbon monoxide poisonous to humans?

   A. It decreases the total hemoglobin concentration of the blood.
   B. It destroys lung tissue.
   C. It blocks the electron transport chain.
   D. Hemoglobin has a greater affinity for carbon monoxide than for molecular oxygen.

163. Which of the following is true of anomers?

   A. They are achiral.
   B. They are mirror images.
   C. They differ in the configuration of the first carbon.
   D. They differ in the configuration of the second carbon.

GO ON TO THE NEXT PAGE.

Passage IV (Questions 164–168)

P elements are a type of *transposable element* found in fruit flies. Transposable elements are self-replicating DNA sequences that are able to insert themselves in random locations within a host's genome. P elements were discovered after scientists noticed that crossing certain strains of flies produced offspring with an unusually high incidence of mutation. This syndrome, known as *P-M hybrid dysgenesis,* occurs only if the inherited P elements are activated. P elements are activated in all offspring when males from strains containing P elements, called P (paternal contributing) strains, are crossed with females from strains lacking P elements, called M (maternal contributing) strains. P elements produce an increased mutation rate by several different mechanisms: 1) Insertion of a P element into the coding region of a gene deactivates that gene; 2) recombination between P elements on different chromosomes or in different regions of a single chromosome can produce inversions, translocations, deletions, or duplications. This high level of mutation produces sterile offspring.

Geneticists have noted that strains of flies descended from wild flies caught at least 30 years ago are almost always M strains, whereas strains descended from flies caught fewer than 10 years ago are usually P strains. Two hypotheses have been proposed to account for this observation.

Hypothesis 1
P elements arose in wild fruit fly populations during the last 10–30 years, and subsequently spread throughout the species. P elements may have originated as viruses. Consequently, only strains derived from recently captured flies possess P elements.

Hypothesis 2
P elements have long existed in wild fruit populations, but have a finite probability of being lost from the genome during each generation. Therefore, strains that have been cultured for many generations are likely to have lost their P elements over the course of time.

164. A researcher puts 9 M-strain flies and 1 P-strain fly into a culture box and grows them for 800 days (100 generations). She finds that most of their descendants are P flies. This observation supports:

A. Hypothesis 1, because the flies with P elements leave more offspring than M-strain flies.
B. Hypothesis 1, because the incidence of P elements in the population has increased.
C. Hypothesis 2, because the P elements have been lost during lab culture.
D. Hypothesis 2, because the flies have been cultured for many generations.

165. If P elements arose by viral infection, as suggested by Hypothesis 1, the virus in question would have been:

A. lytic.
B. lysogenic.
C. a bacteriophage.
D. attenuated.

166. Which of the following would NOT be a plausible mechanism whereby P elements might be "lost" from a fruit fly's DNA, as suggested by Hypothesis 2?

A. Genetic drift
B. Recombination between P elements on a single chromosome, leading to deletion
C. Recombination between P elements on separate chromosomes, leading to translocation
D. Natural selection

END OF TEST.

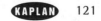 121

167. Which of the following is a potential consequence of P elements in a population?

    A. Increased likelihood of speciation
    B. Increased viability of offspring
    C. Decreased mutation rate
    D. Decreased genetic drift

168. Dysgenesis will be seen in the offspring from a cross between:

    I.   a P-strain female and an M-strain male.
    II. a P-strain male and a female offspring from a cross between a P-strain male and an M-strain female.
    III. two offspring from a cross between an M-strain male and a P-strain female.
    IV. a male from a cross between two P-strain flies and a female from a cross between two M-strain flies.

    A. I and III only
    B. IV only
    C. II and IV only
    D. II, III, and IV only

GO ON TO THE NEXT PAGE.

Passage V (Questions 169–173)

Blood pressure is the force per unit area that blood exerts on the walls of the vessels it travels through. An instrument called a *sphygmomanometer* is used to measure blood pressure in an artery in the arm. A sphygmomanometer is an inflatable cuff attached to a pressure gauge; it is wrapped around the upper arm and inflated with air until blood flow to the artery is completely cut off. The cuff is then gradually deflated until blood begins to flow through the artery again. The initial sounds heard with the stethoscope are those produced when the blood pressure exceeds the pressure exerted by the cuff, and the pressure measured at this point corresponds to the pressure during ventricular contraction (systole). As the cuff is further deflated such that blood flow through the artery is normal, the pressure recorded corresponds to the residual pressure between contractions (diastole). Blood pressure is recorded as systole/diastole. Another measurement often taken is *cardiac output*. Cardiac output is defined as the volume of blood pumped by the left ventricle into systemic circulation per minute. Cardiac output is computed by multiplying heart rate (the number of beats per minute) and stroke volume (the volume of blood pumped by the left ventricle per contraction).

A trained athlete and a nonathlete both perform strenuous exercise (running up and down a flight of stairs) for 1 minute. Diastolic pressure and systolic pressure were measured four times: at rest; immediately following the exercise; 2.5 minutes following the exercise; and 6 minutes following the exercise (see Figure 1).

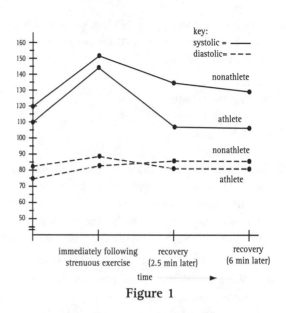

Figure 1

169. What is the athlete's blood pressure at rest (in mmHg)?

    A. 108/83
    B. 83/108
    C. 120/83
    D. 83/120

170. If, during exercise, the nonathlete and the athlete have the same heart rate, but the athlete's cardiac output is greater, then:

    A. the athlete's pulse is greater than the nonathlete's.
    B. the nonathlete's pulse is greater than the athlete's.
    C. the athlete's stroke volume is greater than the nonathlete's.
    D. the nonathlete's stroke volume is greater than the athlete's

GO ON TO THE NEXT PAGE.

171. If a woman's pulse is 20 beats per 15 seconds and her stroke volume is 70 mL per beat, what is her cardiac output?

    A. 1.4 L/min
    B. 1.4 beats/min
    C. 5.6 beats/min
    D. 5.6 L/min

172. Both immediately before and during exercise, there is increased sympathetic activity. As revealed by the slopes of the lines in Figure 1, there is a rise in both systolic and diastolic pressure during exercise. Which of the following best accounts for this observation?

    A. Vasoconstriction of all blood vessels in active muscle
    B. Vasoconstriction of systemic blood vessels except for those in active muscle
    C. Vasodilation of systemic blood vessels except for those in active muscle
    D. Buildup of lactic acid

173. If the athlete normally has a greater cardiac output than the nonathlete, which of the following would most likely occur during strenuous exercise?

    A. The athlete would have a higher systolic pressure than the nonathlete.
    B. The nonathlete would have a higher diastolic pressure than the athlete.
    C. The nonathlete would have a greater buildup of lactic acid in muscle cells than the athlete.
    D. The athlete would have a higher rate of glucose catabolism than the nonathlete.

GO ON TO THE NEXT PAGE.

Passage VI (Questions 174–177)

The different conformations of cyclic alkanes vary significantly in energy, and these energy differences often affect behavior. In cyclohexane, for example, the higher energy conformations are transitory except at high temperatures; the molecule spends most of its time in the lower-energy states.

In cyclic compounds that contain substituents other than hydrogen atoms, the energy differences between conformations are often larger. In some cases, these differences are large enough that even at room temperature, the molecules are permanently fixed in the conformation with the lowest possible energy. In such cases, this lowest-energy conformation may be studied and information about its energy values may be obtained. The table below shows energy differences between the axial and equatorial positions for several different substituent groups.

Table 1

Name	Group	Energy difference (Axial/equatorial)
Bromide	–Br	0.50 kcal/mol
Hydroxyl	–OH	0.95 kcal/mol
Amino	–NH$_2$	1.40 kcal/mol
Methyl	–CH$_3$	1.74 kcal/mol
Isopropyl	–CH(CH$_3$)$_2$	2.15 kcal/mol
t-Butyl	–C(CH$_3$)$_3$	5.00 kcal/mol

174. What is the correct name for the following compound?

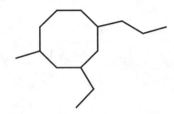

A. 1-ethyl-3-methyl-7-propylcyclooctane
B. 1-methyl-3-ethyl-5-methylcyclooctane
C. l-methyl-3-ethyl-5-propylcyclooctane
D. 3-ethyl-1-methyl-5-propylcyclooctane

175. What is the energy difference between the two conformations of 1-methyl-4-bromocyclohexane shown below?

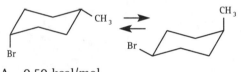

A. 0.50 kcal/mol
B. 1.24 kcal/mol
C. 1.74 kcal/mol
D. 2.24 kcal/mol

GO ON TO THE NEXT PAGE.

176. Which of the following structures is the most stable?

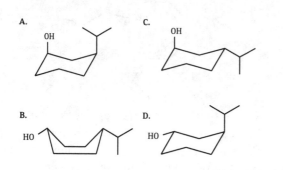

A.

C.

B.

D.

177. Which of the following structures is NOT in its lowest energy conformation?

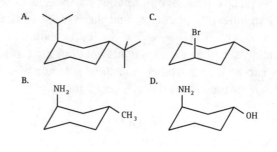

A.

C.

B.

D.

GO ON TO THE NEXT PAGE.

Passage VII (Questions 178–183)

Antibodies are proteins produced by animal immune systems in response to foreign agents, called antigens. The active site of an antibody is called the antigen-binding site; this antigen-binding site "recognizes" the antigen and binds to it, thereby rendering it inactive. Each antibody is specific to a particular antigen; it recognizes this antigen and occasionally closely related ones. Two theories attempt to explain antibody recognition and binding.

Theory 1:

An antibody recognizes its antigen by means of the antigen's chemical composition, via chemical interactions between the antibody's antigen-binding site and the antigen. The specific amino acids in the antigen binding site are what enable the antibody to interact with the antigen. Thus, the chemical composition of the antigen is the crucial factor determining whether binding between antibody and antigen occurs. The physical configuration of the antigen does not affect this interaction.

Theory 2:

An antibody recognizes its antigen by means of the antigen's physical configuration. The chemical composition of the antigen is of lesser importance. The antigen-binding site on the antibody is a "pocket" of characteristic shape into which the antigen fits and binds. The antigen must have the correct configuration, regardless of chemical composition, to be able to fit into and bind to the antigen-binding site of the antibody.

178. If Theory 1 were correct, which of the following structures would be recognized by an antibody produced against p-aminophenole-α-glucoside?

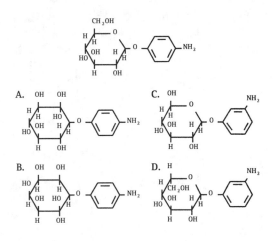

179. Which of the following statements supports Theory 2?

I. The antibody to p-aminobenzenesulfonic acid does not interact with m-aminobenzenesulfonic acid.

II. The antibody to p-aminobenzenesulfonic acid interacts with p-aminohydroxybenzene.

III. The antibody to p-aminobenzenesulfonic acid does not interact with m-aminohydroxybenzene.

A. II only
B. I and II only
C. II and III only
D. I, II, and III

GO ON TO THE NEXT PAGE.

180. In an experiment, benzenesulfonic acid is chlorinated and an antibody is produced against it. According to Theory 2, which of the following structures will interact with this antibody?

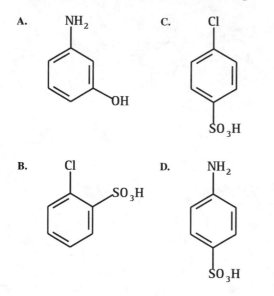

181. Which of the following statements is FALSE?

   A. The fact that two conformational isomers were recognized by the same antibody supports Theory 1 over Theory 2.
   B. The fact that two enantiomers were recognized by the same antibody supports Theory 1 over Theory 2.
   C. The fact that two structural isomers were recognized by the same antibody supports Theory 2 over Theory 1.
   D. The fact that two geometric isomers were not recognized by the same antibody supports Theory 2 over Theory 1.

182. A mouse is injected with *m*-aminobenzenesulfonic acid, and the antibodies that it produces in response are extracted and tested for their ability to bind to different organic compounds. The resulting data are shown below.

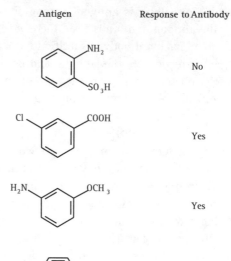

Which of the following statements best describes these results?

   A. The antibody recognizes the chemical composition of the antigens, supporting Theory 1.
   B. The antibody recognizes the physical configuration of the antigens, supporting Theory 2.
   C. The antibody recognizes the chemical composition of the antigens, supporting Theory 2.
   D. The antibody recognizes the physical configuration of the antigens, supporting Theory 1.

183. The antigen-binding site of an antibody:

   A. is nonpolar.
   B. cannot contain disulfide bonds.
   C. cannot be denatured.
   D. represents the antibody's tertiary structure.

GO ON TO THE NEXT PAGE.

184. *In vitro*, intracellular glucose concentration in muscle cells varies as a function of the composition of the growth media. Based on the graph below, which of the following conclusions can be drawn?

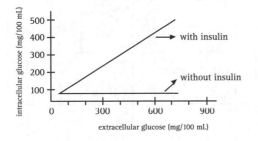

intracellular glucose (mg/100 mL)

with insulin

without insulin

extracellular glucose (mg/100 mL)

A. Insulin decreases intracellular glucose concentration in muscle cells.
B. Muscle cell membranes are practically impermeable to glucose.
C. Glucose transport across muscle cell membranes requires ATP.
D. Insulin stimulates the conversion of glucose into glycogen in almost all body tissues.

185. A patient with insufficient ADH secretion would most likely exhibit an:

A. increased urinary volume.
B. increased urinary osmolarity.
C. increased water reabsorption in the kidneys.
D. increased filtration rate in the kidneys.

186. Which of the following reactions is NOT accompanied by an extension of the carbon chain?

A. $(CH_3)_2CHMgBr + 1. CO_2(g)$
   $2. H_2O / H^+ \rightarrow$
B. $(CH_3)_2CHBr + CH_3CH_2O^- / KOH \rightarrow$
C. $CH_3CH_2Br + KCN / acetone \rightarrow$
D. $CH_3MgBr + 1. R' CH = O$
   $2. H_2O \rightarrow$

187. Which of the following is achiral?

A. $CH_3CH_2CH_2^+$
B. D-glucose
C. $CH_3CBr(OH)CCl(OH)CH_3$
D. $HOOC(CH_3CH_2)C(CH_3)CH = O$

188. How is carbon dioxide typically transported in the blood?

A. In the form of CO_2 gas
B. In the form of HCO_3^-
C. In the form of carbonic anhydrase
D. In the form of H_2CO_3

GO ON TO THE NEXT PAGE.

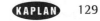 129

Passage VIII (Questions 189–193)

Duchenne muscular dystrophy (DMD) is an X-linked recessive degenerative disorder of the muscle. By comparing the ability of X-linked DNA probes to hybridize with DNA from DMD patients and with DNA from normal individuals, cloned fragments were obtained that correspond to the region of DNA that contains the deletions characteristic of DMD. The deletions occur at different locations in each patient, suggesting that they occurred *de novo*. Analysis of this region of DNA obtained from numerous patients identified large deletions, extending in either direction. The most revealing deletion is located in the center of the isolated region. The sequence of this segment was determined to be:

5' --GCCATAGAGCGA--3'

The normal gene codes for a protein of approximately 500 kD, which has been named *dystrophin*. It is a component of muscle, present in rather low amounts. All patients with DMD have deletions at this locus, and either lack dystrophin or synthesize defective dystrophin.

189. Which of the following sequences of DNA is complementary to the one given in the passage?

   A. 5' --TCGCTCTATGGC--3'
   B. 5' --CGGTATCTCGCT--3'
   C. 5' --CGGUAUCUCGCU--3'
   D. 5' --CGGUUUCUCGCU--3'

190. Based on the chart of the genetic code below and the DNA sequence provided in the passage, what is the missing sequence of dystrophin amino acids in DMD patients with this particular deletion?

second letter

		U	C	A	G	
first letter	U	UUU UUC } Phe UUA UUG } Leu	UCU UCC UCA UCG } Ser	UAU UAC } Tyr UAA Stop UAG Stop	UGU UGC } Cys UGA Stop UGG Trp	U C A G
	C	CUU CUC CUA CUG } Leu	CCU CCC CCA CCG } Pro	CAU CAC } His CAA CAA } Gin	CGU CGC CGA CGA } Arg	U C A G
	A	AUU AUC } Ile AUA AUG Start/Met	ACU ACC ACA ACG } Thr	AAU AAC } Asn AAA AAG } Lys	AGU AGC } Ser AGA AGG } Arg	U C A G
	G	GUU GUC GUA GUG } Val	GCU GCC GCA GCG } Ala	GAU GAC } Asp GAA GAG } Glu	GGU GGC GGA GGG } Gly	U C A G

(third letter)

   A. Ser-Glu-Ile-Pro
   B. Met-Ala-Ile-Glu
   C. Arg-Tyr-Leu-Ala
   D. Ser-Leu-Tyr-Gly

191. Which of the following is the site of transcription in eukaryotic organisms?

   A. Ribosome
   B. Nucleus
   C. Centromere
   D. Cytoplasm

GO ON TO THE NEXT PAGE.

192. If a normal woman whose father had DMD married a normal man, what is the probability that they will have two children with DMD?

    A. 6.25%

    B. 12.5%

    C. 25%

    D. 50%

193. Based on the information in the passage, which of the following can be inferred about the ability of the X-linked DNA probes to hybridize with the DNA from DMD patients as compared to the DNA from normal individuals?

    A. The probes have a greater degree of complementarity with DMD DNA.

    B. The probes have a greater degree of complementarity with normal DNA.

    C. The probes have an equal degree of complementarity with both DMD DNA and normal DNA.

    D. The probes hybridized with the DMD DNA of female patients only.

GO ON TO THE NEXT PAGE.

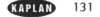

Passage IX (Questions 194–201)

Three pairs of electrons may be transferred among atoms of a phenyl ether by forming an intermediate that facilitates movement of these electrons through a sigmatropic process known as the Claisen rearrangement. A *sigmatropic rearrangement* is a reaction in which an allylic *s* bond at one end of a π-electron system appears to migrate to the other end of the π-electron system. An example of a reaction involving the Claisen rearrangement follows:

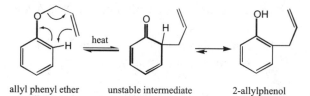

allyl phenyl ether   unstable intermediate   2-allylphenol

In this example, rearrangement occurs by a sigmatropic shift of the allylic group to give an *ortho* dienone, before forming the stable product. However, if the *ortho* position is occupied in an aromatic ring system, migration will primarily occur at the *para* position of the aromatic ring system. This type of rearrangement is not limited to phenyl ethers. A similar reaction can take place with aliphatic unsaturated ethers as well as unsaturated hydrocarbons. With aliphatic unsaturated ethers, the reaction usually stops at the intermediate stage (prior to enolization).

The Cope rearrangement is also a sigmatropic reaction which can be used as a synthetic tool to produce seven- and eight-membered unsaturated rings systems from 1,2 divinylalkanes.

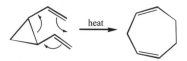

1,2-divinylcyclopropane   cyclohepta-1,4-diene

In other reactions involving the Cope rearrangement, 1,5-dienes are rearranged to produce their 1,5-diene isomers. This transformation occurs with the addition of heat. The Cope/Claisen rearrangement is often visualized as the interaction of two allylic systems, a carbocation and a carbanion.

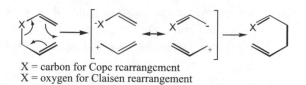

X = carbon for Cope rearrangement
X = oxygen for Claisen rearrangement

The Cope rearrangement is reversible so that the thermodynamically favorable isomer predominates. Evidence that an isomerization occurs is determined from the configuration of the end product. For example, among *meso*-3,4-dimethylhexa-1,5-diene, the diene formed almost exclusively is *cis, trans*-octa-2,6-diene with the addition of heat. A look at the chair and boat configurations of the reaction and intermediate transition geometries gives insight as to why the *cis, trans*-isomer predominates for the *meso* compound. During the transition state, the allylic group is delocalized to provide overlap between the p orbitals and a new bond is formed between carbons 1 and 6.

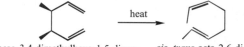

meso-3,4-dimethylhexa-1,5-diene   *cis, trans*-octa-2,6-diene

Both the Cope and Claisen rearrangements are cyclic, concerted, intramolecular reactions that are thermally induced and classified under the [3,3] sigmatropic shift. Depending on steric constraints, the transition states of both rearrangements prefer the chair conformation. Upon analysis of the stereochemical properties of the rearranged product, one may be able to discern which transition state conformation (chair or boat) was favored. While the Cope rearrangement is often used to give stereochemical products different from the starting material, a given molecule may undergo the rearrangement to form a product indistinguishable from the starting material.

GO ON TO THE NEXT PAGE.

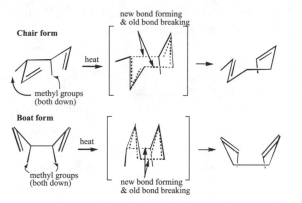

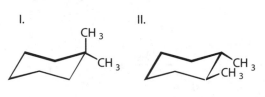

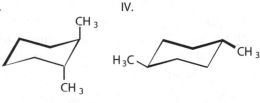

Figure 1. Chair and Boat Structures during the transition state of the Cope Rearrangement of *meso*-3,4-dimethylhexa-1,5-diene.

194. List the following structures in order of increasing stability.

I.

II.

III.

IV.

A. II < IV < III < I
B. IV < II < III < I
C. I < II < III < IV
D. I < III < II < IV

195. What is the product of a Claisen rearrangement of the following allyl vinyl ether?

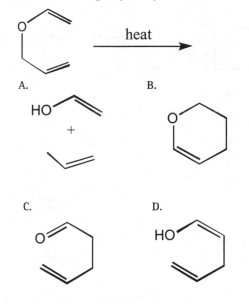

A.

+

B.

C.

D.

196. Which of the following is the MOST LIKELY intermediate of the following "oxyCope" rearrangement?

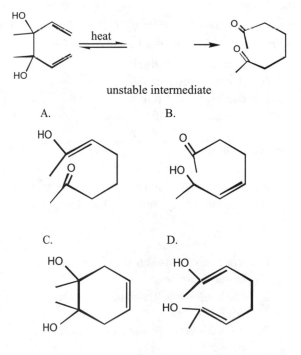

unstable intermediate

A.

B.

C.

D.

GO ON TO THE NEXT PAGE.

197. What is the MOST LIKELY product of the following reaction?

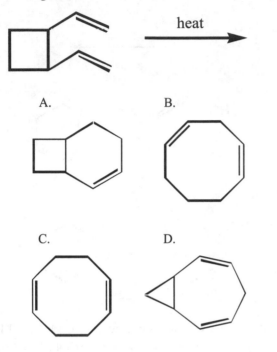

A.

B.

C.

D.

198. What type of relationship exists between the intermediate of the Claisen rearrangement and the product of the allyl phenyl ether reaction?

  A. keto-enol tautomerism
  B. β-keto Claisen condensation
  C. conjugate addition
  D. proton shift

199. What would be the MOST LIKELY product(s) for the Cope rearrangement of *racemic* 3,4-dimethylhexa-1,5-diene assuming the transition state geometry favored the chair form?

  A. trans, trans-hepta-2,6-diene *and* cis, cis-hepta-2,6-diene
  B. trans, cis-hepta-2,6-diene *and* cis, trans-hepta-2,6-diene
  C. cis, trans-octa-2,6-diene *and* trans, cis-octa-2,6-diene
  D. cis, cis-octa-2,6-diene *and* trans, trans-octa-2,6-diene

200. Which of the following reactions would proceed via the boat transition state?

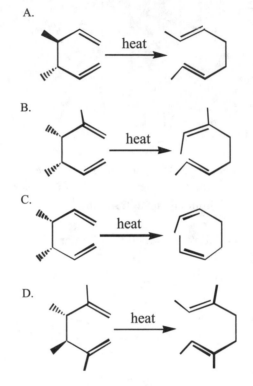

A.

B.

C.

D.

201. Which one of the following structures would MOST LIKELY undergo a Claisen rearrangement to the *para* position?

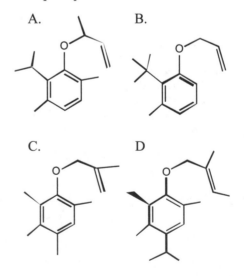

A.

B.

C.

D

GO ON TO THE NEXT PAGE.

Passage X (Questions 202–209)

Recently, scientists have analyzed the contents of what they believe to be the tomb of King Midas residing at Gordion in central Turkey. Amazingly, preservation conditions inside the tomb were extraordinarily good. In fact, molecular archeological techniques were used to identify the ancient foods and beverages supposedly eaten at the funerary feast for King Midas. The analysis revealed that a spicy meal of sheep or goat was eaten at a royal banquet before the burial, while fermented beverages consisting of grape wine, barley beer, and honey mead were also found.

Using Fourier-transform infrared spectroscopy (FT-IR), high performance liquid chromatography (HPLC), and mass spectrometry (MS), the chemical composition of the banquet entrée was determined. Figure 1 shows the FT-IR spectrum of the food residue (dashed line). From the spectrum in Figure 1, the meal consisted of triacylglycerols indicative of sheep or goat fat. The FT-IR absorptions and HPLC revealed that the predominant fatty acids (derived from the triacylglycerols) were saturated palmitic (16:0) and stearic (18:0) acid, and unsaturated oleic (18:1$^{\Delta 9}$) acid. Other compounds such as cholesterol and the saturated acids, caproic (6:0), caprylic (8:0), and capric (10:0) acid, were also present in the food residues.

Figure 1 (solid line) shows the representative FT-IR spectrum of the mixed fermented beverage found in the tomb. The drink was comprised of tartaric acid (a carboxylic acid found in grapes), calcium oxalate ('beerstone', the main precipitate of barley beer), and beeswax (from mead). The characteristic FT-IR functional group absorptions are listed in Table I. Other compounds found in the tomb were the "trans" isomer of oleic acid (olive oil), alkyl phenol derivatives such as cresols (barbecued meat), and terpene type compounds (spices).

Triacylglycerols are comprised of a glycerol backbone with three long chain acyl groups (derived from fatty acids) attached to the backbone via ester bonds. Hydrolysis of triacylglycerols results in the formation of 3 moles of carboxylate salt (fatty acid) and 1 mol of glycerol. The breakdown of the

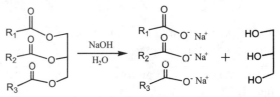

R$_1$, R$_2$, and R$_3$ are long chain alkyl groups (saturated or unsaturated)

triacylglycerols to their corresponding fatty acids produces a rancid odor characteristic of fats and fatty acids, which was observed when the tomb was opened. Terpenes are often fragrant or flavorful compounds made from isoprene subunits often consisting of a specific "head-to-tail" connectivity. Terpenes are recognized by two criteria: 1) a multiple of five carbon atoms in the main carbon skeleton; and 2) the carbon connectivity of the isoprene

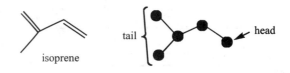

carbon skeleton within each five-carbon unit. In fact, squalene, the precursor to cholesterol, is a

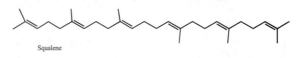

terpene that underogoes cyclization via carbocation intermediates to form a steroid, which eventually forms cholesterol.

[*Fatty Acid Parenthetical Notation*: The fatty acid contains the total number of carbon atoms indicated by the first number in parenthesis. For palmitic acid (16:0), there are 16 total carbons in the chain including the carbon of the carboxylic acid functional group. The second number after the colon represents the number of double bonds in the chain. If the compound is unsaturated the position of the double bond

GO ON TO THE NEXT PAGE.

is indicated behind the number of double bonds in a superscripted number. For example, oleic acid ($18:1^{\Delta 9}$) has one double bond positioned between carbons 9 and 10. All double bonds are '*cis*' unless otherwise indicated.]

Table I. Typical infrared absorptions of some organic functional groups.

Wavenumber (cm⁻¹)	Type of Absorption			
3400	O—H	N—H	C—H	stretching
2250–2100		C≡N	C≡C	stretching
1850–1600	C=O	C=N	C=C	stretching
1600–1000	C—C	C—O	C—N	stretching; various other bending absorptions, fingerprint region
1000–600			C—H	bending
3100–2950	=C—H	=CH₂		stretching
	O—H			O-H stretch of carboxylic acid (strong; broad); also has C-O stretch at 1200–1300 and carboxylate C=O stretch at 1570–1730

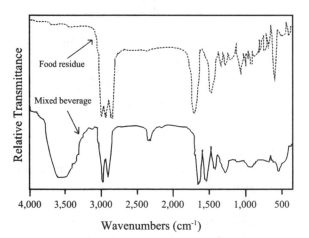

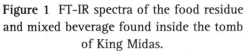

Figure 1 FT-IR spectra of the food residue and mixed beverage found inside the tomb of King Midas.

202. In the FT-IR spectrum of the mixed beverage in Figure 1, the broad absorption at 3250-3750 is primarily due to

   A. the C-H stretching of the aliphatic groups in beeswax.

   B. the O-H stretching of hydroxyl and carboxylic acid groups in tartaric acid.

   C. the C-O stretching of the carboxylic acid group in tartaric acid.

   D. the C=O stretching of the ester group in the beeswax.

203. In the FT-IR spectrum of the food residue there are two fairly large, sharp hydrocarbon absorption bands at 2860 and 2930 cm⁻¹ attributable to long carbon chain C-H stretching. The second largest absorption band at 1690-1730 cm⁻¹ is due to

   A. the C=C stretching of unsaturated fatty acids.

   B. the C-O stretching of carboxylic acids derived from fatty acids.

   C. the C=O stretching of carbonyl groups derived from esters.

   D. the C=C stretching of the unsaturated hydrocarbon chain derived from esters.

204. Lengthening the chain length on a fatty acid raises the corresponding melting point. What does adding a double bond to the carbon chain do to the melting point when comparing fatty acids of similar carbon chain lengths?

   A. the melting point is lowered

   B. the melting point is unchanged

   C. the melting point is slightly raised

   D. the melting point is significantly raised

GO ON TO THE NEXT PAGE.

205. A triacylglycerol is comprised of three different R groups, decanoic acid, hexadecanoic acid, and *cis,cis*-9,12-octadenoic acid, respectively. During hydrolysis of the fat, 1 mole of each carboxylate is formed for each mole of fat. List the carboxylates in order using the parenthetical notation for fatty acids.

    A. (10:0), (16:0), (16:2$^{\Delta 10,14}$)
    B. (12:0), (16:0), (18: 2$^{\Delta 9,12}$)
    C. (8:0), (14:0), (16:2$^{\Delta 9,14}$)
    D. (10:0), (16:0), (18:2$^{\Delta 9,12}$)

206. Which type of reaction best describes the hydrolysis reaction of triacylglycerol in the passage?

    A. Fischer esterification
    B. E1 elimination
    C. Saponification
    D. E2 elimination

207. The following compound belongs to which class of compounds?

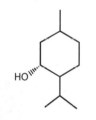

    A. cresols
    B. waxes
    C. steriods
    D. terpenes

208. A monoterpene is a terpene that contains two five-carbon units (10 carbon atoms) derived from isoprene (as shown in the passage). A diterpene contains four five carbon units (20 carbon atoms). How many isoprene subunits are shown in the structure of squalene?

    A. 5
    B. 6
    C. 7
    D. 8

209. Which method would be most useful to determine the number of individual compounds contained in the mixed beverage sampled from the tomb of King Midas?

    A. Nuclear Magnetic Resonance Spectroscopy (NMR)
    B. Mass Spectroscopy (MS)
    C. Fourier Transform-Infrared Spectroscopy (FT-IR)
    D. High Pressure Liquid Chromatography (HPLC)

GO ON TO THE NEXT PAGE.

210. Which of the following enzymes changes disaccharides to monosaccharides?

    A. lactase
    B. kinase
    C. zymogen
    D. lipase

211. A heart beat is initiated by the pacemaker, which is

    A. also known as the atrioventricular (AV) node.
    B. also known as the sinoatrial node.
    C. located in the wall of the right ventricle.
    D. functionally dependent upon nervous stimulation.

212. In the digestive system, all of the following are true EXCEPT

    A. digestive enzymes from the pancreas are released via a duct into the duodenum.
    B. peristalsis is a wave of smooth muscle contraction that proceeds along the digestive tract
    C. in the small intestine, villi absorb nutrients into both the lymphatic and circulatory systems.
    D. the low pH of the stomach is essential for the function of carbohydrate digestive enzymes.

213. Which of the following is true of activity within the kidney?

    A. Nephrons are located only in the cortex of the organ.
    B. Ammonia is converted to urea.
    C. Both glucose and water are actively reabsorbed from the glomerular filtrate.
    D. Antidiuretic hormone causes the reabsorption of water from the collecting tubule.

214. Which of the following statements about blood is false?

    A. Mature red blood cells are not nucleated.
    B. Blood platelets are involved in the clotting process.
    C. The adult spleen is a site of red blood cell development.
    D. White blood cells are capable of phagocytosing foreign matter.

STOP.

IF YOU FINISH BEFORE TIME HAS EXPIRED, CHECK YOUR WORK.
YOU MAY GO BACK TO ANY QUESTION IN THIS PART ONLY.

KAPLAN

Practice Test I Answer Key

Full-Length Practice MCAT

PHYSICAL SCIENCES

1.	A	9.	B	17.	B	25.	A	33.	A	41.	B	49.	A	57.	D
2.	B	10.	B	18.	B	26.	B	34.	B	42.	C	50.	A	58.	A
3.	B	11.	C	19.	B	27.	C	35.	A	43.	C	51.	D	59.	C
4.	C	12.	D	20.	A	28.	A	36.	C	44.	D	52.	C	60.	C
5.	D	13.	B	21.	D	29.	B	37.	B	45.	B	53.	C	61.	C
6.	D	14.	C	22.	C	30.	D	38.	D	46.	B	54.	A	62.	B
7.	A	15.	D	23.	B	31.	B	39.	B	47.	A	55.	B	63.	A
8.	B	16.	A	24.	D	32.	D	40.	A	48.	B	56.	B	64.	D

65. C   73. D
66. D   74. C
67. B   75. D
68. D   76. D
69. A   77. D
70. B
71. B
72. C

VERBAL REASONING

78.	B	84.	B	90.	D	96.	B	102.	D	108.	B	114.	A	120.	D
79.	D	85.	C	91.	B	97.	D	103.	B	109.	C	115.	D	121.	A
80.	A	86.	D	92.	C	98.	A	104.	D	110.	B	116.	C	122.	C
81.	B	87.	C	93.	B	99.	C	105.	A	111.	B	117.	C	123.	A
82.	C	88.	B	94.	A	100.	A	106.	C	112.	B	118.	A	124.	C
83.	D	89.	C	95.	C	101.	C	107.	C	113.	D	119.	A	125.	D

126. D   132. B
127. C   133. B
128. C   134. C
129. C   135. C
130. A   136. D
131. B   137. C

BIOLOGICAL SCIENCES

138.	B	146.	C	154.	C	162.	D	170.	C	178.	D	186.	B	194.	D
139.	B	147.	C	155.	A	163.	C	171.	D	179.	B	187.	A	195.	C
140.	C	148.	D	156.	D	164.	B	172.	B	180.	A	188.	B	196.	D
141.	D	149.	A	157.	D	165.	B	173.	C	181.	C	189.	A	197.	C
142.	A	150.	D	158.	B	166.	C	174.	D	182.	B	190.	D	198.	A
143.	A	151.	C	159.	C	167.	A	175.	B	183.	D	191.	B	199.	D
144.	C	152.	A	160.	D	168.	B	176.	C	184.	B	192.	A	200.	C
145.	B	153.	B	161.	B	169.	A	177.	D	185.	A	193.	B	201.	A

202. B   210. A
203. C   211. B
204. A   212. D
205. D   213. D
206. C   214. C
207. D
208. B
209. D

Score Conversion Chart

Full-Length Practice MCAT

Physical Science		Verbal Reasoning		Biological Science	
Raw Score*	Estimated Scaled Score*	Raw Score*	Estimated Scaled Score*	Raw Score*	Estimated Scaled Score*
0	1	0–24	1	0–10	1
1–14	2	25–27	2	11–21	2
15–20	3	28–30	3	22–25	3
21–26	4	31–33	4	26–30	4
27–32	5	34–36	5	31–35	5
33–38	6	37–40	6	36–40	6
39–42	7	41–43	7	41–43	7
43–47	8	44–47	8	44–47	8
48–51	9	48–49	9	48–52	9
52–55	10	50–51	10	53–55	10
56–59	11	52–53	11	56–60	11
60–62	12	54–55	12	61–62	12
63–66	13	56–57	13	63–66	13
67–74	14	58–59	14	67–71	14
75–77	15	60	15	72–77	15

* This score coversion chart has been derived from a large representative sample of Kaplan students around the country. It will provide you with a score based on your performance compared to others who have taken this exam. Because the exam has been designed to closely match the MCAT content and format specifications, and because so many MCAT test takers prepare with Kaplan, this chart provides a rough estimate of your performance against the population who will sit for the MCAT. No test or score conversion chart can exactly predict actual test-day performance.

Answers and Explanations

Physical Sciences

Passage I (Questions 1–5)

1. A

This is one of those questions that can be answered without using any information from the passage. All we need to know is the relationship between the index of refraction of a medium, the speed of light in a medium, and the speed of light in a vacuum. The definition of the index of refraction is $n = c/v$, where n is the index of refraction of the medium, c is the speed of light in a vacuum, and v is the speed of light in the medium. So we can rearrange the equation to solve for v. We get that $v = c/n$. So the material with the lowest index of refraction will enable light to travel through it at the fastest speed. Therefore, choice A must be correct. It lists the media in order of increasing indices of refraction; so the speed of light in the media will be in decreasing order.

2. B

We are asked to determine the focal length of the eye's lens, in order to focus on an object 20 centimeters away. The equation that relates the focal length of a lens f, to the image distance i, and the object distance o, is: $1/f = 1/o + 1/i$. In the question we are told that the object is 20 centimeters away, but we don't know what the image distance is. If you read the passage carefully, and/or underlined the numbers in the passage, you would have easily found that the distance between the lens and the retina is 2 centimeters. This is essentially the image distance. Note that we haven't converted the distances from centimeters into meters. This is fine, as long as we

use centimeters for *all* the distances. We would have a problem if we started mixing units, using centimeters for some things, and meters for others. Substituting into the equation, we get that $1/f = 1/20 + 1/2$, or $11/20$. Taking the reciprocal of this, we find that the focal length $f = 20/11$. Of the answer choices, this is closest to 1.8 centimeters, which is choice B.

3. B

To answer this question, you must remember that for a multiple-lens system, the reciprocal of the total focal length is equal to the sum of the reciprocals of the focal lengths of the individual lenses. So for a two-lens system, this means that $1/f_t = 1/f_1 + 1/f_2$, where f_t is the total focal length, and f_1 and f_2 are the individual focal lengths of the two lenses. Here we have two lenses, each with a focal length of 5 centimeters, so $1/f_t = 1/5 + 1/5$, which equals $2/5$. Taking the reciprocal, we find that the focal length of the two-lens system equals 2.5 centimeters, which is answer choice B.

4. C

In the passage, we're told that myopia, or nearsightedness, is caused when the image of an object at infinity is brought into focus in front of the retina. In the question, we're told that a myopic person's eye has a relaxed focal length of 1.9 centimeters, and we're asked to determine the maximum distance from the eye at which this person can clearly see an object. This question essentially asks us to calculate the object distance, which is the distance from the eye's lens to the object. We know the focal length is 1.9 centimeters, but we don't know the image distance.

In the passage we are told that the distance from the lens to the retina is 2 centimeters. This is equal to the image distance because the image must be focused on the retina. As mentioned before, $1/f = 1/o + 1/i$. Rearranging this to get an equation in terms of the object distance, we find that $1/o = 1/f - 1/i$. Now, remember our sign conventions: for a converging lens the focal length is positive. Substituting in, we get that $1/o = 1/1.9 - 1/2$, which works out to $1/38$. Taking the reciprocal of this, we get that the object distance o is 38 centimeters.

That's the first part of our answer, and it narrows our choices down to B or C. The second part of the question asks us to calculate the magnification of the image. The equation for magnification m is: $m = -i/o$, where i is the image distance and o is the object distance. Well, we just calculated that the object distance is 38 centimeters, and we know that the image distance is 2 centimeters. Putting these numbers into the equation, we find that the magnification m equals -2 over 38, or -1 over 19. (The fact that this value is much less than 1 tells us that the image is reduced, and the negative sign tells us that the image is inverted.) Therefore, the maximum distance from the eye that an object can be seen clearly is 38 centimeters, and the magnification of an object at this point is $-1/19$. Choice C is correct.

5.   D

This question asks us which of the Roman numeral statements about the image formed in the eye is true. The first statement says that the image formed is real. In the passage we are told that the lens of the eye is a converging lens, and you should remember that for a converging lens, the image is real, provided that the object is placed outside the focal length. Note that all objects clearly viewed by the eye are outside the focal length. We can figure this out from the information in the passage and a little reasoning.

We are told that the focal length of the eye is only 2 centimeters, and we can reason that a young person with normal sight won't be able to focus on objects at a distance of less than 2 centimeters from the eye. Therefore, Statement I is true. So we can eliminate choice C because it doesn't contain Statement I.

Statement II suggests that the image is inverted. Remember that any real image formed by a converging lens is also inverted, so this statement is also true. Now we can eliminate choice A because it doesn't contain Statement II.

Now we have to examine Statement III to choose between answer choices B and D. Statement III says that the image is reduced. To determine whether or not this is true, consider that the retina is about the size of a postage stamp, and so for it to be possible to view an object that is larger than the retina of the eye, the image formed must be reduced. At this point you might say, "Hang on; it is also possible for a converging lens to produce a virtual image." This is true, but only if the object itself is inside the focal length of the eye, and as already mentioned, this is not the case for objects seen by the eye. So Statement III is true, and the correct answer is D.

Passage II (Questions 6–11)

6.   D

When two substances form a maximum-boiling azeotrope, the mixture has a higher boiling point than that corresponding to the vapor pressure predicted by Raoult's Law. You should realize that this increase in boiling point results from a decrease in the vapor pressures of the constituent species. That means that choice D is correct. Choice C, an increase in the vapor pressure of the constituents, would result in a lower boiling point, which is characteristic of a minimum-boiling azeotrope. Choices A and B can be eliminated because the two species being mixed together do not change the characteristic specific heats of each other.

7. A

You're looking for a combination of molecules that would not be strongly attracted to each other. All the choices contain water, which is a highly polar substance. Choice A is the only one in which water is combined with a molecule that is mostly nonpolar and hydrophobic. In a mixture of water and chlorobenzene, the absence of dipole-dipole or hydrogen-bonding attractions would allow them both to escape into the vapor phase more easily than they could if they were in separate, pure solutions.

8. B

Answering this question is simply a matter of understanding boiling point elevation and what is meant by the percent solute by weight. For every mole of solute in a kilogram of solvent, the boiling point is raised by a certain amount. This means that the boiling point is proportional to the molality of a solution. However, molality does not increase linearly with the percent of solute in solution, so choice A is wrong. With that choice out of the way, the easiest way to answer this question is to simply reason your way though it. When the solution becomes 100 percent NaCl by weight, it will have a much higher boiling point than the pure water. Does this change come on gradually or quickly? When you add just a little salt, the boiling point won't change too much because there is very little salt interacting with the water. That eliminates choice C, since it has the greatest degree of boiling point change coming when there is very little salt added. So what happens as you add more and more salt? As the percent salt becomes greater, it takes less and less added salt to increase the solution's boiling point to the same degree. So the graph will show a

steady curve upward. That is choice B, the correct answer. Choice D makes it seem like there is a critical point at about 50 percent salt where the slightest addition of salt kicks the boiling point of the solution up to the pure NaCl boiling point. This is the sort of thing we'd expect to see in a neutralization, not a steady increase in boiling point.

9. B

The key to answering this question is understanding the correct way to read Figure 1. On the x-axis are the mole fractions of A and B, while the y-axis indicates temperature. The lower line on the graph—the one that's concave upward—shows the boiling points of a mixture of A and B at various mole fractions. The two upper lines, the ones that are concave downward, show the mole fractions of A and B in the vapor at any given temperature. The two upper lines—the vapor lines—are the real issue in this question. The vapor that boils off from an azeotrope does not necessarily contain the same mole fraction of A and B that is found in the boiling liquid. In fact, the mole fractions in the vapor will always be different from the mole fractions in the liquid except at the single unique composition where the two curves meet. Since we're concerned with vapor in this question, we'll ignore the lower line completely. We want to know the mole fractions in the vapor at 40 degrees, not the mole fractions in the boiling liquid at 40 degrees. So all we have to do is read the points on the graph where the vapor curve crosses 40 degrees on the y-axis. There are actually two points that correspond to this temperature, so there are two possible compositions of the vapor at 40 degrees. One consists of a mole fraction of A equal to 0.60, and a mole fraction of B equal to 0.40. The other consists of a mole fraction of A equal to 0.80, and a mole fraction of B equal to 0.20. So, 0.40 and 0.20 are the two mole fractions of B possible in the vapor at 40 degrees, and choice B is the correct answer. You could find the compositions of the solutions boiling at 40 degrees that produces these vapor ratios by seeing where the lower, liquid line matches up to 40 degrees. However, that would just be for a point of interest since it isn't part of the question.

10.   B

The passage tells you that if you try to separate the components of an azeotrope by fractional distillation, the best you can do is get one pure component and the azeotrope. In the case of ethanol and water, the best you can get is a 95 percent solution of ethanol. But is the azeotrope minimum-boiling or maximum-boiling, and which species is more volatile? Well, the boiling point of the 95 percent ethanol solution is the temperature at which the azeotrope boils. Since the boiling point is lower than the boiling point of either pure component, this must be a minimum-boiling azeotrope, eliminating choices C and D. Now, think about the distillation; as the mixture is boiling, the vapor above it must have a greater percentage of ethanol than water, because when the vapor is condensed, the resulting solution had a greater percentage of ethanol than the original mixture. That means that ethanol is more likely to enter the gas phase and is therefore the more volatile of the two components. As said in the first paragraph of the passage, an ideal solution will always have a greater percentage of the more volatile component in the vapor. Since this mixture is not ideal, we can't make that assumption, but we can assume that the component that is more abundant in the critical composition is the more volatile of the two components. That makes choice B correct.

11.   C

This is just a matter of remembering the boiling point elevation equation and the designations for molarity and molality. The K_b is called the molal boiling point elevation constant. Its value is different for each solvent. The increase in boiling point is found by multiplying this constant by the molality of the solution. Boiling point elevation, just like freezing point depression, does not depend so much on the identity of the solute as it does on its concentration. As discussed earlier, the change in boiling point is directly proportional to the molality of the solution. That means that choices B and D are out. Since the symbol for molarity, moles per liter solution, is a capital M, and the symbol for molality, moles per kilogram solvent, is a small m, the correct choice is C.

Passage III (Questions 12–17)

12.   D

To answer this question, we need an equation that relates the electric field to the potential difference. This equation is $E = V/d$, where E is the electric field, V is the potential difference, and d is the separation of the plates. In the question stem, we are told that the potential difference between the plates V_{AB} is 20 volts, but we don't have a value for the separation of the plates. For this, we have to go back to the passage. In the first sentence of the second paragraph, we are told that the plates are separated by a distance of 1 centimeter, or 0.01 meters. Substituting into the equation $E = V/d$, we get that $E = 20/0.01$, which equals 2,000, or 2×10^3 volts per meter. This is answer choice D.

13.   B

When a drop is held motionless between the plates, there are two forces acting on the drop: the force of gravity acting downwards, which equals mg; and an equal but opposite force acting upwards, which is due to the electric field. The force due to the electric field is given by $F = qE$, where F is the force, q is the total charge on the drop, and E is the electric field. Both the force F and the electric field E are vector quantities; in other words, they have both magnitude and direction. Therefore, when we use this equation, we keep the sign of the charge. So for a negative charge, the force F is in the opposite direction to the electric field. Since the droplet is stationary, the force due to the electric field must be acting upwards to counteract the force due to gravity. Therefore, the electric field must be in the opposite direction, which is downwards, and choice B is correct.

14. C

In the question stem, we are told that the separation of the two parallel plates is reduced, but the potential difference across the plates is kept constant. We are asked which of the Roman numeral statements is true. Let's go through each of them in turn. Statement I suggests that the electric field increases. We noted earlier that the electric field is given by the equation $E = V/d$, where E is the electric field, V is the potential difference, and d is the separation of the plates. Since the potential difference is kept constant, the electric field E is inversely proportional to the separation of the plates d. Therefore, as we decrease the separation of the plates, the electric field must increase proportionally. So Statement I must be true, and we can eliminate choice D.

Statement II says that the magnetic field increases. Magnetic fields are created by moving charges, currents in wires, and permanent magnets. There is no current flow in our setup, no movement of charges, and therefore no magnetic field. Decreasing the separation of the plates will not change the situation. Therefore, Statement II is untrue.

It's either choice A or C, so let's look at Statement III. This says that the capacitance increases. It's a little tricky, though; you might have ignored this statement since it has nothing to with the passage. However, two plates in parallel form a parallel-plate capacitor, with a capacitance C given by the equation $C = \varepsilon_0 A/d$, where ε_0 is the permittivity of free space, A is the area of overlap of

the two plates, and d is the separation of the plates. ε_0 is a constant, and the area of overlap of the plates is kept constant, so the capacitance of the parallel plates must be inversely proportional to the separation of the plates. In other words, as the separation of the plates decreases, the capacitance must increase. Thus, Statements I and III are true, and the correct answer is C.

15. D

The drop is stationary, so the force due to the weight of the drop acting downwards is exactly balanced by the force due to the electric field directed upwards. The force due to the weight of the drop is given by the equation $F_w = mg$, where m is the mass and g is the acceleration due to gravity. The force due to the electric field is given by the equation $Fe = n\,e\,E$, where n is the total number of excess charges, e is the fundamental unit of charge—which we are told equals 1.6×10^{-19} coulombs—and E is the electric field. We know that $Fw = Fe$, so our force equation becomes: $mg = n\,e\,E$. We don't have a value for the mass of the oil drop, but we do know the volume of the drop, and we are given the density of oil at the end of the passage. So from the equation $\rho = m/V$, where ρ is the density, m is the mass, and V is the volume, we can determine the mass of the drop. Rearranging the equation, we get that $m = \rho V$. Substituting this into our force equation, we find that $\rho V g = n\,e\,E$. We want to find the value of n. Rearranging the equation, we find that $n = \rho V g /(e\,E)$. Putting values in, we get that $n = (800 \times 4 \times 10^{-19} \times 9.8)/(.6 \times 10^{-19} \times 490)$. Doing the math, we find that n equals 40, answer choice D.

16. A

This question is a two-step reasoning problem. We are told that an oil drop carrying a single electron charge falls between the two plates when the electric field is zero. The electric field is then increased from zero to 800 volts per meter, and we are asked to predict what happens to the oil drop. Initially the electric field is zero; the only force acting on the drop is the force due to the weight of the drop, and this force acts directly downwards. So at the beginning, the drop will move downwards under the influence of gravity. As the electric field increases from zero, there is an additional force due to the electric field. So there are now two forces acting on the drop: its weight acting downwards, and the force due to the electric field acting upwards. The force due to the electric field increases gradually as the electric field increases, since the force is directly proportional to the electric field. We have to determine what the magnitude of the electric field would be at the point that the forces become equal, and see whether this is larger than the maximum value of the electric field applied across the plates. Well, at the point that the drop becomes stationary, the force due to the weight of the drop equals the force due to the electric field. So our force equation is $qE = mg$, or, in terms of E, $E = mg/q$. We can approximate g as 10 m/s^2. Substituting in, we get that $E = (5 \times 10^{-16} \times 10)/(8 \times 10^{-18})$, which equals 625 volts per meter. We are told in the question stem that the maximum value of the electric field is 800 volts per meter, which is greater than the field required to hold the drop stationary. So there will be a point when the forces become equal. But the field continues to increase; therefore, there will be a net upwards force acting on the drop when the electric field is greater than 625 volts per meter increasing as the electric field increases. So the drop initially moves down, then stops and reverses direction moving upward. Therefore, the correct answer is choice A.

17.   B

This is a tricky question. We have two forces acting on the oil drop: the force due to its weight acting downwards, and the force due to the electric field acting upwards. Our drop is accelerated towards the top plate, and this tells us that the force in the upwards direction is greater than the force in the downwards direction. In other words, the force due to the electric field is greater than the force due to the weight of the oil. Therefore, the resultant force acting on the oil drop $Fr = Fe - Fw$, where Fw is the force due to the weight of the drop, and Fe is the force due to the electric field. Now, Fe is equal to qE, where q is the total charge, and E is the electric field, and Fw is equal to mg, where m is the mass and g is the acceleration due to gravity. Putting this into the equation for the resultant force, we get that $Fr = qE - mg$. In the question stem we are told that the charge on the drop is 3×10^{-18} coulombs, the electric field equals 4×10^3 volts per meter, and the mass of the drop is 5×10^{-16} kilograms. Substituting into the equation for the resultant force, we get that $Fr = 3 \times 10^{-18} \times 4 \times 10^3 - 5 \times 10^{-16} \times 9.8$. Doing the math, we get that $Fr = 7.1 \times 10^{-15}$ newtons. Well, we have found the resultant force acting on the drop, but the question asks us to find the resultant *acceleration*. To do this, we must use Newton's second law, $F = ma$. Rearranging to get an equation in terms of a, we find that $a = F/m$, so putting our values in we get that $a = (7.1 \times 10^{-15})/(5 \times 10^{-16})$, or 14.2 m/s^2. This is answer choice B.

Discrete Questions

18.   B

The molality of a solution is defined as the number of moles of solute added to 1 kilogram of solvent (you should know that one kilogram of water has a volume of one liter at room temperature). Molarity is the number of moles of solute per liter of total solution. Since you are told that one mole of calcium chloride has been added to one liter of water, the total volume of the solution will be greater than one liter. Noticing this, you should know that molality is a far more convenient concentration unit; choices A and C can be eliminated. Since the question is asking for the calcium concentration and there is only one mole of calcium per mole of calcium chloride, the correct answer is B, one molal.

19. B

In the question stem, we are told that we have two blocks of equal density, but different mass, and therefore different volume. We're asked to determine the ratio of their apparent weights when they're completely submerged in water. Well, there are two forces acting on a block when it is completely submerged in water: its weight, mg, acting downwards, and the buoyant force acting upwards. The apparent weight in water is equal to the actual weight of the block in air, mg, minus the buoyant force.

The buoyant force exerted on a block when it is submerged in water is equal to the weight of water that the block displaces. The weight of water displaced is equal to m_wg, where m_w is the mass of the water displaced, and g is the acceleration due to gravity. Using the equation $m = \rho V$, where m is the mass, ρ is the density, and V is the volume of the block (and therefore the volume of water displaced when the block is completely submerged), we can express the mass of water displaced as being $m_w = \rho V$. We are given that the mass and volume of the first block are m and V, respectively. We are told that the second block has a mass of $2m$ and the same density as the first block. The density of the first block is just m/v, so m/v must equal the mass of the second block over the volume of the second block. The mass of the second block is $2m$, so the volume of the second block must equal $2V$. So the second block displaces twice as much water, and therefore, the buoyant force on the second block is twice as great.

Now we can express the apparent weights of the two blocks when submerged in water. The block

of mass m has an apparent weight of $mg - m_wg$, and the block of mass $2m$, has an apparent weight of $2\ mg - 2m_wg$. So the apparent weight of block one is one-half the apparent weight of block two. Therefore, the correct ratio is 1 to 2, which is answer choice B.

20. A

The alkaline earth elements are those in the second column from the left of the periodic table. The first two columns of the periodic table are the s-block elements, so their valence electrons are in the s-subshell. The alkaline earth elements have two valence electrons, and therefore a complete s subshell in their outer electron shell. They lose these two electrons to gain a valence number of +2. Anyway, all of these valence electron properties aside, the correct answer to the question is the s orbital, choice A.

21. D

This question requires a good understanding of circuit laws. A key law to remember here is that charge is conserved, and as a result, the current that flows through the first parallel combination must also flow through the second parallel combination.

We're told that the reading on ammeter A_1 is 3 amps. You should remember that for resistors in parallel, the sum of the currents through each of the resistors is equal to the total current that enters the parallel combination. The current is split in the ratio of the resistance of the two resistors, and since the resistors in the first parallel combination are equal, the current traveling through each must be equal. We know that the current traveling through one of the resistors is 3 amps, so the current traveling through the other resistor must be 3 amps also. This means that the total current in the circuit equals 3 + 3, or 6 amps.

As we've already said, this 6-amp current also travels through the second parallel combination. This time we have a $1R$ resistor in parallel with a $2R$ resistor, so the current will *not* be split equally among the two resistors. To find how much current goes through the $1R$ resistor, we must first calculate the resistance of the parallel combination. For two resistors in parallel, the reciprocal of the total resistance equals the sum of the reciprocals of the individual resistances. Substituting in, we get that one over the total resistance equals $1/(1R) + 1/(2R)$, which equals $3/(2R)$. Taking the reciprocal of this, we find that the total resistance equals $2R/3$. Now, we can use Ohm's law to determine the voltage across the parallel combination. Ohm's law in equation form is $V = iR$, where V is the potential difference, i is the current, and R is the resistance. Substituting in we get that $V = (6 \times 2R)/3$, or $4R$ volts. To find the current through the $1R$ resistor, and therefore the current through ammeter A_2, we apply Ohm's law again. This time we have the $4R$ volts across the $1R$ resistor, so substituting in we get that $i = 4R/(1R)$, or 4 amps, which is answer choice D.

22. C

Each electron shell can be divided into up to four subshells, designated s, p, d, and f. The s subshell contains 1 orbital, the p subshell contains 3, the d subshell contains 5, and the f subshell contains 7. Since each orbital can hold two electrons, the numbers of electrons that can be held by these four subshells are 2, 6, 10, and 14, respectively. To remember how many electrons are in each subshell, you can look at the periodic table. The elements in the two columns on the left have their valence electrons in the s subshell. Those elements in the six columns on the right also contain electrons in their p subshell. The transition elements in the middle are found in ten columns, representing the 10 electrons that fit into the d subshell. The fourteen rows in the inner transition elements, listed below the rest of the periodic table, show those elements with electrons in the f subshell. So the ratio of f electrons to p electrons is 14 to 6, which is equal to 7 to 3, choice C.

Passage IV (Questions 23–27)

23. B

Metals in their elemental, or free, form can only be oxidized, not reduced. That is, metals in their ground state tend to lose electrons rather than gain them. Therefore, the reaction with HCl proceeds when electrons are lost from the metal, thereby reducing the hydrogen ions to H_2 gas. The other product of the reaction is the metal chloride salt. Now, to be a little more specific, the higher their reduction potential of a species, the more likely it is to be reduced. Thus, the elements with the lowest reduction potential are most likely to be oxidized in this reaction. Therefore the elements at the bottom of the table are more likely to be oxidized. However, all of this information doesn't tell you where the cutoff point is between those metals that well react and those that won't. In any redox reaction, the element with the higher reduction potential will be reduced while the one with the lower reduction potential will be oxidized. You can determine the cutoff point for reactivity by comparing the reduction potentials of these metals with the reduction potential of the hydrogen ions the metal reacts with. Any metal that has a reduction potential lower than the reduction potential of hydrogen will react. Since the reduction potential of hydrogen ions to hydrogen gas is set at zero for all temperatures, those metals with a reduction potential of less than zero can be oxidized by hydrochloric acid. So tin, nickel, and iron will react with the hydrochloric acid, and metallic silver and copper will not. This is answer choice B. Note that the positive reduction potentials of copper and silver indicates a reluctance to oxidize, not a tendency to reduce.

24. D

As just discussed, reduction potentials are a direct measure of the reactivity of a species. The metals with negative reduction potentials are the ones that will react with the HCl to produce the metal chloride salt and hydrogen gas. The lower the reduction potential, the more vigorously it will react. Right away we know that choices A and B are wrong since they don't even react. That leaves C and D. Since iron has the lowest reduction potential, it must be the metal that reacts the best with the HCl. So the correct answer must be D.

25. A

To answer this question, you need to figure out what happens to the metallic zinc in Experiment II. You know that you're starting with HCl, and that a reaction occurs; this means that the hydrogen ion in the HCl must be reduced to molecular hydrogen. Therefore, the zinc will have to be oxidized from zinc metal to Zn^{2+}. Since zinc is oxidized, the zinc electrode must be called the anode and not the cathode, because the electrode at which oxidation takes place is always called the anode. This means that either choice A or choice C must be correct. If you couldn't take this question any farther, at least eliminating two of the four choices improves your odds of guessing dramatically. However, all we need to get the answer is the identity of the cathode. In simple terms, since the cell was set up so that zinc would be oxidized by hydrochloric acid, the second electrode must be a hydrogen electrode since the reduced species in the reaction is the hydrogen ion. Copper was never mentioned, so it doesn't really make sense in the context of the question, although zinc/copper cells are very common in general chemistry problems. The other convenient thing about using hydrogen at the cathode is that the half-cell potential of the hydrogen electrode at 1 molar concentration is always zero, and that helps our calculations. Since hydrogen must be at the cathode and zinc

at the anode, choice A must be the correct answer.

26. B

To answer this question correctly, you need to know the difference between oxidation and reduction. Remember, when an element is reduced, its oxidation number is made lower because it gains negatively charged electrons. A reduction in the oxidation number means that the element itself has been reduced. Oxidation occurs when the oxidation number is increased due to the loss of negatively charged electrons. You should also know that when one species in a reaction is oxidized, another must be reduced. We call the species that is oxidized the reducing agent because it supplies the electrons that are gained by the reduced species. The opposite is true for an oxidizing agent. So, an oxidizing agent is itself reduced, and a reducing agent is itself oxidized. We've already discussed that when hydrochloric acid is added to a metal, the metal is oxidized and the hydrogen ions are reduced. Since the hydrogen ions have caused the zinc to be oxidized, the HCl is an oxidizing agent, and choices C and D are wrong since the HCl participates directly in the reaction, rather than being simply a catalyst or solvent.

27. C

This question is really a gas-laws and stoichiometry problem-solving question. As you should know, a mole of gas occupies 22.4 liters at STP. However, we're not at STP in this experiment. While 25° C, or 298 K, is the temperature used here, the STP temperature is zero Celsius, or 273 K. In order to know how much zinc can be used in this experiment, we need to find out how much hydrogen, in moles, can be contained in a liter bottle at 25° C. So first, we need to determine the volume of a mole of gas at this temperature. The volume of a gas is directly proportional to its temperature in Kelvins; an increase in temperature leads to an increase in volume. So the ratio of the volumes will be equal to the ratio of the temperatures. The temperature has increased from 273 K to 298 K, or by a factor of 1.09. So the volume must increase from 22.4 L to 22.4 L × 1.09, or about 24.4 L. So if one mole is 24.4 L, 1 L must be taken up by 1/24.4 moles, or 0.04 moles. So how many moles of zinc are reacted to produce 0.04 moles of hydrogen gas? Well, the reaction stoichiometry of zinc reactant to hydrogen gas product is 1:1, so 0.04 moles of zinc, which releases two electrons in its oxidation, produces 0.04 moles of hydrogen gas, which needs two electrons to be made from hydrogen ions. So all we need now for the answer is the molar weight of zinc, which we can get from the periodic table. If one mole of zinc is 65 grams, 0.04 moles of zinc is 2.6 grams, which is choice C.

Passage V (Questions 28–32)

28. A

From the passage, we know that a light bulb burns out because its filament is gradually vaporized by intense heat. If the filament is in a vacuum, it will vaporize at a faster rate than it would at normal atmospheric pressure. You can see this if you remember the shape of a phase diagram, which gives the relationship between temperature, pressure, and phase. If you think about the line separating the solid phase from the gaseous phase in that diagram, you'll remember that a reduction in pressure, at constant temperature, can cause a solid to sublimate to the gaseous form. Vacuum bulbs were originally used so as to exclude oxygen from the system so that they wouldn't oxidize the filament, but the vacuum greatly increases the sublimation rate, so it's not an optimal solution to the problem of oxidation. An inert gas won't cause oxidation, of course, but it does slow down the process of sublimation; thus, choice A is correct.

It's true that the presence of a gas removes some heat from the filament, as is stated in choice B, but this isn't the reason for putting gas into the light bulb. The heat of the filament could easily be decreased just by reducing the voltage through the filament, or by using a filament with a lower resistance. But in fact, the filament is intentionally designed to become very hot so that it will produce an intense white light; a lower temperature would mean less intense, redder light. The ultimate purpose of the inert gas is actually to allow the filament to be made hotter without being destroyed too fast by vaporization. Choice C is wrong because the danger of implosion is not the reason for using inert gas in a light bulb. The end of the first paragraph of the passage tells us that the inert gas increases the life of the filament, so there's no reason to go off into speculation about implosion and all that. Of course, light bulbs do sometimes break when subject to vibration, but whether they implode or not when they break is hardly the issue here, since as you probably know, light bulbs burn out—that is, their filaments break—much more often than their bulbs break. Finally, choice D is wrong because the gas normally would absorb very little energy from the electrons, which are moving through the metal of the wire, not in the gas. Even if the gas did absorb energy, it wouldn't be helpful, since we want the energy from the voltage to go into producing heat in the wire, not be dissipated in the gas.

29. B

Exposure to light is known to improve people's moods, while long hours of darkness can cause depression. There is still some question as to whether the improvement in mood is caused simply by exposure to very bright light, or whether exposure to certain wavelengths is also needed. So it's not clear whether some people get depressed in cloudy weather simply because there is less light, or because they need more light of a certain wavelength. The advertiser in this question is claiming that short-wavelength light is needed, and that incandescent lights are therefore inadequate to improve people's moods. You are asked which statement could be used as an argument against this claim, based on the information in the passage. The first paragraph tells you that the visible light produced by an incandescent lamp is just the tip of the iceberg: Most of the radiation is produced in the infrared range. As a filament is heated, it becomes hot enough to radiate energy in the visible wavelengths, starting at the red end of the spectrum and then adding wavelengths of other colors. So incandescent light is stronger on the red side of the spectrum. Infrared radiation, or heat, has longer wavelengths and lower frequency than visible light, while ultraviolet light is of higher frequency and shorter wavelengths. So incandescent light is relatively more intense in the longer wavelengths and less intense in the shorter wavelengths, and so choice A is wrong.

As for choice B, the passage states that the light on a sunny day is least intense in the short wavelengths, while light on a cloudy day is most intense on the blue end of the spectrum, which is the short-wavelength end. Thus, the light on a sunny day is most intense at the long wavelengths, while on a cloudy day the short wavelengths are most intense. So a person could argue that what we need in cloudy weather is more long-wavelength light, and that incandescent lamps would be helpful for that purpose. This could be used as an argument against the advertiser's claim. On the other hand, we don't know if this is really true. On a cloudy day, all light is less intense, so it might turn out to be the short-wavelength light that we need more of after all. However, the advertiser here doesn't provide any evidence to support this position. Since long-wavelength light is most reduced in cloudy weather, judging by the information available in this passage, we can only conclude that people most likely need more light of longer, not short-

er wavelengths, if wavelengths really do matter. Choice B, which says outdoor light is of longer wavelength on a sunny day than a cloudy day, is true, and choice C, which says the opposite, is false. As for choice D, this says that the spectrum produced by an incandescent lamp is irrelevant since the intensity is too low. But that's a weaker argument than choice B, since the advertiser is arguing specifically about the wavelengths produced by incandescent lamps. Actually, D is false, since it's possible, though expensive, to produce very high-intensity light using incandescent lamps.

30. D

Since incandescent lamps produce mostly infrared radiation, and the visible radiation they produce is most intense on the red end of the spectrum, they must produce comparatively little ultraviolet radiation. Fluorescent lamps do produce ultraviolet radiation, but this radiation is absorbed by the phosphorescent coating on the surface of the glass tube, and longer-wavelength visible radiation is emitted. Thus, neither kind of lamp will normally produce dangerous levels of ultraviolet radiation. It *is* possible to produce special lamps of both kinds that do produce ultraviolet—for instance, the lamps used in tanning salons. But ultraviolet radiation is not a danger from the kind of incandescent and fluorescent lamps that are commonly used in people's homes.

31. B

A lamp is an apparatus for converting electrical energy into light energy, so its efficiency is defined as how much visible light it puts out for a given input of electrical power. Like any other system, a lamp is somewhat inefficient. To figure out where that inefficiency enters into the process, you have to use information from the passage. Incandescent lamps produce a great deal of infrared—that is, heat—and only a comparatively small amount of light. Notice the fourth sentence in the first paragraph: This states that *almost all* of the radiation produced by incandescent lamps is in the infrared range. In a fluorescent lamp, on the other hand, all the radiation gets converted to light, although the final frequency of that light is lower than the original frequency, and so there must be some energy lost there. So fluorescent lamps lose some of their energy, but incandescent lamps lose almost all of theirs. Thus the correct answer is B.

32. D

The passage tells you that the wavelengths of light emitted from a fluorescent lamp are controlled by the composition of the phosphor coating the inside of the glass tube. It also tells you that a "warm white" lamp produces more light at the red end of the spectrum than a "cool white" lamp. So, if a manufacturer that made "warm white" lamps wanted to start making "cool white" lamps, all he'd have to do is change the composition of the phosphor to produce more blue-violet light when it absorbed ultraviolet light from the mercury vapor. This is choice D. Choice A is wrong because the phosphor will always emit the same wavelengths of light, regardless of the amount of ultraviolet light. Choice B is wrong because "warm white" and "cool white" lights are defined by the wavelengths of the light they emit, not by the angle at which they emit the light. Choice C is wrong because it is the identity of the phosphor that determines the wavelengths of visible light emitted, not the strength of the electric arc.

Passage VI (Questions 33–39)

33. A

In this question, you are told that the flow in the pipes is laminar, and you are asked to describe the streamlines. Streamlines show the path taken by a fluid as it moves through a pipe. Laminar flow occurs when adjacent layers of fluid slide smoothly over each other. Laminar flow implies ordered and regular flow. So if we have laminar flow, the stream lines are uniform and regular. Answer choice A is therefore correct.

When the flow becomes fast enough, or the fluid flows around an irregularly shaped obstacle, the flow becomes turbulent; in that case, the streamlines of the flow are complex. If you picked choice C, which says the streamlines are far apart, you may have thought that if the streamlines were far apart, the speed of the flow was small, and therefore, the flow would be laminar. Streamlines represent the path taken by fluid. Converging streamlines indicate increasing speed of the fluid, and diverging streamlines indicate decreasing speed of the fluid. However, the relative distance between the streamlines in any one place doesn't really mean anything—it just depends on the number of streamlines you chose to draw. In other words, it's only how the distance between the streamlines *changes* within a drawing that indicates the relative speed.

34. B

At first sight this question looks like it involves a complicated calculation. However, if we break it down and make some reasonable estimations, it's not too difficult. First, we need to find the power generated by the heater. This can be found from the formula power equals voltage squared over resistance. Since the answer choices are mostly in hours, it will be useful to find the power in joules per hour. We therefore find that the power equals $240 \times 240/20$ J/s which equals $240 \times 240 \times 60 \times 60/20$ J/hr. Rather than do any more calculation at this time, it is better to wait until the final answer to see if we get any cancellations. So next, we figure out how much heat is supplied to the water. This equals the mass times the specific heat times the change in temperature which equals 60 × 4200 × 40 J. Now we divide this by the power to find the time. So we have (60 × 4200 × 40 × 20)/(240 × 240 × 60 × 60). First, cancel zeros to get (6 × 42 × 4 × 20)/(24 × 24 × 60 × 60). Next, cancel the 4 and 6 on the top against one of the 24's on the bottom. This gives (42 × 20)/(24 × 6 × 6) or 840/864 hours which equals 0.97 hours. This is closest to 1 hour, choice B.

35. A

First, remember that the resistance of the wire coil in the hot water heating system is given as 20 Ω. In order to answer the question, calculate the total resistance of each circuit until we find the one that equals 20 Ω. Sum the resistors in series to get the total resistance and sum the reciprocal of the resistors in parallel to get the reciprocal of the total resistance. In choice A, the two 20-Ω resistors are in parallel, and therefore, one over their equivalent resistance equals 1/20 + 1/20, which is 2/20 or 1/10. So their equivalent resistance is 10/1 or 10 Ω. The two parallel resistors as a unit are in series with the 10 Ω resistor shown. The total resistance is therefore 10 Ω + 10 Ω, or 20 Ω.

Just to be thorough, look at the other choices. Choice B shows three 30-Ω resistors in series which gives a total resistance of 90 Ω. For choice C, we first add 3 Ω to 9 Ω to get a 12-Ω resistor which is in parallel with a 6-Ω resistor. One over the total resistance is one over 12 plus one over 6 which equals 1/12 + 2/12 or 3/12. The total resistance is therefore 12 /3 or 4 Ω. Choice D gives three 30-Ω resistors in parallel. One over the total resistance equals 1/30 + 1/30 + 1/30 or 3/30 which gives a total resistance of 10 Ω.

36. C

The question asks us what the heat of vaporization for water is. The heat of vaporization is the heat required to turn water at its boiling point of 100°C into steam at the same temperature. Since we must put in heat to turn the water into steam, the steam must have a greater internal energy. When steam condenses back into water, it releases this energy as heat. Choices A and B can, therefore, immediately be ruled out. Choice D is a true statement, but it does not explain what the heat of vaporization is.

37. B

Since the shower is running, the water coming out of the shower opening must be at atmospheric pressure. Therefore, Statements I and II cannot be correct, and by a process of elimination the answer must be choice B. To see why the water will decrease in velocity, we can use Bernoulli's equation. Call the water at the fill level of the storage tank point 1 and the water at the shower opening point 2. Bernoulli's equation gives $P_1 + rv_1^2/2 + rgy_1 = P_2 + rv_2^2/2 + rgy_2$. $P_1 = P_2$ because they are both at atmospheric pressure and the r's cancel, so we get $v_1^2/2 + gy_1 = v_2^2/2 + gy_2$ or after rearranging $v_2^2 - v_1^2 = 2g(y_1 - y_2)$. The continuity equation says that $v_1A_1 = v_2A_2$, where A_1 and A_2 are the cross-sectional areas at points 1 and 2, respectively. The area at the fill level, A_1, is so much larger than the area at the shower opening, A_2, so v_1 must be much smaller than v_2. We can approximate $v_1 = 0$. The final result is therefore $v_2^2 = 2g(y_1 - y_2)$. As the fill level decreases, y_1 and therefore $y_1 - y_2$ gets smaller, so the velocity at the shower opening, v_2, must also decrease.

38. D

This question can be answered quickly with the knowledge that in a closed, static fluid system, the pressure depends only on the depth relative to the highest point in the fluid. The deeper that one looks in the system, the larger the pressure will be. All points of equal height have the same pressure. Therefore, according to the diagram in Figure 1, the pressure is greatest in the basement.

39. B

In order to answer this question, we follow the same logic given in the answer for question 10. Again, let point 1 be the water at the fill level of the storage tank, and now, let point 2 be the water at the hole in the bottom of the tank. And again, we find from Bernoulli's equation that $v_2^2 - v_1^2 = 2g(y_1 - y_2)$. Since the hole in the bottom of the tank is small, we can again assume that the velocity of the fill level in the storage tank is zero. We therefore find for the velocity of the water exiting the hole $v^2 = 2g(y_1 - y_2)$, or $v^2 = 2gh$ where h is $y_1 - y_2$, the height difference between the fill level y_1 and the hole y_2. We are told that $h = 1.25$ m. Substituting $g = 10$ m/s^2, $v^2 = 2$ times 10 times 1.25 or 25. So $v = 5$ m/s.

Discrete Questions

40. A

The equation you need to answer this question was derived by Neils Bohr. It predicts the frequency of light produced when an electron falls from one quantum level to another in a hydrogen atom, though it doesn't work for other kinds of atoms, since those have more complex subshells. The equation states that E equals $-A$ times the quantity $(1/ni^2 - 1/nf^2)$, where ni is the first quantum number of the electron in its initial state and nf is the first quantum number of the electron in its final state. A, which is a constant, is the amount of energy needed to remove an electron from the lowest energy level of a hydrogen atom to a point at an infinite distance away. The negative sign in front of the A is there because the electron in the question is falling *toward* the nucleus of the atom, and therefore is giving off energy. So we have to multiply $-A$ by $1/3^2 - 1/2^2$. This comes to $-A \times -5/36$, which is equal to 0.14 A, choice A.

41. B

We're told that an airplane with a mass of 150,000 kilograms produces a thrust of 200,000 newtons to go from rest to a cruising speed of 720 kilometers per hour. So we're given a mass, force, and speed and we're asked to find the time it takes to reach that speed. We need to find an equation that relates what we need to find to what we're given.

An equation that accomplishes this is the familiar kinematic equation $v = v_0 + a\,t$, where v is the final speed, v_0 is the initial speed, a is the acceleration, which is equal to the force over the mass, and t is the time. The plane starts from rest, so $v_0 = 0$. Solving for t, we find that $t = v/a$. We know $v = 720$ kilometers per hour, but what is the acceleration? As noted earlier, we can calculate the acceleration from Newton's second law, $F = m\,a$, where F is the force, and m is the mass. We know that $F = 200,000$ newtons and $m = 150,000$ kilograms. So we can calculate a by dividing F by m. We get $a = 200,000$ over 150,000, or four-thirds. Now that we have a we can calculate t from the equation $t = v/a$. But before we can substitute our numbers in, we must first convert the speed of the aircraft from kilometers per hour to meters per second. Multiply the speed by the number of meters in a kilometer, and divide it by the number of seconds in an hour; we get that the speed equals $(720 \times 1,000)/3,600$, or 200 meters per second. Plugging that number into our equation, we find that the time t equals v over a or 200 over four-thirds or 150 seconds, which is answer choice B.

You could also use the formula for impulse to answer this question. Impulse, J, is the product of the force, F, and the time over which the force acts, t. It also equals the change in momentum, Dp, which equals the final momentum minus the initial momentum. Therefore, we can say that $J = Dp = Ft$. Since momentum is the product of mass and speed and the aircraft is initially at rest, the initial momentum of the aircraft is zero. So the change in momentum Dp is simply the final momentum of the aircraft. Thus, our equation becomes $mv = Ft$, where m is the mass of the aircraft, and v is the final speed of the aircraft. We are trying to find the time, so rearranging to get an equation in terms of the time t, we get that $t = mv$ over F. Plugging in the values for m and v, we get that $t = (150,000 \times 200)/200,000$, or 150 seconds.

42. C

There are two ways you could do this problem: an easy way if you have the Henderson-Hasselbach equation memorized, and a longer way based on the definition of the acid dissociation constant, K_a, if you don't remember that equation. (If you don't, you'll have to decide if it's worth trying to memorize. It can potentially save you time on the exam, but on the other hand, if you try to memorize it, that's one more equation you could forget or get mixed up. If you understand how to figure out questions like this one based on pK_a, it may take longer, but you'll be less likely to forget how to do it.)

By definition, the pK_a of an acid solution is –log of the acid dissociation constant, or K_a. The acid dissocation constant, in turn, is equal to (the concentration of the hydrogen ion) $\times$ (the concentration of the anion, X-) divided by (the concentration of the undissociated acid, HX). If the concentration of X- and the concentration of HX are equal, they'll cancel each other out. This means that the concentration of hydrogen ion will be equal to the value of the acid constant. In that case, the pH, which is the *negative log* of the hydrogen ion concentration, will be equal to the negative log of the acid constant—that is, equal to the pK_a. So any time the pH is equal to the pK_a, the concentration of X- must also be equal to the concentration of HX. In this example, the pH is not equal to the pK_a, so the concentrations of X- and of HX will not be equal. But you can figure out what they will be just by remembering that the pK_a is the negative log of the acid constant. Since the pH is 6, the hydrogen ion concentration will be 1×10^{-6}. Since the pK_a is 5, the acid constant must be 1×10^{-5}. If you plug these values into the equation for the acid constant, and then divide both sides

of the equation by the hydrogen ion concentration, you find that the concentration of X- divided by the concentration of HX is equal to 1×10^{-5} divided by 1×10^{-6}. This comes to 10^1, or 10. So the concentration of X- must be 10 times the concentration of HX, and choice C is correct.

Now for the other method of answering this question. The Henderson-Hasselbach equation says that for a weak acid solution, the pH equals the pK_a plus the log of the ratio of the concentration of conjugate base to the concentration of acid. For an acid HX, the conjugate base is the X- ion that's formed when the acid dissociates. Now, if the pK_a of an acid is 5, then for its pH to be 6, the log of that concentration ratio must be 1, or in other words, the ratio must be 10. This means that the concentration of conjugate base, and therefore of dissociated acid, must be 10 times the concentration of acid.

43. C

We are told that a metal plate is *completely* illuminated by a monochromatic light source, and we are asked which of the Roman numeral statements would increase the number of electrons ejected from the surface of the metal.

Statement I suggests that increasing the intensity of the light source would increase the number of electrons ejected. Light may be thought of as being made of particles. These light particles are more commonly known as photons, and have an energy given by the equation $E = hf$, where E is the energy, h is Planck's constant, and f is the frequency of the light. The intensity of a light source is the number of photons produced per unit time. Therefore, when we increase the intensity of the light source, we increase the number of photons striking the metal plate, resulting in more electrons being ejected from the metal. Thus Statement I is true, so we can eliminate answer choice D.

Statement II suggests that increasing the frequency of the light source would increase the number of electrons ejected. From the equation $E = hf$, we see that by increasing the frequency of the light, we increase the energy of the incident photons. This means that a photon that strikes the metal will eject an electron with a higher kinetic energy. However, it will not increase the number of electrons ejected, since the number of electrons ejected is proportional to the number of incident photons. Therefore, Statement II is false, and we can eliminate answer choice B. This leaves us with answer choices A and C.

The final statement suggests that increasing the surface area of the metal plate would increase the number of electrons ejected. The key point to remember here is that the metal plate is completely illuminated by the light source. Therefore, by increasing the area of the metal plate, we increase the area on which the light source is incident. This implies that more photons will strike the plate, resulting in an increase in the number of electrons ejected. Since Statements I and III are true, the correct answer must be choice C.

44. D

There are two things you need to know to answer this question. First, in a chemical cell, the flow of electricity through the wire—and thus the flow of electrons—always runs from the anode to the cathode. This is true both in galvanic cells such as this one, where the reaction itself is the source of power, and in electrolytic cells that are powered by an external power source. Thus the cathode receives the electric current that subsequently runs down into the solution. This means that we can eliminate choices A and C, since both of these talk about the electrons moving toward the anode. Second, the cell voltage is measured with a voltmeter, not an ammeter, so choice B is wrong. Again, the direction of the current is from the anode to the voltmeter to the cathode, and thus choice D is correct.

Passage VII (Questions 45–49)

45. B

This question asks us to determine which of the Roman numeral statements would increase the current generated by the pyroelectric device. Statement I suggests that by increasing the rate of change in temperature we would increase the current. To establish whether this is true or not, go back to the passage and look at the equation for the current generated by a pyroelectric material. The current generated is proportional to the change in temperature over the time. In other words, the current is proportional to the rate of change in temperature, so if we increase the rate of change in temperature, we increase the current generated. Therefore Statement I is true, and this allows us to eliminate answer choice C.

Statement II suggests that increasing the area of the electrodes would increase the current. Since the current is proportional to the area of the electrodes, if we increase the area of the electrodes, we must increase the current generated. Since this statement is true, we can eliminate answer choice A, leaving us with choices B and D.

The final statement suggests that increasing the thickness of the thin film would increase the current. But the thickness of the film has nothing to do with the magnitude of the current generated by the pyroelectric device. Thus Statement III is false. Only Statements I and II would increase the magnitude of the current generated, and so the correct answer is choice B.

46. B

The maximum voltage across the resistor will occur when the pyroelectric is first connected. The charge on the pyroelectric is given by i times t or $Q = pA(\Delta T)$. The voltage across the resistor will be equal to the voltage across the pyroelectric since they are connected in parallel. For a

KAPLAN

capacitor $C = Q/V$, where C is the capacitance, Q is the absolute charge on one of the plates, and V is the voltage across the capacitor. Therefore, $V = Q/C$ and we get that $V = pA(\Delta T)/C$.

47. A

We're told in the passage that when the thin film is sandwiched between two parallel plates, it acts as a dielectric. The plates in this case are the metal electrodes. Now, the equation for the capacitance of a parallel plate capacitor is $C = K\varepsilon_o A$ over d, where C is the capacitance, K is the dielectric constant, ε_o is the permittivity of free space, A is the area of the plates, and d is the separation of the plates. By increasing the thickness of the thin film, we effectively increase the separation of the plates. Since the capacitance is inversely proportional to the separation of the plates, increasing the thickness will cause the capacitance to decrease. Therefore, we are looking for a graph that shows that as the thickness of the film increases, the capacitance decreases. The only graph that represents this relationship is the one in choice A.

48. B

This is sort of a trick question. The dielectric constant is a property of a substance. It is the ratio of the capacitance of a capacitor with that substance between the plates to the capacitance of a capacitor with just air between the plates. So the dielectric constant is a property of a substance and does not depend on the dimensions of the capacitor.

49. A

Answer this question by using the formula given in the note at the end of the passage: $2nd = (m + 1/2)\lambda$ where n is the index of refraction, d is the thickness of the film, m is an integer equal to or greater than 0, and k is the wavelength of light. For m equal to 0, we get $d = \lambda/4n$. Putting in the numbers gives d = 480nm/6 which equals 80nm.

Passage VIII (Questions 50–57)

50. A

We're told that the "energy of the clusters" can be derived from the minimum frequency of light required to break down a cluster. The frequency of a photon of light is related to its energy, and clearly if light is required to break down a cluster, energy must be absorbed when the cluster breaks down. That means choice D is wrong. None of the choices describes the energy absorbed when the cluster breaks down, so to answer the question, we have to look for a choice that's equivalent to that value. Clusters are held together by intermolecular forces; therefore, formation of a cluster represents an increase in stability compared to the overall stability of the original component molecules when they existed independently. That's why energy must be added to break down a cluster. Likewise, when a cluster forms, an identical amount of energy will be released. Thus, choice A is correct. Choice B is wrong because once the cluster forms, the energy is gone—it's not in the cluster at all—so it's simply wrong to say that it's shared among the cluster molecules. And the bond energy of the molecules in the cluster, choice C, is the energy needed to break the intramolecular bonds that hold the individual molecules together; this is definitely not related to the energy released when the cluster is formed.

51. D

The stronger the intermolecular forces within a cluster, the more strongly bound together the cluster will be. So you have to compare the strengths of the intermolecular forces for the four answer choices. This is relatively simple, since the table lays out the different possible types of intermolecular forces and their respective energies. All four choices include argon. Since argon is a noble gas and therefore can't form covalent bonds to another atom, it can't form hydrogen bonds and it can't have any intrinsic dipole moment, so we don't expect to find either hydrogen bonds or dipole-dipole forces in any of these clusters. The next strongest intermolecular force in the table is dipole-induced dipole interaction. In order for these to exist, the other molecule of the pair (besides argon) would have to have a dipole moment. Nitric oxide and hydrogen chloride both have dipole moments, so choices A and D are both possibilities. The strength of a dipole-induced dipole interaction depends on how strong a dipole moment is involved, so we need to compare the dipole moments of the two compounds. Hydrogen chloride is made up of unlike elements that are widely separated from one another in the periodic table. Chlorine is highly electronegative and attracts electron density from the hydrogen atom, giving the molecule a strong dipole moment. As for nitric oxide, this molecule consists of two fairly similar elements that are side-by-side in the periodic table. Oxygen is more electronegative than nitrogen, but the difference isn't large, and so the dipole moment here will be much weaker than for hydrogen chloride. Hydrogen chloride has a significantly larger dipole moment than nitric oxide, and the cluster containing hydrogen chloride will be more strongly bound than the cluster containing nitric oxide. As for the other two choices, B shows two argon molecules, which can't have dipole moments. Likewise, choice C shows argon and carbon tetrachloride; the carbon tetrachloride molecule is symmetric and therefore does not have a net dipole moment, even though the individual carbon-chlorine bonds are polar. So both of these clusters will be held together just by dispersion forces, which are relatively weak.

52. C

To solve this question you have to remember the relative energies of different parts of the electromagnetic spectrum. In the electromagnetic spectrum, energy increases along the following sequence: radio waves, microwaves, far-infrared, near-infrared, red light, the rest of the visible spectrum, and finally ultraviolet light. The passage states that the energy required to break a chemical bond is tens of thousands of wavenumbers, or wavelengths per centimeter, while the energy of the strongest cluster bond is on the order of a couple thousand wavenumbers. Since a few thousand wavenumbers correspond to the near-infrared region of the spectrum, it follows that the energy required to break a chemical bond will be considerably higher than the near-infrared. The narrow spectral region of red light is only slightly higher in energy than the near-infrared. Therefore, the only possibility is the choice with the highest energy, the ultraviolet region of the spectrum, choice C.

53. C

Both water and methanol possess dipole moments, since the electronegative oxygen atoms attract electron density from the hydrogen atoms, and both molecules are asymmetrical. They're also both capable of forming hydrogen bonds. Since hydrogen bonding is the strongest form of dipole-dipole interaction, it will be the primary attractive force between these two molecules, so answer choice C is correct. Hydrogen bonds are a type of dipole-dipole interaction, choice A, but remember we're always looking for the best answer. Since choice C describes the interaction more precisely, it's a better answer. As for choices B and D, both of these types of forces will also occur, but they will have much weaker effects, and since you're looking for the strongest interaction, those answers are also wrong.

54. A

Like all the noble gases, neon is often considered an ideal gas, meaning that neon atoms don't interact with each other at all; however, in reality, even neon atoms are weakly attracted to each other. To be exact, neon atoms are subject

 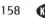

to dispersion forces, as Statement I describes. Dispersion forces, also called London forces, are temporary dipoles caused by momentary unevenness in the electron distribution around atoms. If you didn't know off the top of your head that even noble gases are subject to dispersion forces, you should have been able to guess it from the table, which shows that atoms of argon, another noble gas, are subject to dispersion forces. However, as described in Question 24, noble gas molecules can't have permanent dipole moments, and so Statements II and III are both out. The correct answer choice is therefore A.

55. B

In order for two molecules to undergo dipole-dipole interactions, both of them must be polar—that is, both of them must have dipole moments. Their relative polarities don't matter; for instance, two nitric oxide molecules clearly are equally polar, but they'll still be subject to dipole-dipole interactions, because the slightly more electronegative oxygen atom of one molecule will be attracted to the slightly less electronegative nitrogen atom of another. Therefore, choice C is wrong. Choice A is wrong because the fact that a molecule contains an electronegative element doesn't mean anything, since it doesn't guarantee that a molecule will be polar. For example, carbon tetrachloride contains four chlorine atoms, and chlorine is an electronegative element, but since carbon tetrachloride is symmetric in shape, its four individual dipoles cancel each other out and the molecule is non-polar. And finally, the fact that both molecules contain oxygen certainly doesn't imply that will necessarily have dipole-dipole interactions, so choice D is also wrong.

56. B

The easiest way to answer this is by a process of elimination. Since sulfur dioxide is shown as being involved in dipole-dipole interactions, the sulfur dioxide must have a net dipole moment, and that means it must be asymmetrical. This rules out choice A, linear, and choice D, trigonal planar, both of which are symmetrical shapes. This leaves choices B and C. A T-shaped molecule, choice C, requires four atoms, so sulfur dioxide, which is only triatomic, can't be T-shaped, because it doesn't have enough atoms; this rules out C. The sulfur dioxide molecule must be bent. Therefore, choice B is the correct answer.

57. D

To answer this question you need to know the expression for electromagnetic energy, which states that the energy of a photon is equal to h, Planck's constant, times nu, the frequency of the radiation. Since nu is equal to c, the speed of light, divided by l, the wavelength of the radiation, the equation can be rewritten as E equals h times c over l. Here we're given the wave number, which is the inverse of the wavelength, or the number of wavelengths per centimeter. So we can say that E is h times c times the wavenumber. But be careful here: Since the wavenumber is given per centimeter, you have to express the speed of light, 3×10^8 meters per second, as 3×10^{10} centimeters per second. Then multiplying, you should get $(6.6 \times 10^{-34}) \times (3 \times 10^{10}) \times 1000$, or 2×10^{-20} Joules. This corresponds to answer choice D.

Passage IX (Questions 58–64)

58. A

The energy of a process is always the sum of the final energies minus the sum of the initial energies:

$$\Delta E = \Sigma(\Delta E_f) - \Sigma(\Delta E_i)$$

The balanced combustion reaction for benzophenone (as for all oxygenated hydrocarbons) is

$(C_6H_5)2CO + 15O_2 \rightarrow 13CO_2 + 5H_2O$

The energy of combustion is then the sum of the products' energies of formation minus the sum of the reactants' energies of formation. We incorporate the stoichiometric coefficients in:

$\Delta E_{comb} = 13\Delta E_{f,CO_2} + 5\Delta E_{f,H_2O} - \Delta E_{f,benzophenone} - 15\Delta E_{f,O_2}$

Recall that the energy of formation of an element in its standard state is 0. Therefore we can remove the term with oxygen:

$\Delta E_{comb} = 13\Delta E_{f,CO_2} + 5\Delta E_{f,H_2O} - \Delta E_{f,benzophenone}$

This is choice A.

59. C

The combustion is performed in a heavy canister. When the gaseous products are made, they create additional pressure inside the container, so the pressure is not constant. A crucial measurement of bomb calorimetry is the temperature rise, so the temperature is not constant during the process. The number of moles of substances usually changes during any chemical reaction, therefore the amount of material is not defined to be constant. The only parameter that is essentially constant is the volume inside the bomb, so choice C is the best answer.

60. C

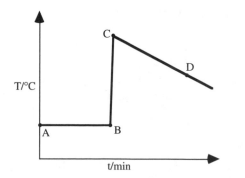

The experiment starts at point B, with ignition, therefore we can eliminate point A from con-

tention. Point B is the initial temperature, T_i, so it cannot be the final temperature T_f, and so choice B is incorrect. Point C is the final temperature T_f after combustion of products. Point D is incorrect, for it is an arbitrary point somewhere along the cooling curve as the calorimeter cools back to room temperature.

61. C

Let us convert grams of benzophenone to moles:

13 x C = 13 $\times$ 12 g/mol
10 x H = 10 $\times$ 1 g/mol
1 x O = 1 $\times$ 16 g/mol
Total benzophenone = 182 g/mol
1 mol/182 g $\times$ 1.3916 g benzophenone can be simplified to 1 mol/200 g $\times$ 1.5 g benzophenone = 0.005 mol/g $\times$ 1.5 g benzophenone = 0.0075 mol benzophenone

From stoichiometry, we set up a proportion of oxygen gas to benzophenone:

? mol O_2/0.0075 mol benzophenone = 15 mol O_2/1 mol benzophenone

We solve the proportion to get 0.1 mol oxygen, which is choice C.

62. B

We use Equation II:
$C_{calorimeter} = -\Delta E/\Delta T$

and solve for the energy required, ΔE:
$\Delta E = -C_{calorimeter}\Delta T$
$= -(2417 \text{ cal/°C})(4.92 \text{ °C})$
$= -12\ 000 \text{ J}$

The negative value indicates energy added to the system. We convert our answer into kJ to match the choices, and end up with 12 kJ, choice B.

KAPLAN

63. A

We assume the system is adiabatic, that is, no energy enters or leaves the system. Then any temperature rise in the system is due solely to that caused by combustion of the sample and iron wire. The other assumption, that pressure is constant, is false, because the bomb is sealed. Thus product gases are created and raise the pressure inside the bomb. Choice A is correct.

64. D

In general, any process for heat exchange uses the relation

ΔE = amount $\times$ heat capacity

We can find the molar heat capacity for iron (the heat capacity for 1 mol Fe) by converting from mass to moles:

C_{Fe} (cal/g) $\times$ molar mass (g/mol) = $C_{mol,Fe}$ (cal/mol)

When we susbstitute in numbers,
1400 cal/g $\times$ 56 g/mol = $C_{mol,Fe}$

Simplifying gives
1500 cal/g $\times$ 60 g/mol = 90 000 cal/mol

The closest answer is 78 kcal/mol or 78 000 cal/mol, which is choice D.

Passage X (Questions 65–71)

65. C

The passage says that the K_{eq} for Equation II increases with temperature, thus hot weather is favored for NO_2 generation. By Le Châtelier's Principle, adding humidity (water) will shift Equation III to the right, favoring production of acids.

66. D

The passage claims that the dissociation energy of N_2O_4 is 57 kJ/mol. This means a mole of pho-

tons with 57 kJ of energy will be able to dissociate a mole of N_2O_4 into 2 moles of NO_2. To find the wavelength from energy use
$E = hc/l$

and rearrange to give
$l = hc/E$
= $(6.63 \times 10^{-34}$ J s$)(3.00 \times 10^8$ m/s$)/(57\ 000$ J/mol$)$
= $(6.63 \times 10^{-34}$ J s$)(3.00 \times 10^8$ m/s$)(6.02 \times 10^{23}$ photons$)/(57\ 000$ J$)$
= 2.1×10^{-6} m

The only photons with at least this energy are mid-infrared or shorter. Thus ultraviolet, choice D, is the only acceptable answer.

67. B

A radical is a species with an unpaired electron. Therefore, when we add up the total number of electrons in a species, we search for that species with an odd number of electrons. The only species listed with an odd number of electrons is choice B, NO_2:

$N_{electrons}$ = 15
$2 \times O_{electrons}$ = 2×8
Total electrons = $15 + (2 \times 8)$ = 31.

Therefore NO_2 is a radical.

68. D

According to the Equation II, N_2O_4 is colorless, while NO_2 is brown. Therefore the production of NO_2 would be accompanied by an increase in the brown color of the mixture, detectable by UV-Visible spectroscopy, choice A. A manometer measures pressure of gases. As Equation II shifts to the right and reaches equilibrium, for every mole of $N_2O_4(g)$ removed, 2 moles of $NO_2(g)$ are created, and the pressure increases. Thus a manometer, choice B, could detect the creation of NO_2. Litmus paper, choice C, detects changes in pH. If the paper were wet, newly created molecules of NO_2 would react with the water (as in Equation III) and form acids, lowering the pH. The only answer remaining is gravimetric analysis, choice D, which detects materials by measuring masses. The mass inside the vessel is constant (Law of Conservation of Matter), and cannot be used to detect formation of NO_2.

69. A

In N2, the oxidation number of N is 0. In NO, the oxidation number of N is +2 (to balance out O's –2). In NO_2, the oxidation number of N is +4 (to balance out the two oxygens' –4). Finally, in HNO_3, the NO_3^- ion has a total charge of –1, and the three oxygens have a total oxidation number of –6, so the nitrogen must have an oxidation number of +5.

70. B

By Le Châtelier's Principle, a system tries to relieve stress placed on it. When a mixture of gases in Equation II is compressed, the system will try to lower the pressure, by reducing the amount of gas in the vessel. This would shift the reaction to the left, creating more dimeric N_2O_4 molecules, which are colorless. The decrease in concentration of brown NO_2 gas would lessen the intensity of the gas mixture's color, choice B.

71. B

We convert grams/km of NO into mol/km of NO:
N = 14 g/mol
O = 16 g/mol
NO = 14 + 16 g/mol = 30 g/mol
mol/km NO = 0.30 g/km ¥ 1 mol/30 g = 0.010 mol/km

Then we convert moles of NO to liters of NO. Remember than standard temperature is 0 °C = 273 K, and standard temperature is 1 atm. We must use kelvins as our temperature unit in the Ideal-Gas Law:
$PV = nRT$
or

$V = nRT/P$
= (0.010 mol)(0.08206 L·atm/mol·K)(273 K)/(1 atm)
= 0.22 L/km which is choice B.

72. C

Convection is the process of energy transfer through mass movement of heated material. Clearly this cannot occur in a vacuum since by definition there are no particles with mass in a vacuum. Likewise the process of conduction requires vibrations of molecules and hence requires molecules. Conduction, then, can't proceed in a vacuum. Radiation, however, is the transfer of energy via electromagnetic waves, and certainly electromagnetic waves propagate through vacuum.

73. D

We're given that the half-life of the radioactive isotope $^{204}_{84}Po$ is 3.8 hours. This means that in a time of 3.8 hours, half of the original nuclei will undergo a-decay. In a time of 7.6 hours (two half lives), only one quarter of the original nuclei will not have undergone decay. This also means that after 7.6 hours, three quarters of the original nuclei will have undergone decay. Every a-decay results in the emission of an a particle. Recall that an a particle is a helium nucleus. Thus, the reduction with mass over time is due to the emission of the α-particles.

To determine the total reduction in mass, we need to find the mass of the a particles emitted. We're given an initial quantity of two moles of $^{204}_{84}Po$, and we've determined that three quarters of these two moles undergo decay. Thus, the quantity decayed is 3/2 moles. Since every decay produces one a-particle, we know that 3/2 moles of a-particles are produced. An α-particle is a helium nucleus, containing two protons and two neutrons, so its mass number is 4. The production of 3/2 moles of helium nuclei means a mass of (4)(3/2) = 6 grams. Thus, 6 grams of the original substance has been emitted in the form of a-particles. The original 2 moles correspond to a mass of (2)(204) = 408 grams. A loss of 6 grams then gives a final mass of 402 grams.

74.   C

In order to solve this problem we'll need to use the Doppler effect equation for sound. The equation is: $f_1 = f(v \pm V_D)/(v \pm V_S)$, where f is the frequency of the sound wave when the source and the detector are both at rest, f_1 is the frequency of the sound wave when either the source or detector is in motion, v is the speed of sound in the medium, V_D is the speed of the detector relative to the medium, and V_S is the speed of the source relative to the medium. In the current problem, the detector (observer) is stationary so $V_D = 0$.

As far as the plus and minus signs in the equation are concerned, you can try and remember them or just use what you know qualitatively about the Doppler effect. Since $V_D = 0$ we only have to worry about the signs in the denominator. We know that when the source is moving away from the observer, the perceived frequency is lower than f, which implies using the + sign. When the source is moving towards the observer, the perceived frequency is greater than f, so we'll need to use the – sign.

When the source is moving away from the observer (observer behind source) the equation becomes $f_{behind} = 1000v/(10000 + 2000)$. When the source is moving towards the observer (observer in front of source) the equation becomes $f_{in\ front} = 1000v/(10000 - 2000)$. We're interested in the ratio of the wavelengths and not the frequencies. Recall that wavelength and frequency are related via $v = \lambda f$, so that $\lambda = v/f$. Thus, we have $\lambda_{behind} = 12000/1000$, and $\lambda_{in\ front} = 8000/1000$. So, finally, we have the ratio $\lambda_{behind}/\lambda_{in\ front} = 12000/8000 = 3/2$.

75.   D

This potential gas law problem can be solved faster through reasoning rather than through calculations. First, if the temperature is higher while the pressure and number of moles are the same, it follows that gas A must occupy a larger volume than does gas B, so choices A and B can be removed. Secondly, since 30°C is only slightly higher than 20°C when we convert to the (mandatory!) Kelvin scale by adding 273, it follows that the volume of gas A will be only slightly larger than that of gas B. Choice D is thus the only sensible answer. (Note in particular that choice C is provided for those who forget that gas law problems must always be done with temperature on the Kelvin scale.)

To use the gas law, PV = nRT, to solve this problem through calculation we can rearrange to solve for each of the volumes, V_A and V_B, then set up the desired ratio as follows:

$V_A = \dfrac{n_A R T_A}{P_A} =$ and $V_B = \dfrac{n_B R T_B}{P_B}$. We know that $n_A = n_B = 1$ mol, $P_A = P_B = 1$ and R is a constant.

Therefore, $V_A : V_B = \dfrac{\frac{n_A R T_A}{P_A}}{\frac{n_B R T_B}{P_B}}$. The pressures, moles, and

Rs all cancel, leaving $V_A : V_B = \dfrac{T_A}{T_B} = \dfrac{(30 + 273)}{(20 + 273)} = \dfrac{303}{293}$.

76.   D

This problem is best answered based on atomic properties and periodic trends. In general, a cation is smaller than a neutral atom of the same element because the removal of electrons decreases the electrostatic repulsion between the remaining electrons, thereby allowing the nucleus to pull them closer, decreasing the ionic radius. Conversely, anions are generally larger than the corresponding neutral atoms because of an increased number of electrons that repel one another. Thus the question can be translated into

"Which of the following elements is most likely to form an anion?" This revised stem can be answered on the basis of periodic trends, in particular the trend in electronegativity which increases toward the upper right corner of the table. Chlorine, Cl, is the most electronegative of the elements listed; it would thus be expected to have the greatest electron affinity, and is thus most likely to take on an electron and become anionic. The four elements in the incorrect choices are all more likely to form cations than anions; their ionic radii will thus be smaller than their atomic radii.

77. D

This question is testing some basic concepts of quantum mechanics. According to the Pauli exclusion principle, no two electrons on a single atom can have an identical set of values for the four quantum numbers n, l, m_l, and m_s. If two electrons occupy the $3s$ orbital then they already have the same values of n (=3), l (=0), and m_l(=0); it is therefore necessary, per Dr. Pauli, that their spin numbers be different, i.e., that they have opposite spins, as stated in choice D. Since there is only one orbital in the $3s$ subshell, choice A is impossible. Choice B grossly distorts the Heisenberg uncertainty principle, which states that one cannot simultaneously determine the momentum and the location of an electron precisely; this principle does not require electrons to absorb energy, as they must to occupy a higher energy subshell. Choice C refers to the oxidation state of the atom which is determined by the total number of electrons attributed to the atom in a compound. This total number of electrons, and the resulting oxidation number, depend on the identity of the element; magnesium, for instance, has an oxidation number of zero when two electrons occupy its $3s$ subshell, while a heavy element like uranium always has two electrons in its $3s$ subshell, regardless of its oxidation state.

Verbal Reasoning

Passage I (Questions 78–84)

78. B

In paragraph four, the author mentions that American unions employ more militant tactics than foreign unions. Thus, American unions would be more likely to use violence during a strike. Choice A is logically eliminated by choice B. As for choices C and D, the author never says whether American or foreign unions are more likely to bargain during a strike.

79. D

Throughout the passage, the author argues that American business institutions reflect basic American values. One of these values is making a profit. Therefore, the author's view would be challenged by the existence of corporations that are less interested in making a profit than in helping people. The author acknowledges that American unions have officials who are highly paid in relation to the rank-and-file membership (A); he acknowledges that American unions tend to be "narrowly self-interested" (B); and he acknowledges that American workers have a rather weak sense of group solidarity (C).

80. A

American society emphasizes individual achievement over class solidarity. So, Statement I is false. Statements II and III, however, are true. The author says that American unions tend to be less concerned with nonunion issues than foreign unions; and he notes that both American business and religious organizations reflect basic American values.

81. B

It would contradict the author's view: Again, the author contends that American unions tend to be "narrowly self-interested" in comparison to foreign unions. An American union that encouraged its members to get involved in nonunion issues like national politics would be inconsistent with this view. Choices A and C are logically eliminated by choice B. Choice D would contradict the author's view.

82. C

The phrase *strong materialistic bent* appears in the context of a discussion of basic American values, one of which is the acquisition of wealth. Choices A and D are beyond the scope of the passage. There is no mention of what European socialists think of aristocrats (A), nor is there any religious criticism of secular values (D). Choice B distorts information in paragraph one.

83. D

The author compares American and foreign labor movements, but he doesn't suggest that foreign labor movements have influenced the American labor movement. Choices A and B are mentioned as influences in paragraph two, while choice C is mentioned as an influence in paragraph three.

84. B

The "traditional value system" refers to those basic values that are reflected in America's institutions. Individual achievement, according to paragraph one, is one of those values. As for choice A, the author contends that class solidarity isn't part of the

American value system. Choices C and D play on details in the passage that have nothing to do with the American value system.

Passage II (Questions 85–91)

85. C

Paragraph one states that algal photosynthesis maintains the high level of oxygen saturation in the reef environment. Choices A, B, and D are all "subjects of scientific puzzlement" discussed in the passage.

86. D

Paragraph three states that *Scleractinia,* the coral producers, account for only 10 percent of the average community. As for choice A, to the contrary, the author proposes in the last sentence of paragraph three that this is the reason for the name "coral reef." Choice B is wrong because paragraph one indicates that the coral portion of the reef plays a large role in reef formation as well as reef "renewability." And C is a true statement and would not contribute to a misnomer.

87. C

Opponents of Darwin's theory believe that the "end of the Ice Age" had more to do with the development of reefs than did the "submergence of volcanic islands." Choice A is a belief held by scientists in general. B is a commonly accepted view concerning reefs. And as for choice D, the crux of the theory held by Darwin's opponents is that the Ice Age played a major role in reef development.

88. B

The theory about reef development is one of transformation; therefore, the reefs would not have developed independently of one another. As for choice A, the passage suggests that each the-

ory may contribute to explaining how reefs develop. With choice C, paragraph three states that corals that "lack an algal presence" exist throughout the world. Choice D is wrong because paragraph one demonstrates that multiple factors contribute to a reef's "amazing renewability."

89. C

The last sentence of paragraph two states that the drillings at Enewetak, which have uncovered volcanic rock, support the theory proposed by Darwin. Choices A and B are both wrong because the passage offers no insight into what effect the recent drillings at Enewetak have on the theory proposed by today's scientists. And D is logically eliminated by C.

90. D

Paragraph two contrasts Darwin's theory to that of its opponents by discussing his focus on the submergence of volcanic islands. As for choice A: To the contrary, Darwin's theory is more persuasive due to recent discoveries at the Enewetak atoll. Choice B is wrong because according to the passage, reefs develop through transformation rather than through separate, distinct processes. With C, the passage implies in paragraph two that both theories of reef development are only "partially correct."

91. B

The last sentence of paragraph one states that scientists are puzzled by the mechanism through which the symbionts stimulate the secretion of calcium carbonate in the other. If a chemical stimulus could be isolated, then the symbiotic relationship would be more clearly understood. Choice A is wrong because paragraph one states that algal photosynthesis is responsible for the high level of oxygen saturation. C is wrong because the components of the reef's protective layer are already known. As for choice D, scientists know that the coral produces the colors and formations seen in reefs.

Passage III (Questions 92–98)

92. C

Paragraph five asserts that *Archaeopteryx lithographica* is a "transitionary" species. In other words, it's neither a genuine reptile nor a genuine bird; it's a mixture of both. Choice A goes contrary to the passage: The consensus of opinion is that *Archaeopteryx lithographica* couldn't fly. Choices B and D are beyond the scope of the passage. The only ancient species discussed in the passage is *Archaeopteryx lithographica*.

93. B

How could scientists hold on to the view that *Archaeopteryx lithographica* represented a "transitionary" species between reptiles and birds if a bird capable of flight already existed before it? Choices A and C are logically eliminated by B. And D focuses on an irrelevant passage detail.

94. A

The passage points out the many differences in skeletal structure between *Archaeopteryx lithographica* and modern birds. For choice B, that *Archaeopteryx lithographica's* tail played a larger role in its daily life than the essentially vestigial tail of a modern bird plays in its daily life is revealed in paragraph four. For choice C, paragraphs one and five make this point. And paragraph four raises the point made in choice D.

95. C

The phrase *wealth of information* appears in the context of a remark about what scientists have learned about birds' ability to fly by studying the fossil remains of *Archaeopteryx lithographica*. Choice A is wrong because no "recent research

projects" are mentioned in the passage. As for B, the passage provides a lot of detail on *Archaeopteryx lithographica's* skeletal structure; but the phrase in question doesn't pertain to this information. And choice D is beyond the scope of the passage. There's no mention of any fossil discoveries in central Germany. The passage says only that *Archaeopteryx lithographica* lived near that area.

96. B

The passage mentions that *Archaeopteryx lithographica* had wings, but couldn't fly. Since modern birds have wings and can fly, it can be inferred that the wings of *Archaeopteryx lithographica* and those of modern birds serve different purposes. Choice A goes contrary to the passage: *Archaeopteryx lithographica* had a much better developed tail than modern birds. Choices C and D are beyond the scope of the passage. The author never compares the intelligence (C) or the size (D) of *Archaeopteryx lithographica* and modern birds.

97. D

The passage indicates that one of the reasons that scientists believe that *Archaeopteryx lithographica* couldn't fly is that it lacked a sternum like the one possessed by modern birds. Thus, if scientists were to find an *Archaeopteryx lithographica* skeleton that contains a sternum, they'd very likely have to reassess their views about its ability to fly. Regarding choices A and B, beliefs about where and when *Archaeopteryx lithographica* lived would not necessarily be affected by the discovery of a sternum. Choice C is wrong because according to the passage, scientists believe that *Archaeopteryx lithographica* possessed birdlike feathers.

98. A

Paragraphs one and five state that the *Archaeopteryx* did indeed possess "birdlike feathers." Choices B and C are both described in paragraph two, while choice D is described in paragraph three.

Passage IV (Questions 99–106)

99. C

Paragraph two discusses the efforts of scientists to catalogue Australia's plants, while paragraph four discusses shifts in Australia's position on the earth's surface over the last 40 million years. There is some supporting evidence or explanation, then, for Statements I and II. Statement III, however, is another matter. The author never claims that "Australia has more plant species than any other continent."

100. A

In paragraph two, the author claims that important discoveries are constantly being made in Australia's rainforests. Thus, he'd surely support further research on those rainforests. As for choice B, the author would most likely condemn any effort to reduce Australian rainforests; he'd likely argue that mankind might lose out on important discoveries if the rainforests were to be tampered with. Choices C and D both distort details in paragraph three.

101. C

The first two sentences of paragraph five make it clear that the author feels that evolution in Australia has been a less violent process than evolution elsewhere. The author never discusses plants on other continents; so, there's no basis for endorsing choice A. B is wrong because the author never expresses the opinion that Australian evolution has yet to receive its due in the scientific community. And D is wrong because according to the passage, the author asserts that Australia has been shifting position on the earth's surface over the last 40 million

years. He doesn't say anything about when evolution began in Australia.

102. D

In paragraph three, the author mentions a "chicken-sized" dinosaur that lived in "a refrigerated world." Clearly, then, the author would agree that "not all dinosaur species lived in warm environments." Choice A is wrong because the author mentions only one Australian dinosaur species; so, we can't say that the author would endorse this statement. You can eliminate choice B because the author never draws any link between dinosaurs and marsupials. As for choice C, the author doesn't give us dates relating to the disappearance of dinosaurs or the emergence of rainforests; so, we can't conclude anything about the author's beliefs on this issue.

103. B

According to paragraph two, scientists have catalogued 18,000 Australian plants. Futhermore, they believe about 7,000 remain to be discovered. Thus, most Australian plants *have been* discovered. Choice A is wrong because paragraph four reveals that Australia has moved between the northern and southern hemispheres. As for choices C and D, paragraphs one and two indicate that the study of Australian plants is yielding important information (C) and that Australian rainforests are different from other rainforests (D), especially with regard to the unique plants found in Australian rainforests.

104. D

Paragraph two makes it evident that the author thinks that Australia's rainforests are important. The phrase "unimportant appendages" is in quotes because the author's disparaging another view of the rainforests' worth. This logically eliminates choice A. And choices B and C distort details in paragraph two.

105. A

In paragraph two, the author asserts that scientists are routinely making important discoveries in Australia's rainforests. Hence, the discovery of a plant that had medicinal uses would support his opinion. Choices B and C are logically eliminated by choice A. And the discovery described in choice D would support the author's opinion.

106. C

Neither of these is ever mentioned in the passage. Choice A is supported by paragraph one; choice B is supported by paragraph five, and choice D is supported by the first sentence of paragraph two.

Passage V (Questions 107–113)

107. C

If more criminals are going in than are coming out of prison under selective incapacitation, prison populations are going to increase. Choice A is wrong because if anything, the information in the stem strengthens this claim. You can eliminate choice B because it represents a claim that is never made. And D is a claim that is never made as well; what the author says is that white-collar criminals may unfairly receive shorter sentences under selective incapacitation.

108. B

This is the point of the next-to-last paragraph. Judges make predictions now when they are sentencing criminals, and a judge's judgment is flawed—even more flawed than statistical prediction, according to the author. Choices A and C are far too extreme to be correct. Choice D contradicts everything the author argues for.

109. C

The author would not agree with this because he thinks that all sentencing has a predictive basis.

Choices A and D can be found in the next-to-last paragraph, and choice B comes from the second paragraph.

110. B

If less privileged offenders cannot evade sanction, this means they must be dangerous repeat offenders, since dangerous repeat offenders are the ones imprisoned under selective incapacitation. Choice A does not follow from the author's statement. Choice C misses the point that harmful middle-class people who commit white-collar crimes would go free under selective incapacitation. No money is involved. And choice D distorts the real point, that some middle-class offenders will go free but deserve incarceration.

111. B

The idea is to minimize all error, but that is not a choice here. B is correct because if you minimize the "false negatives," you minimize the number of crimes committed by mistakenly released criminals.

112. B

This is a paraphrase of the end of paragraph six. As for choice A, some people may not like this, but according to the author more people are worried about "false positives" than about "false negatives." Choice C is an argument for statistical prediction. And choice D is way out-of-bounds.

113. D

The author makes this claim but never backs it up with solid evidence. Choices A and B are claims that the author makes and then explains in detail. C is not a claim made in the passage; as far as we know, first-time offenders could get probation.

Passage VI (Questions 114–120)

114. A

This is the sort of product an ergonomics expert wants; something the user doesn't have to spend a lot of time figuring out. B is wrong because ergonomics is not antitechnology; it just seeks to make technological products user-friendly. Choice C is a distractor that plays on the watch example, and choice D is a distortion of the passage's information on the complexity problem.

115. D

In the first paragraph, the author says that the digital watch became hard to reset since it didn't have a conventional winding mechanism, and that consumers were returning the digital watches as defective in the spring and the fall because they couldn't reset them. According to the author's argument, conventional watches should not come back right after the time changes because they are supposed to be easier to reset. If they come back at that time, the author's argument is undermined. Be careful with choice A: The information in the stem is not by itself enough to weaken the argument because the conventional watches really could be defective.

116. C

The author does make this claim, but doesn't support it with any evidence.

117. C

If the tram was never supposed to be driven in reverse—that is, if it should have had enough room to turn around so that it was always moving ahead—then there would have been no reason for the engineers to design the controls for movement in both directions. It would not have been their fault if the tram was not being used as it was supposed to be. Choices A and D are pretty weak defenses that place the blame on the user, and contradict the passage's argument that the user is not at fault if the technology is poorly designed. Choice B is wrong because the driver never physically switched the pedals.

118. A

Consumers feel that the problem lies with them because they think that they are supposed to be able to use the gadget easily. They think this because they assume the gadget was designed for easy use. With choices B and C, if consumers made either of these assumptions, they wouldn't be blaming themselves. And the assumption in choice D defies common sense.

119. A

If features are added to a product because manufacturers know it will make the product more desirable to the consumer, then the nature of the product is at least partially determined by consumers and their desires. You can eliminate choice B because this does not necessarily mean that the nature of those products has come to be determined by consumers and their needs. Choice C, if anything, strengthens rather than weakens the contention. And choice D is wrong because the fact that consumers need answering machines does not mean that the answering machine was designed with the needs of the consumer in mind.

120. D

Correct choice D is consistent with the author's argument in paragraph three. Choice A is wrong because it's not that the user has to find the correct mental model; it's that the designer has to find out what mental model the user will employ. Choice B is wrong because according to the author, most people who can't figure out high-tech equipment blame themselves, not the designer. And you can eliminate choice C because the author, as stated before, would not place the blame on the user.

Passage VII (Questions 121–126)

121. A

This is in accord with the author's point that one's belief system can lead one to the conclusion that others are suffering from self-deception. Choice B is wrong because the author says that some minor self-deceptions are benevolent. Choice C is a distortion of the idea that true believers may think that others are in part aware that their beliefs are false. And D is way too extreme; obviously some anorexics and alcoholics can be helped.

122. C

Self-deception concerning one's physical fitness may or may not be dangerous, depending on the situation. If it were to be dangerous for some reason, the author would advocate bringing the friend around to the realization that he is deceiving himself. Choice A is incorrect because the false belief about physical fitness may be harmless. Choice B describes intervention without bringing the person to a recognition of the self-deception. And D is incorrect because the author says people can be wrong about other people's beliefs, not their physical fitness.

123. A

See paragraph four: Conspiracy theorists argue that "anyone who disagrees with them. . . has been taken over by the forces they are striving to combat." B is wrong because conspiracy theorists don't give up that easily. Choice C is a distortion of the statement in the final paragraph that calling something trivial or far-fetched counts, for conspiracy theorists, as further evidence of its significance. Choice D provides a little comic relief.

124. C

This is supported by the last sentence of paragraph two. You can eliminate choice A because it's not clear that the unorthodox views of the psyche are harmless. As for choice B, there is no reason the author would jump immediately to this conclusion. Choice D goes contrary to the information in the passage; the person with unorthodox views would very easily establish (at least to himself) the presence of unorthodox views in others.

125. D

The final two paragraphs should have convinced you of this. Choice A misconstrues the meaning of the author's statement that conspiracy theorists believe "there are no accidents." You can eliminate choice B because there is no evidence in the passage that conspiracy theorists doubt their beliefs at all. And C is wrong because the author never says anything against the right to free speech.

126. D

This may have seemed like a ridiculous answer at first, but if Bodin were correct in his accusations, then he wouldn't have been such a lunatic after all, and this would ruin the author's argument. Sure, there are no witches, but the stem says "if true." Choice A is wrong: There could have been townspeople with the same convictions as Bodin, for all we know. This wouldn't weaken the author's argument. Choice B is irrelevant to the argument. You can eliminate C because we assume that this is true anyway, based on the information in the last paragraph.

Passage VIII (Questions 127–132)

127. C

Recent archaeological findings have led researchers to change their view that the oldest Mayan civilization dated back to about 1000 B.C. They now believe it may have dated as far back as 2500 B.C. As for choice A, the findings do not discuss the extent to which the Mayans settled throughout the Yucatan penninsula. B is wrong because researchers have always believed that Mayans used pottery. Choice D goes contrary to the passage: The constricted uniface had distinct designs that researchers believed were Mayan.

128. C

Paragraph two states that "until now, the oldest Maya settlements yielded extensive pottery remains." The paragraph (and passage) continue by suggesting that early inhabitants of the Colha area did not use ceramic pottery and that these inhabitants were most likely Mayans. As for choice A, the passage never indicates that Mayans used the stone tools to create clay pottery. Choice B is wrong because if anything, the passage implies that the cultivation of crops occurred before the development of pottery. Choice D draws a conclusion beyond the scope of the passage.

129. C

The designs on the constricted uniface, its radiocarbon date, and its location of discovery, Pulltrouser Swamp (a known Maya site), all indicate that Mayans may have inhabited the area before 1000 B.C. Choice A is wrong because paragraph four indicates that researchers believe that Mayans exclusively inhabited the Colha area. B makes a statement contrary to the passage: Researchers believe that Mayans, not non-Mayans, inhabited Colha, as stated in paragraph four. Choice D also is contrary to the passage, since paragraph four describes the conclusions drawn by the scientists.

130. A

The correct answer is directly stated in paragraph four. Read this paragraph and you'll see that all the other choices can be logically eliminated.

131. B

The term *archaeological serendipity* refers to the unexpected good fortune the researchers experienced upon making their discoveries. Choice A is too simple. The discovery of stone tools was just one of the components of the archaeological progress made by these scientists. You can eliminate choice C because the term does not refer to a method. And in choice D, the term refers to the archaeologists, not the Mayans.

132. B

Choice B would undermine the idea of "preceramic." In addition, the last sentence of paragraph four claims that researchers have not yet found ceramics in these early residential structures. You can eliminate choice A because archaeologists already believe that the stone tools were used for this purpose. Choice C is wrong because stone tools have already been found dating back to 2500 B.C. D is wrong because pottery has already been found dating back to 1000 B.C. at Mayan sites in the Yucatan penninsula.

Passage IX (Questions 133–137)

133. B

The tsetse fly transmits a deadly parasite, not a chemical. Choice A is wrong because paragraph two states that *trypanosomes* depend on vertebrate blood for nourishment. In choice C, paragraph one states that the tsetse uses vertebrate blood for nourishment, while paragraph two states that the *trypanosome* does as well. Choice D is definitely true, according to the passage.

KAPLAN

134. C

The passage discusses the *trypanosome's* ability to alter its genetic code, not the tsetse fly's. Choices A, B, and D are all mentioned in the passage.

135. C

Choice C is exactly what environmentalists fear would happen if the tsetse fly were controlled to the point of elimination. You can infer choice A from the passage since diseases spread by *trypanosomes* can't be controlled by antibodies or vaccines. Choice B is mentioned in paragraph two, while choice D is directly stated in the first sentence of paragraph four.

136. D

Choice D directly follows the logic of the environmentalists argument in paragraph five. The lizard represents the tsetse fly, the locust represents the cattle, and the agricultural crops represent the African grasslands. Choices A and B both misconstrue the analogy presented in the question stem. Choice C is a nonsense answer.

137. C

The author would most favor an approach that controls, rather than eliminates, the population and that does not harm the environment. Choices A and B imply eradication as well as disregard for the environment. Choice D is wrong because the first sentence of paragraph four mentions that the *trypanosome* cannot be conquered by vaccine; therefore, the author would not encourage continued research.

Writing Sample

THE THREE TASKS

Task One
Analyze a given statement. Define and explore its deeper meaning and describe the implications of the statement.

Task Two
Describe an example that contrasts with the statement as you developed it in the first task.

Task Three
Derive and articulate a method of deciding when the statement should be applied and when it shouldn't.

Characteristics of Holistic Scores

Score: 6

- Fulfills all three tasks
- Offers an in-depth consideration of the statement
- Employs ideas that demonstrate subtle, careful thought
- Organizes ideas with coherence and unity
- Shows a sophisticated use of language that clearly articulates ideas

Score: 5

- Fulfills all three tasks
- Offers a well-developed consideration of the statement
- Employs ideas that demonstrate some in-depth thought
- Organizes ideas effectively, though less so than a Level 6 essay
- Shows above-average command of word choice and sentence structure

Score: 4

- Addresses all three tasks
- Offers a consideration of the statement that is adequate but limited
- Employs ideas that are logical but not complex
- Organizes ideas with coherence but may contain digression(s)
- Shows overall control of word choice and sentence structure

Score: 3

- Overlooks or misinterprets one or more of the three tasks
- Offers a barely adequate consideration of the statement
- Employs ideas that may be partially logical, but may also be superficial
- Shows a fundamental control of word choice and sentence structure
- May present problems in clear communication

Score: 2

- Significantly overlooks or misinterprets one or more of the three tasks
- Offers a flawed consideration of the statement
- Organizes ideas with a lack of unity and/or coherence
- May show repeated mistakes in grammar, punctuation, etcetera
- Contains language that may be hard to understand

Score: 1

- Exhibits significant problems in grammar, punctuation, usage, and/or spelling
- Presents ideas in a confusing and/or disjointed manner
- May completely disregard the given statement

SAMPLE RESPONSE TO STIMULUS 1

"The pursuit of knowledge is always justified."

With the application of the scientific method in fields ranging from atomic physics to social psychology, the human pursuit of knowledge has proved particularly fruitful. The benefits we have derived from science are readily visible now in our everyday lives, not just in the labs of physicists and chemists: we use computers to process information at amazing speeds, we use television to tap into vast electronic and satellite networks to receive news from around the globe, we receive treatment at local hospitals for diseases that would have been fatal mere decades ago. That such success from the scientific pursuit of knowledge has been possible could be evidence to support the argument that "the pursuit of knowledge" in this manner "is always justified."

It is clear, however, after one considers only a couple of the negative aspects of science, that the pursuit of knowledge is not always justified. It should not be allowed, for example, for humans to experiment on other humans in order to gain knowledge, whether or not the experimenter is attempting research for "the good of mankind." This is a sticky problem in medical science because researchers can often only be sure of the effects of a particular drug after testing it out on a sample of humans—animal models can only provide so much information. It certainly is not justifiable, however, to try out new drugs on humans when the possible outcome is so unknown.

In cases such as this, when the pursuit of knowledge could adversely impact on another human or group of humans, the justifiability of research is possible only under certain circumstances: when those whom research could negatively affect have acquiesced after being fully informed of the possible consequences of research. Otherwise, if scientific activity in any way endangers the humans it is intended to help, it thereby loses its purpose and its justifiability and should not be sustained.

ANALYSIS OF SAMPLE RESPONSE TO STIMULUS 1

Holistic Score: 4

needs some explanation or definition

Task 1

With the application of **the scientific method** in fields ranging from atomic physics to social psychology, the human pursuit of knowledge has proved particularly fruitful. The benefits we have derived from science are readily visible now in our everyday lives, not just in the labs of physicists and chemists: we use computers to process information at amazing speeds, we use television to tap into vast electronic and satellite networks to receive news from around the globe, we receive treatment at local hospitals for diseases that would have been fatal mere decades ago. **That such success** from the scientific pursuit of knowledge has been possible could be evidence to support the argument that "the pursuit of knowledge" in **this manner** "is always justified."

good details

nice connection

the scientific method?

Task 2

It is clear, however, after one considers only a couple of the negative aspects of science, that the pursuit of knowledge is not always justified. It should not be allowed, for example, for humans to experiment on other humans in order to gain knowledge, whether or not the experimenter is attempting research for "the good of mankind." This is a sticky problem in medical science because researchers can often only be sure of the effects of a particular drug after testing it out on a sample of humans—animal models can only provide so much information. It certainly is not justifiable, however, to try out new drugs on humans when the possible outcome is so unknown.

clarify

Task 3

In cases such as this, when the pursuit of knowledge **could adversely impact** on another human or group of humans, the justifiability of research is possible only under certain circumstances: when those whom research could negatively affect have acquiesced after being fully informed of the possible consequences of research. Otherwise, if scientific activity in any way endangers the humans it is intended to help, it thereby loses its purpose and its justifiability and should not be sustained.

complex sentence structure

Your organization of ideas and your use of details in this essay are very good. However, the ideas themselves often lack clarity and depth. In particular, you never explain why you focus solely on scientific knowledge, nor do you clarify what "the scientific method" is. Thus, paragraph 1 is weaker than it would be otherwise, given its admirable details. Also, your example for Task 2 needs to be more specific to make sense. You say experimentation on humans "should not be allowed" and trying out new drugs "is not justifiable." Yet in paragraph 3, you say such things can be allowed (under certain conditions). What then, exactly, is the example you mean to describe in paragraph 2?

Biological Sciences

Passage I (Questions 138–144)

138. B

This is one of those outside-knowledge questions. In choice A, the oral cavity contains the salivary glands, which begin chemical digestion with the secretion of salivary amylase, or ptyalin. This enzyme hydrolyzes starch to maltose; so choice A is wrong. The esophagus, choice B, is simply a conduit through which a food bolus passes from the pharynx to the stomach. The bolus is propelled forward by peristalsis, which is the involuntary rhythmic contraction of smooth muscle in the digestive tract. Peristalsis is controlled by the autonomic nervous system. The esophagus has two sphincters that prevent the movement of food in the wrong direction. The lower esophageal sphincter prevents the stomach's acidic juices from entering the esophagus. There are no glands that secrete into the esophageal lumen; so choice B is the right answer. The esophagus is lined by squamous epithelium, which is aglandular tissue. The stomach, choice C, contains numerous glandular cells, such as the parietal cells, which secrete hydrochloric acid; the chief cells, which secrete pepsin; and neuroendocrine cells that secrete gastrin. You should have ruled out the stomach immediately since the passage discusses the secretions of the stomach. The duodenum has mucosal glands called Brunners glands, which secrete mucus to protect the small intestine from the acidity of gastric juices. The rest of the small intestine contains pits known as crypts of Lieberkuhn, which also have mucus-secreting glandular cells. In addition, the intestinal glands secrete aminopeptidase and dipeptidases—enzymes that hydrolyze peptide bonds, and enterokinase, which converts trypsinogen to trypsin. So choice D is incorrect.

139. B

If the ulcer is triggered by bacterial infection, as you are told in the question stem, then the easiest way to eliminate the ulcer would be to eliminate the bacteria. Look for the answer choice that would most effectively eliminate the bacteria without harming the patient. Increasing acetylcholine secretion will stimulate HCl secretion, which we know from the passage is a symptom of ulcers. This would only aggravate the symptoms; thus, choice A is incorrect. Choice B suggests that we inhibit formation of the initiator aminoacyl-tRNA molecule, which is found only in prokaryotes. First of all, from the word tRNA, you should have realized that this choice deals with the process of translation, which is the means by which the genetic information in mRNA is translated into a sequence of amino acids during protein synthesis. Translation occurs at the ribosome, which is comprised of two subunits, one large and one small. Ribosomes attach to the 5' end of mRNA. tRNA is an adapter molecule that pairs the correct amino acid, and when a tRNA is charged with an amino acid, it is called an aminoacyl-tRNA. Each tRNA carries the specific amino acid called for by the mRNA codon to which the tRNA pairs. So as each tRNA molecule base pairs with an mRNA codon, the amino acid chain grows by one residue. This occurs until a termination codon is present in the mRNA.

If the initiator aminoacyl-tRNA of prokaryotic protein synthesis cannot be formed, then translation cannot start, no proteins can be made, and the bacteria will die. Since formylmethionyl-tRNA is the initiator of protein synthesis in prokaryotes only, eukaryotic cells will not be affected. Thus, this seems like it would effectively eliminate the ulcer and not harm the patient. Therefore, choice B is correct. According to choice C, puromycin is an aminoacyl-tRNA analog. This means that it looks like an aminoacyl-tRNA molecule, but it's not. You don't have to know the function of the analog because you're told that it operates on both prokaryotes and eukaryotes. That means that whatever this thing does, it will do it to both the bacterial cells and the patient's cells. Therefore, it will not be the most effective treatment. As for choice D, alleviating one of the symptoms of ulcers—internal bleeding—will not eliminate the bacteria causing the ulcer.

140. C

Peptic ulcers develop when the concentration of gastric juice overwhelms the mucoprotective surface of the digestive tract and the neutralizing secretions of the pancreas. Therefore, anything that increases the production of hydrochloric acid, decreases the protective lining, or decreases these pancreatic secretions would contribute to peptic ulcer disease. Which of the choices does *not* do this? Choice A, excessive gastrin production, is a plausible cause of peptic ulcer disease, since gastrin, which is the hormone secreted by the pyloric glands of the stomach, stimulates the parietal cells to secrete more HCl, especially in response to high stomach pH. In fact, an excess of gastrin is a common cause of ulcers in the disease known as Zollinger-Ellison Syndrome. So, choice A is wrong. Weakness in mucosal barriers, choice B, is also a possible cause of peptic ulcer disease. If mucus secretions are abnormal or diminished in some way, then there is a predisposition to peptic ulcer disease. So, choice B is also wrong. Choice D, an abnormally high density of parietal cells, might also predispose an individual to peptic ulcer disease. While the negative

feedback system of stomach pH helps to protect against this, a correlation does exist between ulcer development and excessive parietal cells. Choice D is therefore plausible, and incorrect.

As stated in the passage, parietal cells release hydrochloric acid in response to gastrin, acetylcholine, and histamine. Histamine stimulates HCl secretion by acting on specific histamine receptors on the outer membrane of parietal cells. If the parietal cell's sensitivity to histamine was decreased, as in choice C, then less acid would be released. Therefore, this is *not* a cause of ulcers. In fact, one of the most common drug therapies for ulcer disease is histamine receptor blockers. Choice C is therefore the only one which is *not* a plausible cause of peptic ulcer disease and is therefore the correct answer.

141. D

The portion of the stomach that contains the majority of the parietal cells is the antrum. A common treatment for severe peptic ulcer disease, after medical therapy has failed, is an antrectomy. Removal of the antrum decreases the amount of acid produced by the stomach and therefore decreases the occurrence of ulcers. Therefore, choice A *would* alleviate peptic ulcer disease, and is therefore incorrect. Choice B describes your common, over-the-counter antacid. These are alkaline substances that act within the stomach to neutralize the acid before it can cause cellular damage. So, choice B is also a viable treatment, and is therefore incorrect. There is another oral drug that acts to reinforce the stomach's mucosal barrier by coating it with a gel-like substance. If it is a weakened mucosal barrier that's responsible for the peptic ulcer disease, then administration of such a drug is also a possible treatment; so choice C is wrong, too.

Choice D, however, is *not* a possible therapy for peptic ulcer disease. Increasing stomach acidity might very well decrease the release of acid via a negative feedback mechanism that is responsive to stomach pH. However, the very nature of this acidity would by itself cause more injury to a digestive tract lining already afflicted with peptic ulcer disease.

142. A

You can find the answer to this question in the passage. The stomach has a special mucoprotective surface to combat its acidic environment. The walls of the stomach consist of a continuous layer of mucous cells that secrete a one-millimeter-thick layer of viscous mucus. This mucus both protects the stomach from its acidic environment and lubricates food. So the stomach does not rely on neutralization to protect itself; it couldn't possibly do this since its enzymes work best at a very acidic pH. Therefore, choice C is wrong. Choice B, the large intestine, is also wrong. By the time the chyme reaches the large intestine, it is fully neutralized. The pancreas, choice A, releases negatively charged bicarbonate ion into the duodenum. This neutralizes the incoming acid and protects the duodenal lining. The pancreas secretes sodium bicarbonate, which combines with the hydrochloric acid to form carbonic acid and sodium chloride. The carbonic acid dissociates into water and carbon dioxide, the carbon dioxide is absorbed into body fluids, and the remaining solution of sodium chloride is neutral. So, choice A is correct. The liver, choice D, synthesizes bile, which emulsifies fats. The liver also detoxifies the poisons of cellular metabolism. In addition, one of the main functions of the liver is the regulation of blood glucose concentration. Though the liver has many other functions as well, not one of them is involved in the neutralization of gastric acidity. Therefore, choice D is incorrect.

143. A

Gastric enzymes, such as pepsin, have optimum activity in an environment with a pH between 2

and 3. Enzymes are proteins; they rely on the appropriate ionic state of their primary amino acid structure for proper function. For example, if the substrate binding site of pepsin is altered by a change in electrical charge, then pepsin would not be able to hydrolyze those peptide bonds for which it is specific. The inherent nature of gastric enzymes make them the most effective in an acidic environment. Extreme acidity, however, can cause denaturation of proteins, which is why there is that complex negative feedback system that maintains a narrow pH range within the stomach. So, choice A is the correct answer.

Choice B is incorrect because it is low pH, not high, that stimulates the release of pancreatic secretions. When acidic chyme enters the duodenum, it stimulates the release of secretin from intestinal mucosa. Secretin enters the bloodstream and acts on the pancreas, causing it to secrete large amounts of pancreatic juice with a high concentration of bicarbonate ion. Secretin is secreted any time the pH in the duodenum falls below 4.5. Choice C is also incorrect. As previously stated, many proteins are denatured by acidity. A low intracellular pH would impair cellular function, not to mention protein function. It is the lumenal pH of the stomach that must be kept low. Choice D is incorrect because first of all, the acidity of the chyme entering the small intestine is neutralized by the bicarbonate ion in the duodenum; by the time it reaches the large intestine, the chyme is no longer acidic. Secondly, nutrient absorption occurs in the small intestine, not the large intestine. The large intestine is involved in the absorption of salts and water.

144. C

To answer this question, you have to understand the concept of a negative feedback mechanism. A negative feedback mechanism is one of the primary methods by which homeostasis is maintained; a change in a physiological variable, such as the pH of the gastric juices or the presence of acidic fluid in the duodenum, triggers a physiological response that counteracts the initial change. Two such mechanisms are described for you in the passage. When excess HCl enters the duodenum, the mucosal glands of the small intestine are stimulated to secrete the hormone secretin, which acts on the pancreas to increase its secretion of fluid high in bicarbonate ion. And bicarbonate ion neutralizes the acidity in the duodenum, thereby protecting the small intestine from the harsh effects of acid. The second mechanism discussed is this: When HCl secretion in the stomach becomes so high that there is a decrease in pH below the minimum of optimal activity for the stomach's enzymes, there is a negative feedback loop involving the hormone gastrin that turns off HCl secretion. This raises the pH of the stomach back to its optimum. Based on this discussion, choices A and B are both wrong because they have their "decreases" and "increases" mixed up. An increase in acid secretion *increases* the rate at which bicarbonate ion is secreted into the duodenum. Likewise, choice D is wrong because a decrease in gastric pH *decreases* acid secretion. But choice C is correct because an increase in gastric pH—that is, when the pH becomes more alkaline—would stimulate an increase in acid secretion until the gastric pH returned to its optimum for peptic enzyme function, which is approximately 2.5.

Passage II (Questions 145–150)

145. B

The fastest way to answer this question is to read each answer choice and find the one that corresponds to the illustrated pathways. Choice A states that the names refer to the two carbon atoms between which the ring is cleaved, with respect to the carboxyl group of benzoate. There *are* two carbon atoms ortho to the carboxyl group, and two

carbon atoms meta to the carboxyl group; however, the two ortho carbons are not adjacent to each other, so saying the ring is cleaved in between them doesn't describe the site of cleavage; the same goes for the two meta carbons. So choice A is wrong. Choice B is more specific: it says that the names refer to the farther of the two carbon atoms between which the ring is cleaved, with respect to the carboxyl group. This is correct: in the meta pathway, the cleavage occurs between the ortho carbon and the meta carbon, and in the ortho pathway, the cleavage occurs between the carbon bearing the carboxyl group and the carbon ortho to it. Choice C says that the names refer to the carbon atom that gets oxidized to an aldehyde group at the time of the ring cleavage. This is incorrect because only in the meta pathway is an aldehyde group formed; in the ortho pathway, two carboxyl groups are formed at the point of cleavage, and no aldehyde group is ever formed at all. Choice D says that the names refer to the carbon atom that gets oxidized to a carboxyl group, but in fact, both pathways produce carboxyl groups at the ortho position during the cleavage step, and neither produces a carboxyl group at the meta position; so, choice D is also wrong.

146. C

This question asks about the name of the enzyme that catalyzes the second step of the meta degradation pathway, but what it's really asking is what type of reaction this is. That's indicated by the first sentence of the question, which tells you that enzymes tend to be named after their chemical function.

The compound with a double bond and hydroxyl group—that is, an enol group—is converted through the second step to a compound with a carbon-oxygen double bond—that is, a keto group. These compounds are isomers, but of a specific sort known as tautomers. So this is an example of keto-enol tautomerism, and the correct choice is C, which is 4-oxalocrotonate tautomerase. The big clue here is that both structures are called 4-oxalocrotonate, even though they are slightly different, and that this reaction is unlike all the others in the pathway in being indicated by double arrows, which designate reversible reactions like tautomerism.

An isomerase, choice A, is an enzyme that converts a compound into its isomer. This is wrong because as mentioned earlier, although the compounds are isomers, they are of a specific type—namely, tautomers. The two other choices suggest types of reactions that don't occur here. A dehydrogenase, choice B, would catalyze a reaction in which a hydrogen atom was removed from a compound. Finally, a hydrolase, choice D, would catalyze a hydrolysis—that is, a reaction in which a water molecule attacks the ring and splits it.

147. C

The difference between the four answer choices and benzoate is that they have extra substituent groups—methyl or ethyl—replacing one or more of the hydrogen atoms in benzoate. The way these might interfere with the degradation process would be if one of the steps could not occur because one of the substituents made it impossible—for example, if one of the steps required a particular carbon atom to have a hydrogen substituent and it didn't.

Choice A has an ethyl group para to the carboxyl group. If you look at all the intermediates in the meta pathway, you can see that particular carbon stays pretty much unchanged throughout the pathway. So, there's no reason to think that this compound would have trouble reacting by this pathway, so choice A is wrong. Choice B has one methyl substituent, ortho to the carboxyl group. In the step where catechol is converted to 2-hydroxymuconic semialdehyde, the carbon atom ortho to the carboxyl group is oxidized to a car-

boxylic acid, while the carbon meta to the carboxyl group is oxidized to an aldehyde. As this ortho carbon has a methyl substituent it can't be converted to a carboxylic acid; however, the other ortho carbon can. To see this, it may help to draw compound B in a different orientation—the mirror image of the orientation that it's printed in. Now the methyl group will be on the left side of the molecule. If you look back at the pathway, you can see that nothing happens to the carbon that the methyl group would interfere with: It gains a hydrogen in step II, but that can still happen even with the extra methyl group. So, this compound can react by the meta pathway, and so choice B is also wrong. Choice C has two methyl substituents, one on each meta carbon. Try applying the same sort of reasoning that we just went through. One or the other of those meta carbons is oxidized to an aldehyde and then to a carboxylic acid. However, this would be impossible with the attachment of a methyl group as the meta carbon would have to form five bonds in both the aldehyde and carboxylic acid. Since choice C can't react by the meta pathway, it is the correct response. Finally, choice D has methyl groups para and ortho to the carboxyl group. We've already seen that a para methyl group won't really effect the reaction, and a methyl group on one of the ortho carbons also won't interfere, as long as the other ortho carbon is free. So choice D would be perfectly capable of reacting.

148. D

To answer this, you need to identify the processes which are occurring in step II of the ortho pathway, namely hydrogenation of a double bond, cleavage of a lactone bond, and subsequent formation of a carboxyl and ketone group. The most effective way to hydrogenate the double bond would be with a mixture of hydrogen and platinum; therefore, choice A can be eliminated right away, since there are no reagents here which would hydrogenate the double bond. The next step would be to cleave the lactone bond between carbon 3 and 6. This would produce β-hydroxyadipate which has a hydroxyl group on carbon 3 and carboxyl group on carbon 6. The lactone bond can be cleaved using aqueous acid or base, making choices B, C, and D equally viable. However, the hydroxyl group that is formed on carbon 3 then has to be oxidized to a ketone and the only reagent which will do this is potassium dichromate, as stated in choice D. In choices B and C, the hydroxyl group would not be converted to a ketone.

149. A

If we look carefully at 4-hydroxy-2-oxovalerate, we can see that cleaving the carbon skeleton between carbons 3 and 4 gives us a pyruvate molecule plus a molecule of ethanol. To get acetaldehyde, that ethanol molecule will have to be oxidized. Thus, choice A is correct. Neither choice B, reduction, choice C, isomerization, nor choice D, enolization, would produce acetaldehyde, so these are all incorrect.

150. D

The main piece of information produced by mass spectroscopy, method I, is the molecular weight of the compounds involved. Since 2-hydroxymuconic semialdehyde contains two more oxygen atoms and one less hydrogen atom than does catechol, the mass spectrum of the two compounds would be clearly different; moreover, the one showing the larger molecular weight would belong to the semialdehyde, and the one with the smaller molecular weight would belong to catechol. So the correct answer choice has to include method I, which means we can eliminate choice C. Method II, NMR or nuclear magnetic resonance spectroscopy, reveals the carbon skeleton of a compound. Specifically, it shows how many different, nonequivalent hydrogen atoms the compound has, and how the carbon atoms they're attached to are connected. Catechol is an

achiral molecule, so it has three sets of equivalent hydrogens and so the compound should produce three different peaks. 2-hydroxymuconic semialdehyde is asymmetric and would produce a lot more different signals. Thus, even without getting into the specific structures of the two molecules and figuring out exactly what those peaks would look like, you'd be able to tell from looking at the spectrum that one was much simpler than the other. Method II also has to be in the correct answer, so you can eliminate choice A. Finally, in infrared spectroscopy, the spectra will indicate the functional groups in each compound. The spectrum of 2-hydroxymuconic semialdehyde would have an aldehyde peak, whereas the spectrum of catechol would not. This means that the answer has to include choice III as well, making choice D correct.

Passage III (Questions 151–158)

151. C

This is simply a matter of correctly reading the measurements on the arterial end of the capillary. As you can see, there are two pressures acting at the arterial end. The one labeled "W" is forcing fluid *out* of the capillary with a force of 35 mmHg, and the one labeled "X" is forcing fluid *into* the capillary with a force of 25 mmHg. You don't have to know which arrow represents which type of force, that is, which represents the hydrostatic pressure differential and which represents the osmotic pressure differential; you just have to determine the net pressure. 35 mmHg out versus 25 mmHg in, means that there is a net flow of 10 mmHg *out of* the capillary at its arterial end. So, choice C is the correct answer.

152. A

The arrow designated "W" on the diagram represents the hydrostatic pressure differential. According to the passage, the hydrostatic pressure differential is the net pressure of the blood and the tissue. Since hydrostatic pressure is greater in the blood, fluid moves out of the capillary into the interstitial space. Since you know that the hydrostatic pressure differential forces fluid out of the capillary, while the osmotic pressure differential draws fluid in, you should have been able to determine from the direction of the arrowheads that the arrows labeled "W" represent the hydrostatic pressure differential, and the arrows labeled "X" represent the osmotic pressure differential. Note that the osmotic pressure differential remains constant along the length of the capillary. This is because the plasma proteins always remain in the bloodstream, maintaining the concentration of solutes in the blood at a fairly stable level. Because the hydrostatic pressure differential is greater than the osmotic pressure differential at the arteriole end, there is a net flow of fluid out of the capillary. Likewise, at the venous end of the capillary, there is a net influx of fluid because the tendency for fluid to enter overpowers the tendency for fluid to exit. However, these net flows are not indicated in Figure 1, which is why both choices C and D are incorrect.

153. B

Since the passage doesn't specifically tell you how respiratory gases are exchanged, you have to rely on your outside knowledge. Respiratory gases are exchanged between the blood and the interstitial fluid via passive diffusion. When oxygenated blood travels through the capillaries to oxygen-poor tissue, the difference in the partial pressure of the oxygen between the blood and the tissues favors the dissociation of oxyhemoglobin. Capillary walls consist of a single layer of endothelial cells. The released oxygen dissolves in the lipid membrane of the endothelial cells and diffuses down its concentration gradient—across the capillary walls into the interstitial fluid surrounding the tissues. In the same man-

ner, carbon dioxide diffuses down its concentration gradient from the tissues into the capillary blood. This exchange of gases occurs as a result of differing concentrations. The process requires no energy, so choice A is incorrect because active transport involves an expenditure of energy, and is usually used when transport must go against a concentration gradient. No carrier molecules are required to transport gases across the capillary wall, so choice C, facilitated diffusion, is incorrect. Choice D is also wrong; exocytosis refers to the fusion of a vesicle with the plasma membrane, thereby releasing the vesicle's contents outside the cell.

154. C

What do we know about the permeability of capillary walls? The cell membrane of the endothelial cells is a lipid bilayer, and like all lipid bilayers, it is permeable to lipids and lipid-soluble molecules. Furthermore, small molecules cross the membrane faster than large ones. The hydrophobic interior of the membrane inhibits ions and polar molecules, which are hydrophilic, from crossing the membrane. However, very small polar molecules, such as water and carbon dioxide, can pass through the membrane because they are small enough to pass between lipids of the membrane. We're told all of this stuff in the passage itself. In addition, we're told that there are pores in the capillary walls through which molecules can pass, if they're small enough to fit through. We're asked to determine what conclusion *cannot* be drawn about the nature of the protein C1INH if it *cannot* pass through capillary walls. Don't worry about the specific functions of this protein, since you're not expected to know anything about C1INH to answer the question. Since it cannot pass through, then it is possible that C1INH is simply too large to pass through the pores in the capillary wall, so choice A is incorrect since this conclusion *can* be drawn. There is also the possibility that C1INH is a large

KAPLAN

polar molecule, which, as just discussed, cannot pass through the membrane because of its size and its hydrophilic nature; therefore, choice B is also incorrect. However, choice C is *not* a conclusion that might be drawn based on the fact that C1INH cannot pass through capillary walls; lipid-soluble molecules *can* pass through the walls. So, choice C is the right answer. Choice D is wrong because it may also account for the inability of substances to pass through the capillary walls. If C1INH moves across the membrane by passive diffusion, then C1INH will move from a region of higher concentration to a region of lower concentration. But if the concentration is equal on both sides, then C1INH will pass through the capillary walls, but there will be a net movement of zero.

155. A

Capillaries are specialized for the exchange of nutrients, fluids, and gases between the circulatory system and the tissues. Since the capillary wall is selectively permeable, allowing only those particles that are soluble in the lipid membrane or those that are small enough to pass through its pores to cross it, it can be said that the capillary wall is semipermeable. So, choice B is incorrect. Choice C is incorrect because capillary walls ARE composed of a single layer of endothelial cells. Choice A, however, that capillary walls are muscular, is incorrect because they do not contain any smooth muscle tissue or elastic tissue, like arteries and veins do.

156. D

This is another question that requires you to interpret Figure 1. The hydrostatic pressure differential tends to drive fluid out of the capillary into the surrounding tissue at both ends of the capillary, while the osmotic pressure differential tends to drive fluid from the tissue into the capillary. As is shown in the figure, these forces oppose each other along the capillary membrane. Even if you

were unable to determine which forces the lines labeled "W" and "X" represent, you still should have seen that the arrows for W and X face opposite directions at either end of the capillary. Therefore, choice D is the correct answer.

Choice A is incorrect; although the hydrostatic pressure differential decreases as it travels along the length of the capillary, dropping from 35 mmHg to 15 mmHg, the osmotic pressure differential remains unchanged throughout the capillary because the solute concentration of the blood remains fairly constant. Choice B is incorrect for the same reasons. Choice C is also incorrect because although these forces work in opposing directions, they do not vary inversely with one another; as previously discussed, the osmotic pressure differential remains relatively constant, while the hydrostatic pressure differential decreases from the arterial end to the venous end.

157. D

Since the arterioles lead directly into the capillaries, an increase in arteriolar pressure will lead to a direct increase in the blood pressure within the capillaries. Choice A is incorrect because closure of precapillary sphincters, which are pieces of smooth muscle surrounding the front end of capillaries, would result in a decrease in the amount of blood that is sent through those capillaries. This would lead to a decrease in blood pressure. Choice B is incorrect because decreased resistance in the veins would ease venous blood flow, which in turn, would decrease blood pressure within the capillaries. Decreased arteriolar pressure would also lead to a direct decrease in capillary blood pressure, so choice C is incorrect.

158. B

Most proteins dissolved in the blood, such as albumin, are essentially confined to the lumen of the capillary because they are too large to pass through the pores in the capillary wall. This basically ensures that the osmolarity of the blood will be higher than the osmolarity of the tissues, which is why the osmotic pressure differential of the blood tends to draw water into the capillary. Therefore, plasma proteins play an important role in maintaining the osmotic pressure differential of the blood. Choice A is incorrect because, as just explained, plasma proteins are usually too large to cross the capillary wall. Choice C is incorrect because plasma proteins do not have any influence whatsoever on the dissociation of oxyhemoglobin into oxygen and hemoglobin. This dissociation is dependent on factors such as blood pH, and the relative partial pressures of oxygen and carbon dioxide in the bloodstream. Choice D is incorrect because the plasma proteins facilitate fluid exchange by maintaining the osmotic pressure differential, not by binding to fluid molecules.

Discrete Questions

159. C

This is your basic endoderm, ectoderm, mesoderm question; that is, a question about the three primary germ layers in a developing mammalian embryo. It's just worded a little differently than you're probably used to seeing. You're simply being asked to determine which of the physiological systems described in the answer choices is derived from ectoderm. Ectoderm gives rise to the epidermis, the lens of the eye, the inner ear, the adrenal medulla, and the nervous system. And since responding to stimuli is a function of the nervous system, choice C is the correct answer. Mesoderm gives rise to the musculoskeletal system, the circulatory system, the excretory system, the gonads, the kidneys, the lining of the body cavity, and the dermis. Endoderm gives rise to the lining of the digestive tract, the lining of the respiratory system, and the liver and pancreas.

160. D

This question tests your understanding of osmosis, which is the passive diffusion of water from regions of low solute concentration to regions of high solute concentration until there isn't any difference in solute concentration between the two regions. An endothelial cell, like most other eukaryotic cells, is surrounded by a water-permeable lipid bilayer membrane and contains a nucleus, mitochondria, endoplasmic reticulum, Golgi apparatus, lysosomes, cytoplasm, and other cellular structures and organelles. Cytosol is the fluid component of cytoplasm, and consists of an aqueous solution with proteins, nutrients, ions, and other solutes dissolved in it. Distilled water has nothing dissolved in it; it has a solution concentration of 0. Therefore, an endothelial cell is said to be hypertonic to a medium of distilled water—that is, it has a higher solute concentration than its surroundings. Furthermore, because of this difference in solute concentration, water will flow into the cell, from a region of low to high solute concentration, eventually causing the cell to lyse. The cell lyses because its membrane cannot withstand the great volume of water entering the cell. An endothelial cell would shrivel if it were placed in a medium to which it was hypotonic; in this instance, water would rush out of the cell into the medium. So choice A is wrong. Choice C is wrong because the cell would remain the same size only if it were placed in a medium to which it was isotonic—say, for instance, if it were placed in a medium of free cytoplasm. Choice B is wrong because cell division has nothing whatsoever to do with osmosis and solute concentration; it is irrelevant to the question.

161. B

Cyclohexane is the most stable structure since there is almost no angle, torsional, or Van der Waals strain. The bond angle of a tetrahedral carbon atom, which is the structure of a carbon with four single bonds, is 109.5° and the closer the actual bond angle is to this number, the more stable the ring. The bond angle in cyclohexane is just about 109.5°, so angle strain is minimized. Also, none of the hydrogens in the ring are eclipsed–the chair conformation ensures that they are all staggered with respect to each other– so torsional strain is avoided. In addition, the hydrogens don't compete for the same position in space, which also eliminates any Van der Waals strain. On the other hand, cyclopropane has a carbon-carbon bond angle that's less than 109.5° and so is subjected to more angle strain. Moreover, the hydrogens are eclipsed and so the molecule undergoes a great deal of torsional strain. As a result, choice A is incorrect. Choices C and D–cyclononane and cyclodecane–can assume a number of conformations, none of which can minimize all three types of strain. For instance, a conformation that minimizes torsional strain results in an increase in angle strain.

162. D

Carbon monoxide is poisonous to humans because it binds more readily to hemoglobin than does oxygen; that is, hemoglobin has a greater affinity for carbon monoxide than for oxygen. Carbon monoxide is a gas formed by the incomplete combustion of carbon, and it's toxic because it readily forms carbonmonoxyhemoglobin, or COHb. COHb cannot bind to oxygen. In fact, hemoglobin's affinity for carbon monoxide is 210 times greater than its affinity for oxygen. Therefore, when carbon monoxide enters the bloodstream and binds to hemoglobin, the amount of hemoglobin capable of carrying oxygen decreases; however, the total concentration of hemoglobin in the blood remains unaffected. So, choice A is wrong. But carbon monoxide does decrease the amount of oxygen that is released to the tissues, causing anemic hypoxia. Anemic hypoxia is the condition when the arterial partial pressure of oxygen remains the same

but the amount of hemoglobin available for binding oxygen is reduced. Since the arterial partial pressure of oxygen remains the same, the chemoreceptors in the carotid arteries and aorta do not become stimulated, and hence do not stimulate an increase in respiration. Choices B and C are wrong, because carbon monoxide does not destroy lung tissue, nor does it block the electron transport chain, thereby preventing ATP formation.

163. C

You should know that a monosaccharide in an aqueous solution will form two isomeric cyclic hemiacetals or anomers. The difference between the two hemiacetals is the orientation of the substituents around the first carbon. In the a-anomer, the hydroxyl substituent on C1 is oriented down from the plane of the molecule, *trans* to the substituent on C5, while in the β-anomer, it is oriented up, *cis* to the functionality on C5. The point is that anomers are diastereomers that differ only in their configuration around the first carbon, so choice C is correct. Choice A is wrong because most of the other carbons in a carbohydrate, beside the one in the carbonyl group, are chiral, so that anomers are usually chiral. Choice B is wrong because mirror images have opposite configurations around *all* their chiral carbons, not just around one. Finally, open-chain monosaccharides which differ in configuration around the *second* carbon are called epimers, not anomers, so choice D is also incorrect.

Passage IV (Questions 164–168)

164. B

Choice A says the experiment supports Hypothesis 1, because the flies with P elements leave more offspring than the flies without P elements. This is a natural selection argument; that is, it says that the P-strain flies have a selective advantage: They reproduce more than the M-strain flies. Is this true? There's no evidence for it. This is really a trick question. Normally, if you found that the frequency of a trait increased over time, you might assume that it was evolutionarily favorable; but that's not the only way it could happen—for instance, it could also be due to migration or selective mating. In any case, we're told that the offspring of these crosses have a lot of mutations and as a result are often sterile. And if many P-strain flies are sterile, then they certainly wouldn't be expected to leave more offspring then M-strain flies. So it doesn't sound like P elements should be favored evolutionarily. As a matter of fact, they're not: the reason why the P elements spread is that they're really good at spreading—much better than your average gene, because they can self-replicate and insert themselves all over a fly's DNA. So choice A is wrong. Choice B also says Hypothesis 1 is supported, because the incidence of P elements has increased. The incidence HAS increased, and that does support Hypothesis 1, because that hypothesis requires the P elements to spread. So this looks like the correct answer. But check the other two choices anyway, in case one of them is better. Persuasive argument passages tend to have a lot of questions about the reasoning of the theories they discuss that can sometimes seem pretty subjective; you need to be particularly careful in choosing your answers and checking all the choices. Choice C says that the observation that after 100 generation almost all of the flies are P-strain flies supports Hypothesis 2, because P elements are lost during culture. However, we can see that P elements aren't lost during culture; they are gained, so choice C must be wrong. Finally, choice D says that Hypothesis 2 is supported because the flies have been cultured for many generations. It's true that in the experiment the flies were cultured for many decades. However, since P strains have been around for decades, a long culture time doesn't necessarily

disprove Hypothesis 1. And, according to Hypothesis 2, strains cultured for many generations are expected to lose their P elements, which as already said, does not happen in this instance; so choice D is wrong as well. So choice B is indeed the correct answer.

165. B

The question asks what type of virus could possibly have been the original form of P elements, assuming that Hypothesis 1 is correct and P elements recently arose from viral infection. A lysogenic virus, choice B, is one that infects a cell, integrates itself into its DNA, and then sits there for some amount of time before it does anything; that is, before it re-emerges and takes over the host cell's genetic and protein-synthesizing machinery. This ability to integrate itself into the cell's DNA is a property that P elements share, which is our clue that this is the correct answer. How about the other choices? A lytic virus, choice A, is one that infects a cell, immediately takes over the cell's "machinery" to replicate more viruses, and then kills the cell by lysing it so that the new viruses get released. A bacteriophage, choice C, is a virus that attacks only bacteria—but this hypothetical virus must have been able to infect fruit flies, not bacteria, so choice C must also be wrong. Finally, an attenuated virus, choice D, is a virus that has somehow been weakened—by mutation, for instance—to make it safe to inject it into someone as a vaccine. Since we're not talking about vaccines, choice D must be wrong. It's probably just thrown in here because it's a term that you might associate with viruses and so you might be inclined to pick it if you were in a hurry.

166. C

Here you have to figure out the different ways whereby P elements might be "lost" from a fruit fly's DNA, and which answer choice is *not* a plausible mechanism for this loss. Choice A is genetic drift. Genetic drift is a shift in gene frequency due to chance. That is, if you start out with a 50–50 frequency of two alleles for a particular gene, in the next generation, just by chance, there might wind up being a 49–51 distribution, and then in the next generation 48–52, and so on, until finally you might lose one of the alleles altogether. Genetic drift becomes noticeably only in small populations over periods of many generations. But here we're talking about lab populations, which are pretty small compared to a wild population, and we're talking about 30 years, which is a lot of generations for a fruit fly; so it is plausible that genetic drift could take place. And this *could* lead to the loss of P elements, just like any other genes. Because P elements tend to be present in multiple copies in an organism's genome, they are less likely to be lost to genetic drift, but it could still happen. Now look at choice B. This says P elements might be lost through recombination within a chromosome, which could lead to a deletion. This was mentioned in the passage, so you know that it's a plausible mechanism. If recombination occurred between two P elements on the same chromosome, part of each P element would be lost, or deleted, along with any DNA between them. So choice B is also incorrect. Choice C says that P elements might be lost due to recombination *between* separate chromosomes that causes a translocation. Translocation is when a chromosomal fragment joins up with a nonhomologous chromosome, resulting in a hybrid chromosome that contain parts of the two original ones. Translocation doesn't involve loss of DNA, just reassortment, so this *wouldn't* cause a loss of P elements, and C is therefore the correct answer. Finally, choice D, natural selection, refers to the selective reproduction rates in individuals within a population that have traits that confer an advantage on that individual. So, since P elements often cause mutations, including inviability and sterility, the reproduction rates would

most likely be lower in P strains. Therefore, over many generation, the strain may be selected against. This means that fewer and fewer P elements are found in the population, until they disappear entirely. So choice D does explain how P elements can be lost from a population.

167. A

P strains of fruit flies have a higher mutation rate, and higher mutation rate should lead to more genetic variation and therefore to an increased likelihood of speciation; that is, the evolution of genetically distinct species. In fact, though you weren't told this in the passage, there is difficulty in interbreeding between P-strain flies and M-strain flies, which will tend to increase the chance of genetic divergence within the whole Drosophila melanogaster species; this also increases the likelihood that it will undergo radiation into multiple species. Choice B is wrong because most mutations that have a significant effect are bad for the organism, which means that they will *decrease*, not increase, offspring viability. And besides, we're told that decreased viability is one of the consequences of having P elements. Choice C is wrong because, as we're told, P elements increase the mutation rate. Choice D is wrong because genetic drift doesn't have anything to do with the appearance of new mutations, which is the main effect of P elements—it acts on all alleles, old and new—so the P elements shouldn't affect genetic drift.

168. B

The first thing that you should notice about this question is that it is a Roman numeral question. These are more difficult in that more than one choice can be correct, and you need to pick out all the choices that apply. To solve these types of questions, you need to examine each choice and decide whether it is correct or not. Often times, after you have identified one correct item, it is possible to eliminate several choices by crossing out those that do not contain the item that you have just identified as correct.

All you need to do to answer this question is decide in which crosses the offspring will have dysgenesis. From the passage you know that P–M hybrid dysgenesis only occurs if the inherited P elements are activated. And that activation can occur *only* if a P strain male is crossed with an M-strain female. Look at the choices with this in mind. Roman numeral I crosses a P-strain female and an M-strain male. This does not cause dysgenesis, so Roman numeral I is incorrect and any choices that contain this item can be eliminated. Therefore, choice A is incorrect. In Roman numeral II, the cross is between a P-strain male and a female from a cross between a P-strain male and an M-strain female. This female offspring will have dysgenesis and thus be sterile. Therefore, no offspring can be produced from the cross in item II, and no dysgenesis can occur. So item II is incorrect. From this piece of information, we can eliminate choices C and D. Therefore, choice B is the correct answer. Let's look at items III and IV. In item III, a cross between an M-strain male and a P-strain female will produce P offspring with inactivated P elements, and thus no dysgenesis. So when these two P offspring are crossed, their offspring will also be P-strain flies with inactivated P elements and thus, no dysgenesis. Therefore, Roman numeral III is incorrect. In Roman numeral IV, two P-strain flies will produce another P-strain fly, and two M-strain flies will produce another M-strain fly. So the cross of these offspring is simply a P-strain male crossed with an M-strain female, which you know will cause dysgenesis. Therefore, Roman numeral IV is a correct response, and choice B is the correct answer.

Passage V (Questions 169–173)

169. A

As you're told in the passage, blood pressure is the measure of the hydrostatic force that the blood exerts on the walls of blood vessels, and is recorded as systole over diastole in millimeters of mercury. Systole is the pressure exerted during contraction of the ventricles, and diastole is the pressure exerted during the period between successive contractions. To determine the athlete's blood pressure at rest, which is what you're asked to do, you simply need to read Figure 1, first for systolic pressure, then for diastolic pressure. Systolic pressure for the athlete at rest is approximately 108 mmHg, and diastolic pressure is approximately 83 mmHg. Since blood pressure is expressed as systole over diastole, the correct answer is 108/83, which is choice A.

170. C

To solve this question, all you've got to do is plug the values into the equation for cardiac output that is given to you in the passage. As we're told, the heart rate, or pulse, is the number of heartbeats per minute. Stroke volume is defined as the volume of blood pumped out of the left ventricle per contraction. Cardiac output is defined as the total volume of blood that the left ventricle pumps out of the heart per minute, and can be determined by multiplying the heart rate by the stroke volume. The only thing that's just a little bit tricky about this question is that choices A and B use the word pulse instead of heart rate; but you still should have gotten the right answer from the equation itself. Choices A and B must be wrong because the question tells us that pulse, or heart rate, is the same for both the athlete and the nonathlete. Thus, if the athlete and the nonathlete have the same heart rate, but the athlete's cardiac output is the greater of the two, then the athlete's stroke volume must be greater than the nonathlete's stroke volume, which is choice C.

171. D

As discussed in the previous explanation, cardiac output is defined as the total volume of blood pumped by the left ventricle per minute, and can be calculated by multiplying the heart rate, which is the pulse, with the stroke volume, which is the volume of blood pumped out of the left ventricle per contraction. We're told that the woman's pulse is 20 beats per 15 seconds and that her stroke volume is 70 mL per beat. We cannot simply multiply these two numbers to get the cardiac output because cardiac output is measured in units of L/min. Hence, we must first convert 20 beats/15 seconds into minutes; we simply multiply this number by 60 sec/min, which yields 80 beats/min. Likewise, 70 mL equals 0.070 L. So, cardiac output equals 80 beats/min × 0.070 L/beat, which equals 5.6 L/minute, which is choice D.

172. B

This question requires you to apply your outside knowledge of the sympathetic division of the autonomic nervous system in accounting for the phenomenon described in the question stem. As revealed by the upward slopes of all four lines in Figure 1 during exercise, there is an increase in arterial pressure immediately before and during exercise. This is caused by sympathetic nervous stimulation. When the body is readying itself for action, the sympathetic division of the autonomic nervous system takes over. It stimulates the heart to increase its heart rate and pumping strength so that it can supply the active skeletal muscle with more blood, and hence, with more oxygen. To increase the blood supply to active muscle during exercise, the blood vessels in the muscles themselves become dilated, while the blood vessels elsewhere in the body are con-

stricted. Vasodilation increases the blood flow through those vessels supplying the active muscle, and vasoconstriction of other systemic blood vessels diverts blood to the tissue that needs it most. For example, vessels that supply blood to the digestive tract are constricted during activity. Thus, choice B is correct, and choices A and C are incorrect. Choice D, the build-up of lactic acid, occurs during the initial stages of strenuous exercise when glucose metabolism and ATP production outpaces the oxygen supply delivered to muscle. When this occurs, the cells switch from aerobic respiration to anaerobic respiration. Lactic acid is one of the waste productions of anaerobic respiration and can build up in muscle cells, causing fatigue. The build-up occurs because the conversion of lactic acid to pyruvic acid requires oxygen.

173. C

The question stem tells us that the athlete normally has a higher cardiac output than the nonathlete. And from the passage you know that cardiac output is defined as the volume of blood pumped by the left ventricle into systemic circulation per minute. This means that the athlete is pumping more blood, and hence delivering more oxygen per minute to his muscles than the nonathlete. Since the athlete normally has a higher cardiac output, we can look at Figure 1 for choices A and B. It reveals that during exercise, the athlete has a lower systolic pressure than the nonathlete and a higher diastolic pressure than the nonathlete. Since choices A and B state the opposite, they are both incorrect. Recall that the athlete's muscles are receiving more oxygen per minute than the nonathlete's. This means that the athlete's muscle cells will be able to produce more energy by aerobic respiration than the nonathlete's per given time. The nonathlete will have to resort to anaerobic respiration more than the athlete. From introductory biology you should remember that the end product of anaerobic respiration in eukaryotic cells is lactic acid. Therefore, you would expect the nonathlete to have a higher concentration of lactic acid in his muscles than the athlete, since the nonathlete is using anaerobic respiration more than the athlete. Therefore, choice C is the correct answer. Choice D is incorrect because the nonathlete would have to have a higher rate of glucose catabolism than the athlete, because his only source of energy during anaerobic respiration is through the catabolism of glucose. Remember that catabolism is the breakdown of glucose to pyruvic acid via glycolysis.

Passage VI (Questions 174–177)

174. D

This question is about how to name cyclic hydrocarbons, so you have to know the rules of the IUPAC system. This is a cyclic alkane with eight carbon atoms in the ring, so it's a cyclooctane. All three of its substituents are alkyl groups, so none of them will automatically take precedence over the other in the numbering. This means we have to list the substituent groups in alphabetical order, but their numbers must add up to the lowest possible sum. The three groups are listed alphabetically as ethyl, methyl, then propyl. This means choices B and C can be eliminated. Finally, the numbers in choice A add up to a larger sum than the numbers in choice D, so choice D is the correct response.

175. B

To answer this question, we have to use the table of energy differences that's given in the passage. The two compounds have two substituents, a bromide group and a methyl group. If we consider the transition between the left and right configurations, the bromide group goes from being axial to equatorial, and the methyl group

goes from being equatorial to being axial. If we look up the differences for both of these groups, we see that it's 0.5 kilocalories per mole for the bromide group and 1.74 kilocalories per mole for the methyl group. Now we have to remember a key fact: the axial position is of higher energy than the equatorial position. So the change in the position of bromide represents a *loss* of 0.5 kilocalories per mole, and the change in the position of methyl represents a *gain* of 1.74 kilocalories per mole. So, since we're told to assume that these values are additive, the overall difference between the two conformations is minus 0.5 kilocalories per mole plus 1.74 kilocalories per mole, or 1.24 kilocalories per mole which corresponds to choice B, the correct answer.

176. C

The most stable conformation for a substituted cyclohexane is a chair conformation in which all of the substituents are oriented equatorially. None of the choices here has that sort of conformation, but in comparing the stability of the choices, it's useful to remember that the closer a structure is to that state, the lower its energy. Choice B can be eliminated right away because it's a boat conformation, and there's a big energy difference between the chair and boat conformations. The other three choices are all chair positions. Choice A has both its substituents in axial positions, whereas choices C and D each have one substituent that's axial and one that's equatorial; thus, choice A will be less stable than either C or D and can also be eliminated. As for the difference between C and D, look at the table of energy differences. The energy difference between conformations for a hydroxyl group is 0.95 kilocalories per mole, and for an isopropyl group it's 2.15 kilocalories per mole. So there's more stability to be gained by having the isopropyl group equatorial than in having the hydroxyl group equatorial. Thus, choice C will be more stable than choice D, making it the correct answer.

177. D

Choice A has an isopropyl group and a tertiary butyl group. Looking at the table, we see that the energy difference between conformations is higher for the tertiary butyl group than for the isopropyl group, so the more stable conformation should have *tert*-butyl in an equatorial position. Choice A has that conformation, so it is in its lowest energy conformation and it's an incorrect choice. Likewise, choice B has an amino group and a methyl group; the energy difference is greatest for methyl, so it should be equatorial. So, choice B is also in its most stable conformation making it an incorrect response. In choice C, the energy difference for methyl is greater than for bromide but the methyl group is equatorial, so C is also wrong. Finally, choice D has an amino group and a hydroxyl group. The energy difference for the amino group is greater than for hydroxyl; however, the amino group is axial and so this is not the compound's lowest energy conformation, making choice D the correct answer.

Passage VII (Questions 178–183)

178. D

This question assumes that Theory 1 is valid, and based on that assumption we have to find the structure that would most likely bind to the antibody produced against para-aminophenol-alpha-glycoside. Theory 1 states that an antibody recognizes an antigen based on chemical composition, so we have to find a compound with the same chemical composition, and the only one is choice D. All of the other choices are lacking the methyl alcohol group, so they're all incorrect.

179. B

This one requires us to understand the basic concepts of the second theory, which states that antigen recognition is based on the physical configu-
ration of the antibody. Statement I gives two non-interacting compounds—*para*-aminobenzenesulfonic acid and *meta*-aminobenzenesulfonic acid—which have the same functional groups but different structures. This contradicts Theory 1 and supports Theory 2; therefore, Statement I must be part of the correct answer, and we can eliminate choices A and C. Statement II gives the compounds *para*-aminobenzenesulfonic acid and *para*-aminohydroxybenzene. These have similar structures but different substituent groups. The statement says that these antibodies interact with each other, which also supports Theory 2; therefore, Statement II should also be part of the correct answer. Finally, let's look at Statement III. This gives two non-interacting compounds—*para*-aminobenzenesulfonic acid and *meta*-aminohydroxybenzene—which are different in both structure and chemical composition. This statement doesn't help distinguish between the two theories at all, since it would be predicted by either theory, so it's incorrect. Since only Statements I and II are true, the correct answer is choice B.

180. A

The first thing we need to figure out here is what the product will be when benzenesulfonic acid is chlorinated. The -SO_3H group is a deactivating *meta* director, so the main product will be *meta*-chlorobenzenesulfonic acid. According to Theory 2, if two antigens have the same physical configuration, an antibody produced against one will be able to bind to the other, regardless of the chemical compositions. So the correct choice should be another meta compound, and since choice A is the only compound among the choices that has a meta configuration, it's the correct answer. Choices B and C are wrong because they have the same chemical composition as *meta*-chlorobenzenesulfonic acid, but different structures. Choice D differs from *meta*-chlorobenzenesulfonic acid in both chemical composition and in structure, so it's also wrong.

181. C

Structural isomers are compounds that have the same formulas but different atomic connectivities. Since structural isomers are different in their connectivity, the fact that they were recognized by the same antibody would support Theory 1, not Theory 2, since Theory 1 states that "the physical configuration of the antigen does not effect this interaction." Therefore, choice C is false, making it the correct response. All of the other answer choices are true. Conformational isomers and enantiomers both describe pairs of compounds that differ in the spatial arrangement of their atoms. So, if one antibody recognized two conformational isomers or two enantiomers, it would support Theory 1 over Theory 2. Geometric isomers differ in the arrangement of atoms about a double bond, so if they were *not* recognized by the same antibody, that certainly would support Theory 2 over Theory 1.

182. B

To begin with, we can eliminate two choices right away. Choice C says that Theory 2 is about chemical composition and choice D says that Theory 1 is about physical configuration; both of these assertions are false, so we can eliminate them immediately. Then, to evaluate the other two choices, we have to look at the data from the experiment. We're told that an antibody is produced to an antigen, *meta*-aminobenzenesulfonic acid, and that this antibody is then tested for reactivity with other antigens. The first antigen tested, *ortho*-aminobenzenesulfonic acid, and the fourth antigen tested, *para*-aminobenzenesulfonic acid, both have the same chemical composition, but a different physical configuration than the original antigen; neither one produced any response. The second one, *meta*-chlorobenzoic acid, and the third one, *meta*-aminomethoxybenzene, have different chemical compositions but the same physical configurations; these both *do* produce responses. Thus, the antibody responds

to physical configuration and not chemical composition, and so it supports Theory 2. So, choice A is incorrect and choice B is the correct answer.

183. D

This question asks about the antigen binding site of an antibody, but what it's mainly about is protein structure. As it says at the beginning of the passage, antibodies are proteins, and all of the answer choices relate to the characteristics of proteins. The amino acids in the active site of an antibody, which is its antigen binding site, interact chemically with the antigen. Antibodies that bind different sorts of antigens will have different amino acids in their binding sites. For instance, we might expect nonpolar antigens to bind to antibodies that have lots of nonpolar amino acids in their antigen binding sites, and likewise highly polar antigens would probably bind to antibodies that have lots of polar amino acids in their binding sites. Thus, there's no reason to suppose that the antigen binding site of an antibody is always nonpolar, so choice A is wrong. Choice B is wrong because, again, we would expect different antibodies to have different structures, so there's no reason to rule out the possibility that some of them might contain disulfide bonds. (Remember that disulfide bonds are formed between two cysteines, either on one protein chain or between protein chains, and contribute to the three-dimensional structure of the protein.) Choice C says the antigen binding site cannot be denatured. Denaturation is the disruption of a protein's three-dimensional structure due to heat, leading to loss of function; all proteins can be denatured, and so choice C is incorrect. Finally, choice D says that the antigen binding site represents the tertiary structure of the antibody. The tertiary structure of a protein is its three-dimensional shape, which is determined by interactions between its constituent amino acids, including hydrogen bonds, disulfide bonds, and various van der Waals forces. This three-dimensional structure, in turn, determines a protein's ability to interact with its environment and with its substrate, which in the case of an antibody means its ability to interact with its antigen. Thus the three-dimensional structure of an antibody is what gives it its ability to bind antigens, and so choice D is correct.

Discrete Questions

184. B

You're asked to draw a conclusion based on the experimental results depicted in the graph when muscle cells are grown in various glucose concentrations in the absence and presence of insulin. So first, let's look at the graph. Extracellular glucose concentration is plotted on the x-axis and intracellular glucose concentration is plotted on the y-axis. In the absence of insulin, the intracellular glucose concentration does not change at all, despite high extracellular concentrations. Practically no glucose enters the cell, even though its concentration gradient favors the movement of glucose into the cell. In the presence of insulin, there is an increase in intracellular glucose concentration, up to 500 mg/100 mL. The glucose moved into the muscle cell in the presence of insulin. In fact, there is a directly proportional relationship between the extracellular glucose concentration and the intracellular glucose concentration in the presence of insulin; that is, as one increases, so does the other. So what we've basically determined from the graph is, first of all, no insulin equals no increase in intracellular glucose; and secondly, insulin equals increase in intracellular glucose. Choice A says that insulin decreases intracellular glucose concentration in muscle cells. Well, that contradicts what we've just determined from the graph; insulin *increases,* not decreases, intracellular glucose. So, choice A is incorrect. Choice B says that muscle cell membranes are practically impermeable to glucose. Does our

data support this conclusion? Yes, it does; the control experiment supports it. Despite being grown in media of increasingly higher glucose concentration, intracellular glucose remained unchanged, indicating that although the glucose gradient favored the movement of glucose into the cell, glucose was somehow being prevented from entering it. And if glucose cannot freely cross a cell membrane, then the membrane is said to be impermeable to glucose. So choice B looks like our right answer, but let's look through the remaining two for good measure. Choice C says that glucose transport across muscle cell membranes requires ATP. When glucose transport across the cell membrane does occur, which is in the presence of insulin, transport occurs along glucose's concentration gradient; you don't find glucose leaving the cell, which would be transport *against* its gradient. Energy, or ATP, is required only to move substances against their concentration gradient, so choice C cannot be concluded based on the experimental data. In fact, it is known that insulin causes the facilitated diffusion of glucose across muscle cell membranes. Facilitated diffusion is when a carrier molecule facilitates the diffusion of a substance across a membrane *along* the substance's concentration gradient, not *against* it. Finally, choice D says that insulin stimulates the conversion of glucose into glycogen in almost all body tissues. This is, in fact, a true statement. Insulin is secreted by the pancreas in response to high blood glucose and stimulates the uptake of glucose and its conversion into glycogen in most body tissues, especially muscle, liver, and fat tissue. However, this cannot be concluded from the graph. The graph does not deal with what happens to the glucose after insulin stimulates its transport into muscle cells. You might know what happens after the glucose enters the cell, but the question asks you to draw a conclusion based solely on the information given in the graph. So, choice D is also incorrect.

185. A

ADH, or antidiuretic hormone, also known as vasopressin, is secreted by the posterior pituitary gland in response to high plasma osmolarity. ADH acts on the kidneys to increase their water reabsorption, thereby decreasing the plasma's solute concentration by diluting it with water. Increasing water reabsorption in the kidneys decreases the volume of urine excreted and increases urine osmolarity. A person with insufficient ADH production would therefore be expected to suffer from the opposite effects—decreased water reabsorption in the kidneys, which leads to an increase in urinary volume, a decrease in urine osmolarity, and an increase in plasma osmolarity. Looking at the answer choices, we see that choice A, increased urinary volume, is one of the effects we've just listed, while choices B and C are the effects of normal ADH secretion. Choice D, increased filtration rate in the kidneys, is a function of blood pressure; it is not under direct hormonal control. So, choice A is the correct answer.

186. B

In the presence of ethoxide ion, which is strongly basic, alkyl halides will readily undergo bimolecular elimination to form alkenes. No carbons are either added or removed, so the length of the carbon chain stays constant, and choice B is correct. All the other choices show reactions in which the length of the carbon chain increases. In choice A, the Grignard reagent is treated with gaseous carbon dioxide, and the resulting intermediate is hydrolyzed to form a carboxylic acid. Because carbon dioxide has been added to the molecule, this product has one extra carbon. In choice C, the cyanide ion, a strong nucleophile, displaces bromide from the primary alkyl halide in typical SN_2 fashion, adding an extra carbon. Finally, choice D is the familiar Grignard reaction. In this case, a Grignard reagent, CH_3MgBr is reacted with an aldehyde; washing with water results in a secondary alcohol with an additional carbon, so choice D is incorrect.

187. A

Chiral molecules always contain at least one chiral atom, usually a carbon atom bonded to four different substituents—while achiral compounds contain no such atom. An exception to this is *meso* compounds, which contain chiral carbons—so you would expect the molecule to be optically active—but they also possess a plane of symmetry and so they are achiral and optically *inactive*. Choice A has no carbons bonded to four different substituents—the left-hand carbon is connected with three hydrogens and one carbon, the middle carbon is connected with two hydrogens and two carbons and the right-hand positively charged carbon carries just three substituents. Therefore, choice A is correct. Choice B is wrong because glucose contains several chiral carbons. In choice C, both central carbons are bonded to four different substituents and there is no plane of symmetry in this molecule; hence, it is chiral. Finally, choice D is also chiral as the central carbon is attached to four different substituents—a carboxyl, methyl, ethyl, and carbonyl carbon.

188. B

Carbon dioxide is typically transported as bicarbonate ion, HCO_3^-, in the bloodstream. Carbon dioxide, which is a waste product of cellular metabolism, diffuses out of tissue into blood plasma. Some of the carbon dioxide remains dissolved in the plasma, in the form of CO_2 gas, but most of it diffuses into red blood cells; so choice A is wrong. Some of this carbon dioxide becomes loosely associated with hemoglobin, forming $HbCO_2$; however, most of the carbon dioxide that has diffused into the red blood cell, which is most of all of the carbon dioxide in the blood, combines with water in the red blood cells, forming carbonic acid, H_2CO_3. This reaction is catalyzed by the enzyme carbonic anhydrase; so choice C is wrong. The carbonic acid then dissociates into hydrogen ion and bicarbonate ion; so choice D is wrong and choice B is correct. The hydrogen ions, for the most part, bind to hemoglobin molecules, thereby preventing a sharp decrease in blood pH. Once this blood has reached the capillaries of the lung, this process is reversed. Bicarbonate ion and hydrogen ion reassociate to form carbonic acid, which is then reconverted into carbon dioxide and water by the same enzyme, carbonic anhydrase. The carbon dioxide diffuses out of the capillaries and is expired via the respiratory tract.

Passage VIII (Questions 189–193)

189. A

There are two things that you need to remember to determine the sequence of the DNA that is complementary to the segment of DNA given in the passage. The first is that DNA strands are situated antiparallel to one another in a DNA helix, meaning that the 3′ end of one strand is paired with the 5′ end of the other strand. The next important point is that in DNA there is complementary pairing of the nitrogenous bases; that is, adenine always pairs with thymine, and cytosine always pairs with guanine. Taking this information into account, we can start from the 3′ end of the given strand, which will correspond to the 5′end of the complementary strand, and match up the bases with their complements. Therefore, the complementary DNA strand will be TCGCTC-TATGGC in the 5′ to 3′ direction. So, choice A is the right answer. Choice B is wrong because it has the wrong polarity, but the right sequence. By the way, you should have immediately ruled out choices C and D because they both contain uracil, which is found only in RNA.

190. D

To answer this question, you have to have an understanding of both transcription and translation. Transcription is the process by which mRNA is synthesized from a DNA template. The mRNA

is thus complementary in sequence to this segment of DNA. A key thing to remember is that, as in DNA synthesis, mRNA synthesis occurs in the 5′ to 3′ direction only. First, let's determine the mRNA strand that's transcribed; starting at the 3′end of the DNA segment given in the passage, the resulting mRNA would be 5′-UCGCUCUAUG-GC-3′, considering that in RNA, uracil, rather than thymine, pairs with adenine; RNA does not contain thymine. Next, this strand must be translated from a sequence of bases into a sequence of amino acids. The bases are arranged in a series of triplets, known as codons, and each codon specifies a single amino acid. There are 64 possible codons, three of which are noncoding and signal termination, and one, AUG, that both signals for the start of synthesis and codes for the amino acid methionine. Synthesis begins at this codon only. But, since we're told in the passage that this is only a fragment of the DNA coding for the protein dystrophin that is missing in DMD patients, we can assume that the initiation codon AUG is found somewhere else in the gene. So we can just start translating from left to right, beginning to end.

So, looking at our strand of mRNA, we see that the codons are UCG, CUC, UAU, and GGC. Now, look at the list of mRNA codons in the chart of the genetic code to determine which amino acids they code for. The first codon, UCG, corresponds to serine. The second codon, CUC, corresponds to leucine. The third codon is UAU, which corresponds to tyrosine. And the fourth codon is GGC, which codes for glycine. Thus, the resulting polypeptide is Ser-Leu-Tyr-Gly, or choice D.

191. B

This is one of those questions that could have been answered without even reading the passage. As previously discussed, transcription is the process whereby the information coded in the base sequence of DNA is transcribed onto a strand of mRNA. Since transcription directly involves the DNA, it must take place where the DNA is located—in the nucleus—so choice B is the right answer. After the mRNA is processed inside the nucleus, it exits through pores in the nuclear membrane and goes to a ribosome—the site of translation. So, choice A is incorrect. A centromere is the specialized site that joins two sister chromatids together during mitosis and meiosis; thus, choice C is wrong. Choice D, cytoplasm, is wrong because it is translation, not transcription, that occurs in the cytoplasm. Be careful not to confuse transcription with translation.

192. A

This is your basic genetics question. From the passage you know that DMD is an X-linked recessive disorder. This means that the gene for DMD, which we'll call D, is found on the X chromosome. Remember that men have one X chromosome and one Y chromosome, while women have two X chromosomes. From the question stem you know that the woman is normal but her father had DMD. This means that here genotype must be X^{D}X. Why? Because she inherited one X chromosome from her mother and one from her father. Since you know that her father had DMD, his genotype must have been X^{D}Y. So the only X chromosome he could have passed on to his daughter contained the gene for DMD. And because the woman is normal, the X chromosome from her mother must have been normal. From the question stem you also know that the man is normal. This means that his genotype is XY. So crossing the X^{D}X woman with the XY male yields four possibilities: X^{D}X, XX, X^{D}Y, and XY. So there is a 25 percent chance that this couple will have a child with DMD. But the question stem asks for the probability of this couple having two children with the disease. So how do you figure this out? Multiply the probability of having a DMD child with the probability of having a DMD child. This is the same way you would figure out the probability of getting two heads in a row when you toss

a coin. In other words, 0.25 × 0.25, which is 0.0625. Thus, there is a 6.25% chance that this couple will have two children, both with DMD. Therefore, choice A is the correct answer.

193. B

From the passage you know that one of the initial steps in isolating the gene for DMD was comparing the ability of X-linked DNA probes to hybridize with DNA from DMD patients and with DNA from normal individuals. From this comparison, cloned fragments were obtained that correspond to the region of DNA that contains the deletions characteristic of DMD. This means that DMD DNA contains fewer bases than normal DNA due to these deletions. So a probe will not be able to bind as well to DMD DNA as it can to normal DNA, because normal DNA contains more bases that are complementary to the sequence of bases in the probes. This means that the probes have a *greater* degree of complementarity with normal DNA than with DMD DNA. Thus, choices A and C are incorrect, and choice B is the correct answer. Choice D is wrong because both males and females have an X chromosome to which the probe could hybridize.

Passage IX (Questions 194–201)
194. D

When discerning the stability of substituent groups on a six-membered cyclic chair conformation, it is necessary to look at the position of the substituent group. There are two groups on each carbon atom in the ring and the geometry of the substituent group can be axial or equatorial.

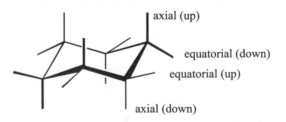

The axial position is more sterically hindered and has greater repulsion with the other axial groups than the equatorial group. The equatorial position allows for least repulsion of the larger substituent group. The structure 1,1-dimethylcyclohexane (I) will have the most steric hindrance because the substituent groups are on the same carbon atom. The 1,2-dimethyl cyclohexane structure (III) will be less stable than the other 1,2-dimethylcyclohexame (II) because structure III has both methyl groups in the axial position with is higher in energy than the equatorial groups. The 1,4-dimethylcyclohexane (IV) will be most stable because both methyl groups are in the equatorial position and they are separated by three bonds. So the order of increasing stability is I (least stable) < III < II < IV (most stable).

195. C

Three pairs of electrons are transferred among the atoms shown below. This is a Claisen rearrangement (as described in the latter part of the first paragraph addressing the reaction with aliphatic unsaturated ethers) to form the aldehyde (carbonyl group) and alkene shown in the product of the rearrangement of the allyl vinyl ether. The reaction stops here prior to enolization. Enolization occurs in the example given in the passage because the phenol (enol) form is aromatic and more stable than the corresponding carbonyl form (ketone). Most carbonyl compounds are considerably more stable than their corresponding enols.

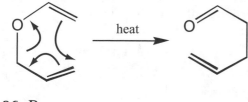

196. D

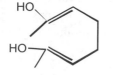

An "oxyCope" reaction is a sigmatropic variant of the Cope rearrangement. It reacts just as a Cope rearrangement, but it has an oxy group which forms an unstable enol. Upon the addition of heat, three electrons are transferred as shown in the reaction and a dienol is formed, which is unstable and readily undergoes tautomerization to the carbonyl (ketone) compound.

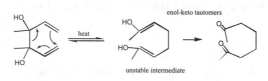

197. C

Three pairs of electrons are transferred as shown with 1,2-divinylcyclopropane to form cis, cis-cyclohepta-1,4-diene. 1,2-divinylcyclobutane forms an eight-membered cyclodiene. The asterick denotes the relative position of the carbon atom compared to the position of the double bonds during the rearrangement.

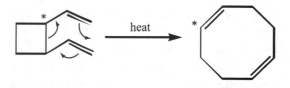

198. A

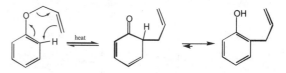

Tautomers are structural isomers that are conceptually related by the shift of a hydrogen and one or more π bonds.

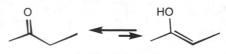

enolization (tautomers)

The enol form of the tautomer is generally not as stable as the carbonyl compound. However, the enol form of the tautomer of 2-allylphenol is more stable because an aromatic ring is formed during enolization. Phenol is an enol and it is aromatic. The β-keto Claisen condensation involves the enolate ions of esters. Conjugate addition is a type of reaction of conjugated dienes including the Diels-Alder reaction.

199. D

A meso compound is an achiral compound with asymmetric atoms and it has an internal plane of symmetry if you were to divide the molecule in half and both halves are structurally identical. A racemic mixture contains equal amounts of two enantiomers.

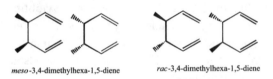

meso-3,4-dimethylhexa-1,5-diene   *rac*-3,4-dimethylhexa-1,5-diene

According to the chair transition state in Figure 1 of the passage, the meso compounds (when both methyl groups are either both up or both down) form cis, trans-octa-2,6-diene or trans, cis-octa-2,6-diene. The racemic mixture (when one methyl group is up and the other methyl group is down) would rearrange to form the cis, cis-isomer or the trans, trans-isomer.

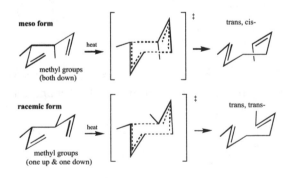

200. C

In order to determine the answer to this question, the reader will have to visualize or draw out each of the following reactions using the boat reaction shown in Figure 1. Reaction A would proceed via the chair transition state as shown in Figure 1. Reaction B would also use the chair conformation during the transition state to form a cis, trans-product. Reaction C can be visualized as having both methyl groups down and according to the passage it would form the cis, cis-isomer if the boat transition state was utilized during the reaction. Reaction D results in a trans, trans-isomer and could only be formed using the chair transition state.

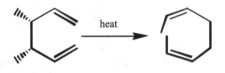

Reaction C

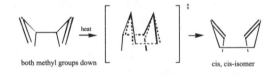

If reaction A were to utilize the boat transition state the answer would be shown below which is not the trans, trans- product shown in the answer of problem 7.

Reaction A (if it reacted via boat)

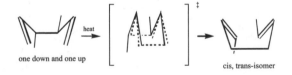

If reaction B utilized the boat transition state the answer would be a cis,trans-isomer, but not the one shown as the product of the reaction.

Reaction B (if it reacted via boat)

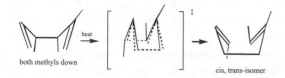

both methyls down   cis, trans-isomer

If reaction D were to utilize the boat transition state the answer would be a trans, cis- isomer, not the trans, trans- product shown in the reaction.

Reaction D (if it reacted via boat)

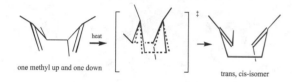

one methyl up and one down   trans, cis-isomer

Discrete Questions

201. A

Structure A has substituent groups in both *ortho* positions and one in the *meta* position. According to the first paragraph discussing the Claisen reaction, rearrangement generally occurs at the *ortho* position, but may occur at the *para* position and can even migrate from the *ortho* position to the *para* position. Compound B has an open *ortho* position. There could also be some formation of the *para* isomer, but the *ortho* isomer would predominate. Compounds C and D have neither the *ortho* nor the *para* position available for rearrangement and would be unlikely structures to undergo the Claisen rearrangement.

Passage X (Questions 202–209)

202. B

In Table I of the passage, the absorption bands of the specific stretchings are listed. The table states that O-H stretches can be in the range, 2800-3400 cm^{-1}. And further down in the table it states that the O-H stretch of a carboxylic acid is strong and broad (range 2800-3400 cm^{-1}), which best fits the range seen on the beverage spectrum (3250-3750 cm^{-1}). The broad band is due to the O-H stretching of the hydroxyl and carboxylic acid groups in tartaric acid. Its structure is shown below. Answer A

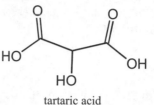

tartaric acid

could not be the correct answer because the aliphatic absorption (C-H) is shown as several large sharp peaks at 2900-3050 cm^{-1}. The C-O stretching in Answer C would correspond to an absorption band in the 1000-1600 cm^{-1} range. Answer D would require that the absorption stretching be between 1600-1850 cm^{-1}.

203. C.

In the second paragraph of the passage, it is stated that the food residue contains triacylglycerols from sheep or goat fat. Triacylglycerols have three ester bonds along with long hydrocarbon carbon chains. The large absorption band at 1690-1730 cm^{-1} could be due to C=O or C=C stretching as shown in Table I. However, since there was not a significant amount of unsaturation in the fatty acids analyzed from the food residue, the carbonyl C=O stretch of the ester would best explain the large absorption. Answers A and B would both require a large broad absorption in the 2800-3400 cm^{-1} range, which is not observed in the food residue spectrum.

204. A

Adding a double bond to an alkane lowers the melting point of the corresponding alkene. For example, hexane has a melting point of –95.3°C, whereas the melting point of 1-hexene is –139.8°C. The melting points of long chain fatty acids are also significantly affected. For example, stearic acid, which is *n*-octadecanoic acid (18:0), has a melting point of 69.6°. Adding a double bond to the corresponding fatty acid, oleic acid (18:1$^{\Delta 9}$), lowers the melting point to 16°C. Adding another double bond lowers the melting point even further. Linoleic acid (18:2$^{\Delta 9,12}$) has a melting point of 5°C.

205. D

According to the hydrolysis of the triacylglycerol reaction embedded within the passage and the fatty acid footnote, the corresponding fatty acids would be formed. If the triacylglycerol were comprised of the decanoic acid (10:0), hexadecanoic acid (16:0), and cis,cis-9,12-octadenoic acid (18:2$^{\Delta 9,12}$), which are capric acid, stearic acid, and linoleic acid, respectively, then the order of carboxylate formation would be (10:0), (16:0), (18:2$^{\Delta 9,12}$).

206. C

Answer A is not correct, because Fischer esterification, also called acid catalyzed esterification, is the formation of ester bonds. The reaction shown in the passage is the hydrolysis of the ester bond. E1 elimination (answer B) is an unimolecular elimination reaction resulting in the formation of a double bond. Saponification (answer C) is the base catalyzed ester hydrolysis shown in the passage. The carboxylate salts are formed during saponification because of the basic conditions. Answer D, E2 elimination is a b-elimination reaction, which results in the formation of a double bond.

207. D

According to the last part of the passage, terpenes are compounds composed of isoprene subunits as designated in the terpene figure embedded within the passage. It does not have to contain a double bond, rather, it must contain the connectivity of the 5 carbon atoms in the arrangement shown (head and tail). In answer A, cresols are aromatic phenols with a methyl group as a second substitutent on the benzene ring. Waxes (answer B) are long chain esters (only one ester moeity). Steriods are a class of connected six-membered rings with one five membered ring as shown below. The fragrant compound shown is menthol (oil of peppermint), a terpene. It has a total of 10 carbon atoms and two head-to-tail 5 carbon isoprene subunits.

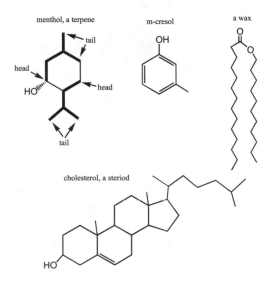

208. B

In the last paragraph of the passage, it is stated that each terpene must contain a multiple of five carbon atoms in the main carbon skeleton and the connectivity of the five carbons must be in the arrangement as shown (may or may not contain a double bond). Squalene contains 30 total carbon atoms and when divided by five carbon atoms, there are 6 five carbon isoprene subunits in the terpene, squalene.

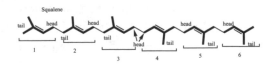

209. D

NMR amd MS are techniques that are used to elucidate the exact structure of a "isolatably pure" compound. FT-IR is qualitatively used to identify functional groups present in a pure compound or even a mixture of compounds. HPLC and chomatography in general, are used to separate and isolate a mixture of compounds according to their solvent polarity and ability to move through a column based on the compound's affinity toward that column. Each compound has its own retention time and elution pattern. Therefore, HPLC would be the most logical choice to identify the number of individual compounds contained in the mixed beverage. When identifying and characterizing the actual structures of the individual compounds, all methods are used to ascertain the compound's identity.

Discrete Questions

210. A

Lactase breaks lactose into glucose and galactose. Answer choice B is incorrect because kinase is an enzyme that phosphorylates its substrate. Answer choice C is incorrect because zymogen is an enzyme that is secreted in an inactive form. The zymogen is cleaved under certain physiological conditions to the active form of the enzyme. Important examples of zymogens include pepsinogen, trypsinogen, and chymotrypsinogen, which are cleaved in the digestive tract to yield the active enzymes pepsin, trypsin, and chymotrypsin. Answer choice D is incorrect because lipase breaks down lipids into free fatty acids.

211. B

The heartbeat is initiated by the sinoatrial (SA) node located in the wall of the right atrium and travels through the atria. It is regulated but not controlled by the accelerator nerve (sympathetic)

and the vagus nerve (parasympathetic). It is then picked up by the AV node which signals the bundle of His (AV bundle) which transports the contraction through the ventricles via the Purkinje fibers. Answer choice A is incorrect because while the AV node does have contractile ability and controls the contraction of the ventricles, it does not control the contraction of the entire heart and is not as regular as thc signal from the SA node. Answer choices C and D are not correct because the SA node is located in the wall of the right atrium and is not functionally dependent upon nervous stimulation as this tissue initiates the heartbeat although it can be modified by the nervous system.

212. D

The low pH of the stomach is essential for the function of the enzymes that break down proteins into their amino acids. Answer choice A is true: amylases, lipases, and bicarbonate are released through the pancreatic duct. Answer choice B is true: peristalsis propels food and waste through the system. Answer choice C is true because glucose and amino acids are picked up by the blood while fats are picked up by lacteals, which are special vessels that connect with the lymphatic system.

213. D

ADH is released by the posterior pituitary gland and causes the collecting tubule to be more permeable to water. Therefore, more water is absorbed and urine becomes more concentrated. Answer choice A is incorrect because in the nephrons, the glomerulus, Bowman's capsule, and the proximal and distal convoluted tubule are in the cortex while the loop of Henle and the collecting tubule are in the medulla. Answer choice B is incorrect because ammonia is transformed into urea in the liver and excreted by the kidney. Answer choice C is incorrect because salts, glucose, and amino acids are reabsorbed by active transport while water is reabsorbed by diffusion.

214. C

In the adult, all hematopoiesis occurs in the bone marrow. In the fetus, hematopoiesis occurs in the fetal liver. The spleen acts as a reservoir for red blood cells and filters the blood. Answer choice A is true because mature red blood cells are not nucleated in order to create more space for hemoglobin. Answer choice B is incorrect because blood platelets are crucial for the clotting of blood, and answer choice D is incorrect because certain white blood cells such as macrophages and neutrophils engulf foreign matter.

Full-Length
Practice Test II

MCAT Overview

PHYSICAL SCIENCES

Time	100 minutes
Format	77 multiple-choice questions: approximately 10–11 passages with 4–8 questions each; 12–17 stand-alone questions (not passage-based)

VERBAL REASONING

Time	85 minutes
Format	60 multiple-choice questions: approximately 9–10 passages with 6–9 questions each

WRITING SAMPLE

Time	60 minutes
Format	2 essay questions (3 tasks per essay)

BIOLOGICAL SCIENCES

Time	100 minutes
Format	77 multiple-choice questions: approximately 10–11 passages with 4–8 questions each; 12–17 stand-alone questions (not passage-based)

INSTRUCTIONS FOR TAKING THE FULL-LENGTH PRACTICE TEST

Before taking this Full-Length Practice Test, find a quiet place where you can work uninterrupted. Make sure you have a comfortable desk and several No. 2 pencils.

Use the answer grid on the following page to record your answers. Time yourself according to the time limits shown at the beginning of each section.

You'll find the answer key, the score converter, and detailed answer explanations following the test.

Good luck.

MARK ONE AND ONLY ONE ANSWER TO EACH QUESTION. BE SURE TO FILL IN COMPLETELY THE SPACE FOR YOUR INTENDED ANSWER CHOICE. IF YOU ERASE, DO SO COMPLETELY. MAKE NO STRAY MARKS.

RIGHT MARK: ● WRONG MARKS: ⊘ ⊗ ◉

1 Ⓐ Ⓑ Ⓒ Ⓓ
2 Ⓐ Ⓑ Ⓒ Ⓓ
3 Ⓐ Ⓑ Ⓒ Ⓓ
4 Ⓐ Ⓑ Ⓒ Ⓓ
5 Ⓐ Ⓑ Ⓒ Ⓓ
6 Ⓐ Ⓑ Ⓒ Ⓓ
7 Ⓐ Ⓑ Ⓒ Ⓓ
8 Ⓐ Ⓑ Ⓒ Ⓓ
9 Ⓐ Ⓑ Ⓒ Ⓓ
10 Ⓐ Ⓑ Ⓒ Ⓓ
11 Ⓐ Ⓑ Ⓒ Ⓓ
12 Ⓐ Ⓑ Ⓒ Ⓓ
13 Ⓐ Ⓑ Ⓒ Ⓓ
14 Ⓐ Ⓑ Ⓒ Ⓓ
15 Ⓐ Ⓑ Ⓒ Ⓓ
16 Ⓐ Ⓑ Ⓒ Ⓓ
17 Ⓐ Ⓑ Ⓒ Ⓓ
18 Ⓐ Ⓑ Ⓒ Ⓓ
19 Ⓐ Ⓑ Ⓒ Ⓓ
20 Ⓐ Ⓑ Ⓒ Ⓓ
21 Ⓐ Ⓑ Ⓒ Ⓓ
22 Ⓐ Ⓑ Ⓒ Ⓓ
23 Ⓐ Ⓑ Ⓒ Ⓓ
24 Ⓐ Ⓑ Ⓒ Ⓓ
25 Ⓐ Ⓑ Ⓒ Ⓓ
26 Ⓐ Ⓑ Ⓒ Ⓓ
27 Ⓐ Ⓑ Ⓒ Ⓓ
28 Ⓐ Ⓑ Ⓒ Ⓓ
29 Ⓐ Ⓑ Ⓒ Ⓓ
30 Ⓐ Ⓑ Ⓒ Ⓓ
31 Ⓐ Ⓑ Ⓒ Ⓓ
32 Ⓐ Ⓑ Ⓒ Ⓓ
33 Ⓐ Ⓑ Ⓒ Ⓓ
34 Ⓐ Ⓑ Ⓒ Ⓓ
35 Ⓐ Ⓑ Ⓒ Ⓓ
36 Ⓐ Ⓑ Ⓒ Ⓓ
37 Ⓐ Ⓑ Ⓒ Ⓓ
38 Ⓐ Ⓑ Ⓒ Ⓓ
39 Ⓐ Ⓑ Ⓒ Ⓓ
40 Ⓐ Ⓑ Ⓒ Ⓓ

41 Ⓐ Ⓑ Ⓒ Ⓓ
42 Ⓐ Ⓑ Ⓒ Ⓓ
43 Ⓐ Ⓑ Ⓒ Ⓓ
44 Ⓐ Ⓑ Ⓒ Ⓓ
45 Ⓐ Ⓑ Ⓒ Ⓓ
46 Ⓐ Ⓑ Ⓒ Ⓓ
47 Ⓐ Ⓑ Ⓒ Ⓓ
48 Ⓐ Ⓑ Ⓒ Ⓓ
49 Ⓐ Ⓑ Ⓒ Ⓓ
50 Ⓐ Ⓑ Ⓒ Ⓓ
51 Ⓐ Ⓑ Ⓒ Ⓓ
52 Ⓐ Ⓑ Ⓒ Ⓓ
53 Ⓐ Ⓑ Ⓒ Ⓓ
54 Ⓐ Ⓑ Ⓒ Ⓓ
55 Ⓐ Ⓑ Ⓒ Ⓓ
56 Ⓐ Ⓑ Ⓒ Ⓓ
57 Ⓐ Ⓑ Ⓒ Ⓓ
58 Ⓐ Ⓑ Ⓒ Ⓓ
59 Ⓐ Ⓑ Ⓒ Ⓓ
60 Ⓐ Ⓑ Ⓒ Ⓓ
61 Ⓐ Ⓑ Ⓒ Ⓓ
62 Ⓐ Ⓑ Ⓒ Ⓓ
63 Ⓐ Ⓑ Ⓒ Ⓓ
64 Ⓐ Ⓑ Ⓒ Ⓓ
65 Ⓐ Ⓑ Ⓒ Ⓓ
66 Ⓐ Ⓑ Ⓒ Ⓓ
67 Ⓐ Ⓑ Ⓒ Ⓓ
68 Ⓐ Ⓑ Ⓒ Ⓓ
69 Ⓐ Ⓑ Ⓒ Ⓓ
70 Ⓐ Ⓑ Ⓒ Ⓓ
71 Ⓐ Ⓑ Ⓒ Ⓓ
72 Ⓐ Ⓑ Ⓒ Ⓓ
73 Ⓐ Ⓑ Ⓒ Ⓓ
74 Ⓐ Ⓑ Ⓒ Ⓓ
75 Ⓐ Ⓑ Ⓒ Ⓓ
76 Ⓐ Ⓑ Ⓒ Ⓓ
77 Ⓐ Ⓑ Ⓒ Ⓓ
78 Ⓐ Ⓑ Ⓒ Ⓓ
79 Ⓐ Ⓑ Ⓒ Ⓓ
80 Ⓐ Ⓑ Ⓒ Ⓓ

81 Ⓐ Ⓑ Ⓒ Ⓓ
82 Ⓐ Ⓑ Ⓒ Ⓓ
83 Ⓐ Ⓑ Ⓒ Ⓓ
84 Ⓐ Ⓑ Ⓒ Ⓓ
85 Ⓐ Ⓑ Ⓒ Ⓓ
86 Ⓐ Ⓑ Ⓒ Ⓓ
87 Ⓐ Ⓑ Ⓒ Ⓓ
88 Ⓐ Ⓑ Ⓒ Ⓓ
89 Ⓐ Ⓑ Ⓒ Ⓓ
90 Ⓐ Ⓑ Ⓒ Ⓓ
91 Ⓐ Ⓑ Ⓒ Ⓓ
92 Ⓐ Ⓑ Ⓒ Ⓓ
93 Ⓐ Ⓑ Ⓒ Ⓓ
94 Ⓐ Ⓑ Ⓒ Ⓓ
95 Ⓐ Ⓑ Ⓒ Ⓓ
96 Ⓐ Ⓑ Ⓒ Ⓓ
97 Ⓐ Ⓑ Ⓒ Ⓓ
98 Ⓐ Ⓑ Ⓒ Ⓓ
99 Ⓐ Ⓑ Ⓒ Ⓓ
100 Ⓐ Ⓑ Ⓒ Ⓓ
101 Ⓐ Ⓑ Ⓒ Ⓓ
102 Ⓐ Ⓑ Ⓒ Ⓓ
103 Ⓐ Ⓑ Ⓒ Ⓓ
104 Ⓐ Ⓑ Ⓒ Ⓓ
105 Ⓐ Ⓑ Ⓒ Ⓓ
106 Ⓐ Ⓑ Ⓒ Ⓓ
107 Ⓐ Ⓑ Ⓒ Ⓓ
108 Ⓐ Ⓑ Ⓒ Ⓓ
109 Ⓐ Ⓑ Ⓒ Ⓓ
110 Ⓐ Ⓑ Ⓒ Ⓓ
111 Ⓐ Ⓑ Ⓒ Ⓓ
112 Ⓐ Ⓑ Ⓒ Ⓓ
113 Ⓐ Ⓑ Ⓒ Ⓓ
114 Ⓐ Ⓑ Ⓒ Ⓓ
115 Ⓐ Ⓑ Ⓒ Ⓓ
116 Ⓐ Ⓑ Ⓒ Ⓓ
117 Ⓐ Ⓑ Ⓒ Ⓓ
118 Ⓐ Ⓑ Ⓒ Ⓓ
119 Ⓐ Ⓑ Ⓒ Ⓓ
120 Ⓐ Ⓑ Ⓒ Ⓓ

121 Ⓐ Ⓑ Ⓒ Ⓓ
122 Ⓐ Ⓑ Ⓒ Ⓓ
123 Ⓐ Ⓑ Ⓒ Ⓓ
124 Ⓐ Ⓑ Ⓒ Ⓓ
125 Ⓐ Ⓑ Ⓒ Ⓓ
126 Ⓐ Ⓑ Ⓒ Ⓓ
127 Ⓐ Ⓑ Ⓒ Ⓓ
128 Ⓐ Ⓑ Ⓒ Ⓓ
129 Ⓐ Ⓑ Ⓒ Ⓓ
130 Ⓐ Ⓑ Ⓒ Ⓓ
131 Ⓐ Ⓑ Ⓒ Ⓓ
132 Ⓐ Ⓑ Ⓒ Ⓓ
133 Ⓐ Ⓑ Ⓒ Ⓓ
134 Ⓐ Ⓑ Ⓒ Ⓓ
135 Ⓐ Ⓑ Ⓒ Ⓓ
136 Ⓐ Ⓑ Ⓒ Ⓓ
137 Ⓐ Ⓑ Ⓒ Ⓓ
138 Ⓐ Ⓑ Ⓒ Ⓓ
139 Ⓐ Ⓑ Ⓒ Ⓓ
140 Ⓐ Ⓑ Ⓒ Ⓓ
141 Ⓐ Ⓑ Ⓒ Ⓓ
142 Ⓐ Ⓑ Ⓒ Ⓓ
143 Ⓐ Ⓑ Ⓒ Ⓓ
144 Ⓐ Ⓑ Ⓒ Ⓓ
145 Ⓐ Ⓑ Ⓒ Ⓓ
146 Ⓐ Ⓑ Ⓒ Ⓓ
147 Ⓐ Ⓑ Ⓒ Ⓓ
148 Ⓐ Ⓑ Ⓒ Ⓓ
149 Ⓐ Ⓑ Ⓒ Ⓓ
150 Ⓐ Ⓑ Ⓒ Ⓓ
151 Ⓐ Ⓑ Ⓒ Ⓓ
152 Ⓐ Ⓑ Ⓒ Ⓓ
153 Ⓐ Ⓑ Ⓒ Ⓓ
154 Ⓐ Ⓑ Ⓒ Ⓓ
155 Ⓐ Ⓑ Ⓒ Ⓓ
156 Ⓐ Ⓑ Ⓒ Ⓓ
157 Ⓐ Ⓑ Ⓒ Ⓓ
158 Ⓐ Ⓑ Ⓒ Ⓓ
159 Ⓐ Ⓑ Ⓒ Ⓓ
160 Ⓐ Ⓑ Ⓒ Ⓓ

161 Ⓐ Ⓑ Ⓒ Ⓓ
162 Ⓐ Ⓑ Ⓒ Ⓓ
163 Ⓐ Ⓑ Ⓒ Ⓓ
164 Ⓐ Ⓑ Ⓒ Ⓓ
165 Ⓐ Ⓑ Ⓒ Ⓓ
166 Ⓐ Ⓑ Ⓒ Ⓓ
167 Ⓐ Ⓑ Ⓒ Ⓓ
168 Ⓐ Ⓑ Ⓒ Ⓓ
169 Ⓐ Ⓑ Ⓒ Ⓓ
170 Ⓐ Ⓑ Ⓒ Ⓓ
171 Ⓐ Ⓑ Ⓒ Ⓓ
172 Ⓐ Ⓑ Ⓒ Ⓓ
173 Ⓐ Ⓑ Ⓒ Ⓓ
174 Ⓐ Ⓑ Ⓒ Ⓓ
175 Ⓐ Ⓑ Ⓒ Ⓓ
176 Ⓐ Ⓑ Ⓒ Ⓓ
177 Ⓐ Ⓑ Ⓒ Ⓓ
178 Ⓐ Ⓑ Ⓒ Ⓓ
179 Ⓐ Ⓑ Ⓒ Ⓓ
180 Ⓐ Ⓑ Ⓒ Ⓓ
181 Ⓐ Ⓑ Ⓒ Ⓓ
182 Ⓐ Ⓑ Ⓒ Ⓓ
183 Ⓐ Ⓑ Ⓒ Ⓓ
184 Ⓐ Ⓑ Ⓒ Ⓓ
185 Ⓐ Ⓑ Ⓒ Ⓓ
186 Ⓐ Ⓑ Ⓒ Ⓓ
187 Ⓐ Ⓑ Ⓒ Ⓓ
188 Ⓐ Ⓑ Ⓒ Ⓓ
189 Ⓐ Ⓑ Ⓒ Ⓓ
190 Ⓐ Ⓑ Ⓒ Ⓓ
191 Ⓐ Ⓑ Ⓒ Ⓓ
192 Ⓐ Ⓑ Ⓒ Ⓓ
193 Ⓐ Ⓑ Ⓒ Ⓓ
194 Ⓐ Ⓑ Ⓒ Ⓓ
195 Ⓐ Ⓑ Ⓒ Ⓓ
196 Ⓐ Ⓑ Ⓒ Ⓓ
197 Ⓐ Ⓑ Ⓒ Ⓓ
198 Ⓐ Ⓑ Ⓒ Ⓓ
199 Ⓐ Ⓑ Ⓒ Ⓓ
200 Ⓐ Ⓑ Ⓒ Ⓓ

201 Ⓐ Ⓑ Ⓒ Ⓓ
202 Ⓐ Ⓑ Ⓒ Ⓓ
203 Ⓐ Ⓑ Ⓒ Ⓓ
204 Ⓐ Ⓑ Ⓒ Ⓓ
205 Ⓐ Ⓑ Ⓒ Ⓓ
206 Ⓐ Ⓑ Ⓒ Ⓓ
207 Ⓐ Ⓑ Ⓒ Ⓓ
208 Ⓐ Ⓑ Ⓒ Ⓓ
209 Ⓐ Ⓑ Ⓒ Ⓓ
210 Ⓐ Ⓑ Ⓒ Ⓓ
211 Ⓐ Ⓑ Ⓒ Ⓓ
212 Ⓐ Ⓑ Ⓒ Ⓓ
213 Ⓐ Ⓑ Ⓒ Ⓓ
214 Ⓐ Ⓑ Ⓒ Ⓓ

Physical Sciences Test

Time: 100 minutes
Questions 1–77

DIRECTIONS: Most of the questions in the following Physical Sciences test are organized into groups, with a descriptive passage preceding each group of questions. Study the passage, then select the single best answer to each question in the group. Some of the questions are not based on a descriptive passage; you must also select the best answer to these questions. If you are unsure of the best answer, eliminate the choices that you know are incorrect, then select an answer from the choices that remain. Indicate your selection by blackening the corresponding oval on your answer document. A periodic table is provided below for your use with the questions.

Periodic Table of the Elements

1 H 1.0																	2 He 4.0
3 Li 6.9	4 Be 9.0											5 B 10.8	6 C 12.0	7 N 14.0	8 O 16.0	9 F 19.0	10 Ne 20.2
11 Na 23.0	12 Mg 24.3											13 Al 27.0	14 Si 28.1	15 P 31.0	16 S 32.1	17 Cl 35.5	18 Ar 39.9
19 K 39.1	20 Ca 40.1	21 Sc 45.0	22 Ti 47.9	23 V 50.9	24 Cr 52.0	25 Mn 54.9	26 Fe 55.8	27 Co 58.9	28 Ni 58.7	29 Cu 63.5	30 Zn 65.4	31 Ga 69.7	32 Ge 72.6	33 As 74.9	34 Se 79.0	35 Br 79.9	36 Kr 83.8
37 Rb 85.5	38 Sr 87.6	39 Y 88.9	40 Zr 91.2	41 Nb 92.9	42 Mo 95.9	43 Tc (98)	44 Ru 101.1	45 Rh 102.9	46 Pd 106.4	47 Ag 107.9	48 Cd 112.4	49 In 114.8	50 Sn 118.7	51 Sb 121.8	52 Te 127.6	53 I 126.9	54 Xe 131.3
55 Cs 132.9	56 Ba 137.3	57 La* 138.9	72 Hf 178.5	73 Ta 180.9	74 W 183.9	75 Re 186.2	76 Os 190.2	77 Ir 192.2	78 Pt 195.1	79 Au 197.0	80 Hg 200.6	81 Tl 204.4	82 Pb 207.2	83 Bi 209.0	84 Po (209)	85 At (210)	86 Rn (222)
87 Fr (223)	88 Ra 226.0	89 Ac† 227.0	104 Unq (261)	105 Unp (262)	106 Unh (263)	107 Uns (262)	108 Uno (265)	109 Une (267)									

*	58 Ce 140.1	59 Pr 140.9	60 Nd 144.2	61 Pm (145)	62 Sm 150.4	63 Eu 152.0	64 Gd 157.3	65 Tb 158.9	66 Dy 162.5	67 Ho 164.9	68 Er 167.3	69 Tm 168.9	70 Yb 173.0	71 Lu 175.0
†	90 Th 232.0	91 Pa (231)	92 U 238.0	93 Np (237)	94 Pu (244)	95 Am (243)	96 Cm (247)	97 Bk (247)	98 Cf (251)	99 Es (252)	100 Fm (257)	101 Md (258)	102 No (259)	103 Lr (260)

GO ON TO THE NEXT PAGE.

Passage I (Questions 1–5)

A continuous spectrum of light, sometimes called blackbody radiation, is emitted from a region of the Sun called the photosphere. Although the continuous spectrum contains light of all wavelengths, the intensity of the emitted light is much greater at some wavelengths than at others. The relationship between the most intense wavelength of blackbody radiation and the temperature of the emitting body is given by Wien's law, $\lambda = 2.9 \times 10^6/T$, where λ is the wavelength in nanometers and T is the temperature in Kelvins.

As the blackbody radiation from the Sun passes through the cooler gases in the Sun's atmosphere, some of the photons are absorbed by the atoms in these gases. A photon will be absorbed if it has just enough energy to excite an electron from a lower energy state to a higher one. The absorbed photon will have an energy equal to the energy difference between these two states. The energy of a photon is given by $E = hf = hc/\lambda$, where $h = 6.63 \times 10^{-34}$ J•s is Planck's constant and $c = 3 \times 10^8$ m/s is the speed of light in a vacuum.

The Sun is composed primarily of hydrogen. Electron transitions in the hydrogen atom from energy state $n = 2$ to higher energy states are listed below along with the energy of the absorbed photon.

Final Energy State	Energy ($\times 10^{-19}$ J)
$n = 3$	3.02
$n = 4$	4.08
$n = 5$	4.57
$n = 6$	4.84
$n = \infty$	5.44

1. If the temperature of the Sun's photosphere is 5,800 K, what wavelength of radiation does the Sun emit with the greatest intensity?

    A. 2 nm
    B. 50 nm
    C. 500 nm
    D. 4,500 nm

2. From the data in the table, what is the approximate wavelength of a photon emitted in the electron transition from energy state $n = 4$ to energy state $n = 3$?

    A. 5 nm
    B. 30 nm
    C. 100 nm
    D. 2,000 nm

3. The energy absorbed by a hydrogen atom as its electron undergoes a transition from the $n = 1$ energy state to the $n = \infty$ state is: (Note: The $n = 1$ energy state is the ground state of hydrogen.)

    A. infinite.
    B. equal to the binding energy of the electron.
    C. equal to the energy of a zero frequency photon.
    D. smaller than the energy absorbed in the $n = 2$ to $n = \infty$ transition.

GO ON TO THE NEXT PAGE.

4. At the center of the visible spectrum is light with a wavelength of $\lambda = 550$ nm. What is the frequency of this light?

    A. 9.0×10^8 Hz
    B. 1.8×10^{12} Hz
    C. 5.4×10^{14} Hz
    D. 1.8×10^{16} Hz

5. If a star suddenly doubles in size but remains at the same temperature, how does its continuous spectrum change?

    A. The peak intensity occurs at the same wavelength.
    B. The peak intensity occurs at a longer wavelength.
    C. The peak intensity occurs at a shorter wavelength.
    D. The intensity peak narrows.

GO ON TO THE NEXT PAGE.

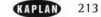

Passage II (Questions 6–12)

The lead-acid battery, also called a lead storage battery, is the battery of choice for starting automobiles. It contains six cells connected in series, each composed of a lead oxide cathode "sandwiched" between two lead anodes. Insulating separators are placed between the electrodes to prevent internal short-circuits. Aqueous sulfuric acid is the electrolyte.

When the battery is being discharged, the following reaction takes place.

$$Pb(s) + PbO_2(s) + 2 H_2SO_4(aq) \rightarrow$$
$$2 PbSO_4(s) + 2 H_2O$$

Reaction 1

The electrode reactions, both written as reductions, are shown in Table 1.

Table 1

Half-reaction	$E^\circ(V)$
$PbO_2(s) + SO_4^{2-}(aq) + 4H^+$ $(aq) + 2e^- \rightarrow PbSO_4(s) + 2H_2O$	1.69
$PbSO_4(s) + 2e^- \rightarrow Pb(s) +$ $SO_4^{2-}(aq)$	–0.36

As a car operates, the battery is recharged by electricity produced by the car's alternator, an AC generator whose ultimate power source is the car's internal combustion engine. In spite of this, batteries eventually lose their power. The battery is said to be "dead" when Reaction 1 has proceeded completely to the right.

6. How many cells would be required to produce a 20-volt lead-acid battery of the type described in the passage?

A. 5
B. 10
C. 15
D. 20

7. Which reaction takes place at the anode as the battery is discharging?

A. The first half-reaction, proceeding to the left
B. The first half-reaction, proceeding to the right
C. The second half-reaction, proceeding to the left
D. The second half-reaction, proceeding to the right

8. Where does oxidation occur in the lead storage battery?

A. At the lead oxide cathodes
B. At the lead oxide anodes
C. At the lead cathodes
D. At the lead anodes

9. Which of the following occurs as the battery is being recharged?

A. An increase in the concentration of H+ ions
B. An increase in the amount of $PbSO_4$ and lead
C. An increase in the concentration of H_2O
D. A decrease in the amount of PbO_2

GO ON TO THE NEXT PAGE.

10. The graph below shows the change in potential versus time of a 12 V lead storage battery during discharge.

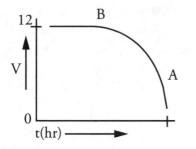

Which of the following is true?

A. The electrolyte density at point A is greater than it is at point B.

B. The electrolyte density at point A is less than it is at point B.

C. The electrolyte density at point A is the same as that at point B.

D. The electrolyte density at points A and B cannot be compared without more information.

11. Currents as small as 0.1 A can be fatal to humans. If the typical resistance of the human body is 10 kΩ, what is the minimum voltage that could be fatal?

A. 0.1 V
B. 1 V
C. 100 V
D. 1000 V

12. Often in cold weather the battery goes "dead." Thermodynamic data confirms that the voltage of most electrochemical cells decrease with decreasing temperature. If the battery is warmed to room temperature, it often recovers its ability to deliver normal power. The battery appeared "dead" because:

I. the resistance of the electrolyte had decreased.
II. the viscosity of the electrolyte had increased.
III. the viscosity of the electrolyte had decreased.

A. I only
B. II only
C. I and II only
D. I and III only

GO ON TO THE NEXT PAGE.

Passage III (Questions 13–17)

The resistance of a resistor is defined as the ratio of the voltage drop across it to the current passing through it. The resistance of a resistor can be measured using the circuit illustrated in Figure 1.

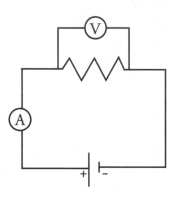

Figure 1

In the above circuit, a variable voltage source with negligible internal resistance is connected to a resistor. The voltage across the resistor is measured by a voltmeter and the current through the resistor is measured by an ammeter.

Additional resistors may be added to the circuit. The total resistance can be calculated as follows: If R_1 and R_2 are two resistances of two resistors, then the total resistance is given by $R_{total} = R_1 + R_2$ when the resistors are connected in series, and by $1/R_{total} = 1/R_1 + 1/R_2$ when the resistors are connected in parallel.

Circuits similar to the one above are used in the common household appliance known as the toaster. The rate by which energy in the form of heat is dissipated by the resistor equals I^2R, where I is the current that passes through the resistor and R is the resistance of the resistor. Energy is dissipated in a resistor because moving electrons collide with atoms in the resistor causing the atoms to vibrate.

13. The variable voltage supply in the circuit in Figure 1 is replaced by a battery connected in series with the resistor and ammeter. The battery has a small internal resistance. How will the circuit be affected?

    A. The current measured by the ammeter at a specific voltage will be larger in the circuit with the battery.
    B. The current measured by the ammeter at a specific voltage will be smaller in the circuit with the battery.
    C. The resistance of the resistor at a specific voltage will be larger in the circuit with the battery.
    D. The resistance of the resistor at a specific voltage will be smaller in the circuit with the battery.

14. In which direction do the electrons travel and in which direction does the current flow in the circuit in Figure 1?

    A. The electrons travel clockwise, and the current flows counterclockwise.
    B. The electrons travel clockwise, and the current flows clockwise.
    C. The electrons travel counterclockwise, and the current flows clockwise.
    D. The electrons travel counterclockwise, and the current flows counterclockwise.

15. In order for the ammeter to have a very small effect on the current flowing through the resistor, the ammeter should:

    A. be connected to the resistor with insulated wire.
    B. be connected nearest to the positive terminal of the voltage source.
    C. have a very low resistance.
    D. be sensitive to currents flowing either way around the circuit.

GO ON TO THE NEXT PAGE.

16. As current passes through a resistor, the temperature of the resistor will increase. Which of the following is a reason the temperature increases?

    A. The average kinetic energy of the atoms in the resistor increases as a result of the collisions with the electrons in the current.
    B. The average potential energy of the atoms in the resistor increases as a result of the collisions with the electrons in the current.
    C. The average kinetic energy of the electrons in the current increases as a result of the collisions with the atoms in the resistor.
    D. The average potential energy of the electrons in the current increases as a result of the collisions with the atoms in the resistor.

17. What is the energy delivered to a piece of toast in one second when it is inside a toaster in which a 4×10^{-3}-A current passes through a 10-kΩ resistor?

    A. 0.04 J
    B. 0.16 J
    C. 2.5 J
    D. 40 J

GO ON TO THE NEXT PAGE.

 217

Passage IV (Questions 18–23)

It is critical that human blood be kept at a pH of approximately 7.4. Decreased or increased blood pH are called acidosis and alkalosis respectively; both are serious metabolic problems that can cause death. The table below lists the major buffers found in the blood and/or kidneys.

Table 1

Buffer	pK_a of a typical conjugate acid:[1]
$HCO_3^- \rightleftharpoons CO_2 + H_2O$	6.1
Histidine side chains	6.3
$HPO_4^{2-} \rightleftharpoons H_2PO_4^-$	6.8
Organic phosphates	7.0
N-terminal amino groups	8.0
$NH_3 \rightleftharpoons NH_4^+$	9.2

[1]For buffers in many of these categories, there is a range of actual pK_a values.

The relationship between blood pH and the pK_a of any buffer can be described by the Henderson-Hasselbach equation:

$$pH = pK_a + \log([\text{conjugate base}]/[\text{conjugate acid}])$$

Equation 1

Bicarbonate, the most important buffer in the plasma, enters the blood in the form of carbon dioxide, a by-product of metabolism, and leaves in two forms: exhaled CO_2 and excreted bicarbonate. Blood pH can be adjusted rapidly by changes in the rate of CO_2 exhalation. The reaction given below, which is catalyzed by carbonic anhydrase in the erythrocytes, describes how bicarbonate and CO_2 interact in the blood.

$$CO_2 + H_2O \rightleftharpoons H^+ + HCO_3^-$$

Reaction 1

18. If the pH of blood were to increase to 7.6, what would be the likely outcome?

    A. An increase in carbonic anhydrase activity
    B. A decrease in carbonic anhydrase activity
    C. An increase in the rate of CO_2 exhalation
    D. A decrease in the rate of CO_2 exhalation

19. The equilibrium as shown in Reaction 1 is most likely to proceed through which of the following intermediates?

    A. H_2CO_3
    B. $2H^+$ and CO_3^{2-}
    C. CO_2 and H_3O^+
    D. CO_2 and H_2

20. What would be the order of conjugate acid strength in the following buffers?

    A. Histidine side chains = organic phosphates $> NH_4^+$
    B. $NH_4^+ >$ organic phosphates $>$ histidine side chains
    C. Histidine side chains $>$ organic phosphates $> NH_4^+$
    D. $NH_4^+ >$ organic phosphates = histidine side chains

GO ON TO THE NEXT PAGE.

21. The following graph shows the titration of 0.01 $M\,H_3PO_4$ with 10 M NaOH. Within which area of the titration curve will the concentration of $H_2PO_4^-$ become equal to that of HPO_4^{2-}?

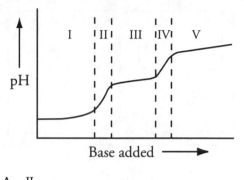

Base added ⟶

A. II
B. III
C. IV
D. V

22. How does the titration of a weak monoprotic acid with a strong base differ from the titration of a strong monoprotic acid with a strong base?

A. The equivalence point will occur at a higher pH.
B. The equivalence point will occur at a lower pH.
C. The equivalence point will occur at the same pH.
D. Whether the equivalence point is higher or lower depends on the particular acids used.

23. What would be the nature of the compensatory change that would take place in response to acidosis caused by organic acids?

A. Breathing rate would increase and total blood CO_2/HCO_3^- concentration would increase.
B. Breathing rate would increase and total blood CO_2/HCO_3^- concentration would decrease.
C. Breathing rate would decrease and total blood CO_2/HCO_3^- concentration would increase.
D. Breathing rate would decrease and total blood CO_2/HCO_3^- concentration would decrease.

GO ON TO THE NEXT PAGE.

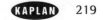

Questions 24 through 28 are NOT based on a descriptive passage.

24. The mouthpiece of a telephone handset has a mass of 100 g, and the earpiece has a mass of 150 g. To balance the handset on one finger, that finger must be: (Note: Assume the bridge connecting the mouthpiece and the earpiece has a negligible mass.)

A. one and one half times farther from the earpiece than from the mouthpiece.
B. two times farther from the earpiece than from the mouthpiece.
C. one and one half times farther from the mouthpiece than from the earpiece.
D. two times farther from the mouthpiece than from the earpiece.

25. The reaction below is not spontaneous at any temperature.

$$2ICl(g) \rightarrow I_2(g) + Cl_2(g)$$

Which of the following is TRUE?
A. $\Delta H > 0, \Delta S > 0$
B. $\Delta H > 0, \Delta S < 0$
C. $\Delta H < 0, \Delta S > 0$
D. $\Delta H < 0, \Delta S < 0$

26. Which of the following is the reason that water boils at a much higher temperature than hydrogen sulfide?

A. The intramolecular O–H bonds are stronger than the intramolecular S–H bonds.
B. The enthalpy of vaporization of water is less than that of hydrogen sulfide.
C. The relative molecular mass of water is less than that of hydrogen sulfide.
D. The intermolecular O–H bonds are stronger than the intermolecular S–H bonds.

27. In the figure below, aqueous solutions A and B are separated by a semipermeable membrane. Which of the following will occur?

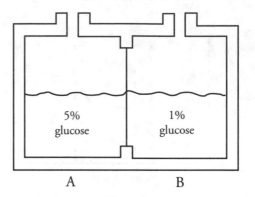

5% glucose   1% glucose

A   B

A. Glucose molecules will move from side B to side A.
B. Glucose molecules will move from side A to side B.
C. Both water and glucose molecules will move from side A to side B.
D. Water molecules will move from side B to side A.

28. What is the normality of a solution containing 49g of H_3PO_4 (MW 98) in 2000 mL of solution?

A. 0.25
B. 0.50
C. 0.75
D. 1.50

GO ON TO THE NEXT PAGE.

Passage V (Questions 29–33)

Band theory explains the conductivity of certain solids by stating that the atomic orbitals of the individual atoms in the solid merge to produce a series of atomic orbitals comprising the entire solid. The closely spaced energy levels of the orbitals form bands. The band corresponding to the outermost occupied subshell of the original atoms is called the valence band. If partially full, as in metals, it serves as a conduction band through which electrons can move freely. If the valence band is full, then electrons must be raised to a higher band for conduction to occur. The greater the band gap between the separate valence and conduction bands, the poorer is the material's conductivity. Figure 1 shows the valence and conduction bands of a semiconductor, which is intermediate in conductivity between conductors and insulators.

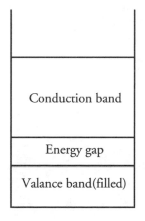

Figure 1

When silicon, a semiconductor with tetrahedral covalent bonds, is heated, a few electrons escape into the conduction band. Doping the silicon with a few phosphorus atoms provides unbonded electrons that escape more easily, increasing conductivity. Doping with boron produces holes in the bonding structure, which may be filled by movement of nearby electrons within the lattice. When a semiconductor in an electric circuit has excess electrons on one side and holes on the other, electron flow occurs more easily from the side with excess electrons to the side with holes than in the reverse direction.

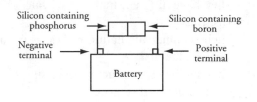

Figure 2

29. Why is iron a good conductor of electricity?

  A. Its 3*d* electrons only partially fill the valence band.
  B. The band gap is small.
  C. The 4*s* and 3*d* orbitals form a filled valence band.
  D. The energy levels of the atomic orbitals are closely spaced.

30. How could heat be expected to increase the conductivity of a semiconductor?

  I. By reducing collisions between moving electrons
  II. By breaking covalent bonds
  III. By raising electrons to a higher energy level

  A. I only
  B. III only
  C. I and III only
  D. II and III only

GO ON TO THE NEXT PAGE.

31. Why do phosphorus and boron atoms enhance the conductivity of silicon?

    A. Their electronegativity differs from that of silicon.
    B. They have different numbers of valence electrons.
    C. Their semimetallic nature makes them good semiconductors.
    D. They are better conductors than silicon even as pure substances.

32. The energy gap for pure silicon is about 1.1 electron volts. If a 1.5 volt electrical potential is connected across a sample of silicon:

    A. the electrons would jump to the conduction band and the silicon would conduct.
    B. the holes in the silicon lattice would move.
    C. the energy gap would be lowered.
    D. the silicon would not conduct.

33. If the semiconductor orientation in Figure 2 were reversed so that the boron-doped silicon were on the left and the phosphorus-doped silicon on the right, what could be said about the electron flow of the new setup?

    A. The electron flow is easier in the new direction than that of Figure 2.
    B. The electron flow is the same in either direction.
    C. The electron flow is harder in the new direction than that of Figure 2.
    D. The electrons cannot flow.

GO ON TO THE NEXT PAGE.

Passage VI (Questions 34–38)

A helium-neon gas discharge laser as shown in Figure 1 below generates a coherent beam of monochromatic light at a wavelength of 632.8 nm.

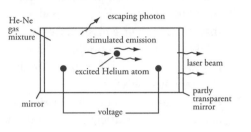

Figure 1

A discharge current of electrons is created in the tube by an applied voltage. When these electrons collide with the helium atoms, they can excite ground-state helium electrons to an energy level of 20.61 eV. The excited electrons cannot decay back to the ground state by emitting a photon because such a transition does not conserve angular momentum. Instead, if the excited helium atom collides with a neon atom, a ground-state electron in the neon atom can be excited to an energy level of 20.66 eV, and the helium electron can return to its ground state.

The above process occurs quite often in the tube until the percentage of neon atoms with electrons in the 20.66-eV energy level is greater than the percentage of neon atoms with electrons in lower levels. This condition is called a population inversion. An excited electron in one of the neon atoms can then spontaneously decay by emitting a photon of wavelength 632.8 nm in a random direction. The photon will stimulate the same transition in another excited atom. The photon radiated by this stimulated emission process travels in the same direction as the original photon. The resulting light is then reflected back and forth inside the tube until it escapes through the partially transparent mirror. (Note: A photon's energy in eV is given by $E = 1240/\lambda$, where λ is the photon's wavelength in nm. The helium and neon ground state energies are both 0 eV.)

34. What is the energy of the photon with wavelength 632.8 nm?

   A. 0.05 eV
   B. 1.96 eV
   C. 20.61 eV
   D. 20.66 eV

35. A population inversion exists when:

   A. the percentage of neon atoms with electrons in the ground state is greater than the percentage of neon atoms with electrons in higher energy levels.
   B. the percentage of neon atoms with electrons in a higher energy level is greater than the percentage of neon atoms with electrons in lower energy levels.
   C. the percentage of neon atoms with electrons in a higher energy level is equal to the percentage of neon atoms with electrons in the ground state.
   D. all the neon atoms have electrons in the ground state only.

GO ON TO THE NEXT PAGE.

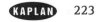 223

36. A helium atom with an electron in the 20.61-eV energy level collides with a neon atom with an electron in the ground state. The result is that the helium electron returns to the ground state, and the ground state neon electron is excited to an energy level of 20.66 eV. What is the minimum kinetic energy lost by the helium atom?

    A. 0.05 eV
    B. 1.96 eV
    C. 10.30 eV
    D. 20.61 eV

37. A laser produces light with a wavelength of 200 nm at a power of 6.2×10^{15} eV/s. How many photons per second does this laser deliver?

    A. 1.0×10^{15}
    B. 2.0×10^{15}
    C. 4.0×10^{15}
    D. 10.0×10^{15}

38. Why is stimulated emission of photons necessary in order to produce a coherent beam of light instead of spontaneous emission alone?

    A. Stimulated emission produces photons of higher energy than those produced by spontaneous emission.
    B. Stimulated emission produces photons that travel in the same direction as the photon that induces their emission.
    C. Stimulated emission produces photons with longer wavelengths than those produced by spontaneous emission.
    D. Either spontaneous or stimulated emission alone would be sufficient to produce laser light.

GO ON TO THE NEXT PAGE.

Passage VII (Questions 39–44)

One of the most common methods that scientists use to determine the age of fossils is known as carbon dating. ^{14}C is an unstable isotope of carbon that undergoes beta decay with a half-life of approximately 5,730 years. Beta decay occurs when a neutron in the nucleus decays to form a proton and an electron which is ejected from the nucleus.

^{14}C is generated in the upper atmosphere when ^{14}N, the most common isotope of nitrogen, is bombarded by neutrons. This mechanism yields a global production rate of 7.5 kg per year of ^{14}C, which combines with oxygen in the atmosphere to produce carbon dioxide. Both the production and the decay of ^{14}C occur simultaneously. This process continues for many half-lives of ^{14}C until the total amount of ^{14}C approaches a constant.

A fixed fraction of the carbon ingested by all living organisms will be ^{14}C. Therefore, as long as an organism is alive, the ratio of $1^{14}C$ to ^{12}C that it contains is constant. After the organism dies, no new ^{14}C is ingested, and the amount of ^{14}C contained in the organism will decrease by beta decay. The amount of ^{14}C that must have been present in the organism when it died can be calculated from the amount of ^{12}C present in a fossil. By comparing the amount of ^{14}C in the fossil to the calculated amount of ^{14}C that was present in the organism when it died, the age of the fossil can be determined.

39. The bones of a living adult human contain about 8 grams of ^{14}C at any given time. If a prehistoric human skeleton is found to contain 1 gram of ^{14}C, how long ago did the person die?

A. 5,730 years
B. 17,190 years
C. 34,380 years
D. 45,840 years

40. If the production rate of ^{14}C were to increase to 10 kg per year:

A. the number of ^{14}C atoms decaying per minute would increase.
B. the number of ^{14}C atoms decaying per minute would decrease.
C. the weight of ^{14}C on the earth would increase indefinitely.
D. the percentage of ^{14}C in living organisms would not change.

41. The method of carbon dating used to determine age depends upon the assumption that:

A. the half-life of ^{14}C changes when it is ingested.
B. all ingested ^{14}C is incorporated into the body.
C. the half-life of ^{14}C depends on the type of molecule in which it resides.
D. the half-life of ^{14}C does not depend upon conditions external to the nucleus.

GO ON TO THE NEXT PAGE.

42. In determining the age of the galaxy, a technique similar to carbon dating is used on stars with the radioactive isotope ^{232}Th, which has a half-life of 10^{10} years. ^{14}C is less suitable for this application because:

A. its half-life is too long.
B. ^{14}C is more abundant in stars.
C. ^{14}C is unstable.
D. its half-life is too short.

43. In generating ^{14}C in the upper atmosphere, a ^{14}N nucleus combines with a neutron to form a ^{14}C nucleus and:

A. a proton.
B. an electron.
C. a ^{4}He nucleus.
D. a neutron.

44. After a ^{14}C nucleus decays, the electron that is emitted enters lead and is stopped. What percentage of its kinetic energy does the electron transfer to lead?

A. 25%
B. 33%
C. 50%
D. 100%

GO ON TO THE NEXT PAGE.

Passage VIII (Questions 45–49)

Arsenic is widely distributed in sulfide ores of many metals and is obtained as a by-product of copper smelting. The element, as well as many compounds of arsenic—for example arsine, AsH_3—are extremely poisonous. Arsenic compounds, as might be expected, have found use in herbicides and pesticides, but have also been successful in some pharmacological agents. The first useful antisyphilitic agent, Salvarsan or 3,3′-diamino-4,4′-dihydroxyarsenobenzene dihydrochloride, is an arsenic compound. The element sublimes at 600°C, forming tetrahedral molecules, As_4. Arsenic is a metalloid, possessing properties characteristic of both metals and non-metals. Ordinarily arsenic is a gray colored metallic-looking solid, but the vapor is yellow in color, has a garliclike odor, and is very poisonous. If the arsenic vapor is cooled rapidly, an unstable yellow crystalline allotrope consisting of As_4 molecules is produced.

The Marsh test, based on the instability of arsine, is a very sensitive test for the presence of arsenic. This test is commonly employed in the detection of arsenic poisoning—either before or after death. The apparatus for the Marsh test is shown in Figure 1.

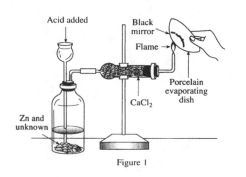

Figure 1

Typically, a sample, usually hair, is taken from a person suspected of being the victim of arsenic poisoning. This sample is then treated in such a way so as to produce arsenic oxide, As_4O_6. The oxide is then placed into the apparatus shown in Figure 1 and reacted according to Reaction 1.

$As_4O_6 + 12\ Zn(s) + 24\ H^+(aq) \rightarrow 4\ AsH_3(g) + 12\ Zn^{2+}(aq) + 6H_2O$

Reaction 1

When the evolved arsine is ignited it decomposes into its elements. The arsenic vapor is rapidly cooled when it encounters the porcelain evaporating dish and deposits a black mirror of arsenic on the bottom, indicating the presence of arsenic in the original sample.

45. The phase diagram for arsenic is shown below. At what point does liquid arsenic exist?

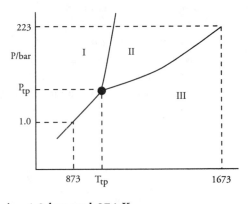

A. 1.0 bar and 874 K
B. 1.0 bar and 1673 K
C. 223 bar and 1672 K
D. 223 bar and 873 K

GO ON TO THE NEXT PAGE.

46. What is the most likely purpose of the calcium chloride in Figure 1?

A. To remove water from the evolved arsine gas.
B. To remove HCl from the evolved arsine gas.
C. To react with the zinc ion making the reaction go to completion.
D. To react with the evolved arsine gas.

47. If equal masses of gray arsenic and yellow arsenic are allowed to completely react with oxygen at 298 K and constant pressure to form As_4O_6, which would produce more heat and why?

A. The yellow, because it is less stable than the gray.
B. The gray, because it is more stable than the yellow.
C. Both would produce the same amount of heat because they form the same product.
D. Both would produce the same amount of heat because they are the same element.

48. The Marsh test takes advantage of the fact that arsine is not very soluble in water. Since arsenic is below nitrogen on the periodic table, it would be expected that arsine, like ammonia, would be very soluble in water. What is the most likely reason for this difference in solubility?

A. Arsine has a higher molecular weight than ammonia.
B. Arsine has a smaller dipole moment than ammonia.
C. Arsine is less basic than ammonia.
D. Arsine is less stable than ammonia.

49. A common ore of arsenic is called orpiment, As_2S_3. What is the oxidation state of arsenic in orpiment?

A. −3
B. 0
C. +3
D. +6

GO ON TO THE NEXT PAGE.

50. What is the shape of a molecule of NH_3?

    A. Trigonal planar
    B. Pyramidal
    C. Tetrahedral
    D. Trigonal bipyramidal

51. A deep sea research module has a volume of 150 m^3. If ocean water has an average density of 1,025 kg/m^3, what will be the buoyant force on the module when it is completely submerged in the water? (Note: The acceleration due to gravity is 9.8 m/s^2.)

    A. 9.8 N
    B. 60 N
    C. 1×103 N
    D. 1.5×106 N

52. If a spring is 64 cm long when it is unstretched and is 8 percent longer when a 0.5–kg mass hangs from it, how long will it be with a 0.4–kg mass suspended from it?

    A. 66 cm
    B. 68 cm
    C. 70 cm
    D. 74 cm

53. Which of the following will halve the magnitude of the electrostatic force of attraction between two charged particles?

    A. Doubling the distance between the particles
    B. Halving the charge on each particle
    C. Halving the charge on one of the particles only
    D. Placing a positively charged particle midway between the particles

54. Which of the following is true when ice melts?

    A. The changes in both enthalpy and entropy are positive.
    B. The changes in both enthalpy and entropy are negative.
    C. The change in enthalpy is positive; the change in entropy is negative.
    D. The change in enthalpy is negative; the change in entropy is positive.

GO ON TO THE NEXT PAGE.

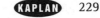

Passage IX (Questions 55–59)

When softball players take batting practice, they often use a machine called an "automatic pitcher," which is essentially a cannon that uses air pressure to launch a projectile. In a prototype automatic pitcher, a softball is loaded into the barrel of the cannon and rests against a flat disk. This disk is locked into place, and a high air pressure is built up behind it. When the disk is released, the softball is pushed along the barrel of the cannon and ejected at a speed of v_0.

Figure 1 shows the batter and automatic pitcher. The angle of the barrel to the horizontal is θ. The unit vectors i and j point in the horizontal and vertical directions respectively.

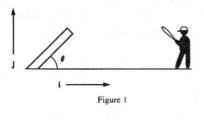

Figure I

Figure 1

The height above the ground y of the softball as a function of time t is shown in Figure 2, where $t = 0$ at Point A, $t = t_B$ at Point B, and $t = t_C$ at Point C. The softball is ejected from the barrel of the cannon at Point A; it reaches its maximum height at Point B; and the batter hits the softball at Point C. (Note: Assume that the effects of air resistance are negligible, unless otherwise stated.)

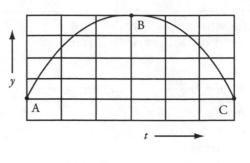

Figure 2

55. What physical quantity is NOT the same at Point C as it is at Point A?

    A. The velocity of the softball
    B. The speed of the softball
    C. The gravitational potential energy of the softball
    D. The horizontal component of the velocity of the softball

56. What is the acceleration of the softball t seconds after it exits the barrel?

    A. $-g$ j
    B. $-v_0/t$ i
    C. $-v_0/t$ j
    D. $-v_0/t$ i $- g$ j

57. How will v_0 change if the impulse on the softball remains the same but its mass is doubled?

    A. It will decrease by a factor of 4.
    B. It will decrease by a factor of 2.
    C. It will not change.
    D. It will increase by a factor of 2.

GO ON TO THE NEXT PAGE.

58. What is the ratio of the horizontal distance travelled by the softball at Point B to the horizontal distance travelled at Point C?

   A. 5:1
   B. 4:1
   C. 3:3
   D. 1:2

59. How does the work done by the automatic pitcher change as the angle of the barrel to the horizontal increases?

   A. The work done increases, because the softball's maximum height increases.
   B. The work done decreases, because the softball lands closer to the cannon.
   C. The work done does not change, because the air pressure behind the disk is unchanged.
   D. The work done does not change, because gravity is a conservative force.

GO ON TO THE NEXT PAGE.

Passage X (Questions 60–65)

There are two opposing theories of light: the particle theory and the wave theory. According to the particle theory, light is composed of a stream of tiny particles that are subject to the same physical laws as other types of elementary particles. One consequence of this is that light particles should travel in a straight line unless an external force acts on them. According to the wave theory, light is a wave that shares the characteristics of other waves. Among other things, this means that light waves should interfere with each other under certain conditions.

In support of the wave theory of light, Thomas Young's double slit experiment proves that light does indeed exhibit interference. Figure 1 shows the essential features of the experiment. Parallel rays of monochromatic light pass through two narrow slits and are projected onto a screen. Constructive interference occurs at certain points on the screen, producing bright areas of maximum light intensity. Between these maxima, destructive interference produces light intensity minima. The positions of the maxima are given by the equation $d\sin\theta = n\lambda$, where d is the distance between the slits, θ is the angle shown in Figure 1, the integer n specifies the particular maxima, and λ is the wavelength of the incident light. (Note: $\sin\theta \approx \tan\theta \approx \theta$ for small angles.)

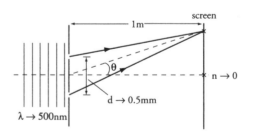

Figure 1

60. What is the angle θ for the third maximum ($n = 3$)?

    A. 3×10^{-5} radians
    B. 3×10^{-3} radians
    C. 0.3 radians
    D. 0.3 degrees

61. Which of the following supports the particle theory of light?

    A. The energy of light is quantized.
    B. Light exhibits interference.
    C. Light is subject to the Doppler effect.
    D. No particle can have a speed greater than the speed of light.

62. A beam of electrons can also produce an interference pattern. Which one of the following expressions gives a consistent definition of an electron's "wavelength" if it has a total energy given by E? (Note: h = 6.6×10^{-34} J•s is Planck's constant and v is the speed of the electrons.)

    A. hvE
    B. hE/v
    C. hv/E
    D. E/hv

GO ON TO THE NEXT PAGE.

63. Which of the following is sufficient information to determine the approximate speed of a ray of light in water?

    A. The angle of incidence and the angle of refraction of the light ray as it enters water from air
    B. The wavelength in water and the wavelength in air of the light ray as it enters water from air
    C. The speed of light in a vacuum and the density of water
    D. The speed of light in a vacuum and the index of refraction of water

64. Light waves can be described in terms of frequency f and wavelength λ or in terms of wave number k and angular frequency ω. These quantities are related by the following equations:

$$k = 2\pi/\lambda \text{ and } \omega = 2\pi f$$

Which equation below accurately describes the speed of the wave v in terms of k and ω ?

    A. $v = f\lambda$
    B. $v = \omega + k$
    C. $v = \omega/k$
    D. $v = \omega k$

65. According to the modern theory of light, a beam of light may be described either as a stream of particles or as a wave, depending on the circumstances. Which of the following correctly states a connection between the two descriptions?

    A. The number of light particles that pass by per second is proportional to the frequency of the light wave.
    B. The mass of each particle of light is proportional to the intensity of the light wave.
    C. The size of each particle of light is proportional to the wavelength of the light wave.
    D. The energy of each particle of light is proportional to the frequency of the light wave.

GO ON TO THE NEXT PAGE.

Passage XI (Questions 66–72)

A researcher investigated the equilibrium between CO_2, C, and CO as a function of temperature. The equation is given below.

$$CO_2(g) + C(s) \rightleftharpoons 2\ CO(g)$$

Carbon dioxide, at 298 K and 1 atm, and an excess of powdered carbon were introduced into a furnace, which was then sealed so that pressure would increase as the temperature rose. The furnace was heated to and held constant at a predetermined temperature. The pressure within the furnace chamber was recorded after it had remained unchanged for one hour. The table below shows the pressures recorded for a series of temperatures together with the pressures expected if no reaction had taken place.

Table 1

T(K)	P_r (P recorded after reaction, in atm)	P_e (P expected without reaction, in atm)
900	3.4	3.0
950	3.8	3.2
1000	4.3	3.4
1050	5.0	3.5
1200	7.2	4.0

66. When the system stabilized at 1200 K, a sample of helium was injected into the furnace. What should happen to the amount of carbon dioxide in the system?

A. It should increase.
B. It should decrease.
C. It should be completely converted to carbon monoxide.
D. It will remain the same.

67. What can be said about the value of $\Delta S°$ of the reaction?

A. It is positive.
B. It is negative.
C. It is zero.
D. It cannot be determined from the information given.

68. How many pi bonds are in the carbon dioxide molecule?

A. 0
B. 1
C. 2
D. 3

69. Which of the following is NOT necessarily true about the equilibrium reaction between CO_2, C, and CO?

A. The standard entropy change is positive.
B. A decrease in pressure at constant temperature would shift the equilibrium to the right.
C. Addition of CO will shift the equilibrium to the left.
D. The standard Gibbs' free energy change is negative.

GO ON TO THE NEXT PAGE.

70. Which of the following shows the correct Lewis structure of carbon monoxide?

A.

$:C{=}\ddot{O}$

B.

$\ddot{C}{=}\ddot{O}$

C.

$:C{\equiv}O:$

D.

$:C{\equiv}\ddot{O}$

71. How are the values of Pe calculated?

A. $(T/273)(1\ atm)$
B. $(T/298)(1\ atm)$
C. $[(T - 273)/273](1\ atm)$
D. $[(T - 298)/298](1\ atm)$

72. If 0.6 g of elemental carbon are consumed during a trial, how many grams of CO are produced?

A. 0.8
B. 1.4
C. 1.6
D. 2.8

GO ON TO THE NEXT PAGE.

73. Light traveling from air into a new medium is refracted away from the normal. This medium might be:

    A. glass.
    B. water.
    C. steel.
    D. a vacuum.

74. Which expression correctly expresses the K_{sp} of a solution of X_mY_n?

    A. $[X^{m+}]^n[Y^{n-}]^m$
    B. $[X^{n+}]^m[Y^{m-}]^n$
    C. $([X^{m+}]^n[Y^{n-}]^m)/X_mY_n$
    D. $([X^{n+}]^m[Y^{m-}]^n)/X_mY_n$

75. Which of the following species exists as a resonance hybrid?

    A. HCN
    B. H_2CO_3
    C. NO_2^-
    D. ClO^-

76. If the reaction between Q and R is third order overall, what is the value of x in the table below?

Trial	Concentration of Q (M)	Concentration of R (M)	Initial rate (M/sec)
1	1.00	1.00	6×10^{-8}
2	2.00	1.00	12×10^{-8}
3	2.00	x	48×10^{-8}

    A. 2.00
    B. 3.00
    C. 4.00
    D. 6.00

77. The temperature of an iron bar is raised, and it expands. If the temperature of a second iron bar, which is initially twice as long as the first bar, is raised by twice as much, what is the ratio of the change in length of the first bar to the change in length of the second bar?

    A. 1:1
    B. 1:2
    C. 1:4
    D. 2:1

STOP.

IF YOU FINISH BEFORE TIME HAS EXPIRED, CHECK YOUR WORK.
YOU MAY GO BACK TO ANY QUESTION IN THIS PART ONLY.

Verbal Reasoning Test

Time: 85 minutes
Questions 78–137

DIRECTIONS: There are nine passages in this Verbal Reasoning test. Each passage is followed by several questions. After reading a passage, select the one best answer to each question. If you are not certain of an answer, eliminate the alternatives that you know to be incorrect and then select an answer from the remaining alternatives. Indicate your selection by blackening the corresponding oval on your answer document.

Passage I (Questions 78–85)

Although nihilism is commonly defined as a form of extremist political thought, the term has a broader meaning. Nihilism is in fact a complex
Line intellectual stance with venerable roots in the histo-
5 ry of ideas, which forms the theoretical basis for many positive assertions of modern thought. Its essence is the systematic negation of all perceptual orders and assumptions. A complete view must account for the influence of two historical crosscur-
10 rents: philosophical skepticism about the ultimacy of any truth, and the mystical quest for that same pure truth. These are united by their categorical rejection of the "known."

The outstanding representative of the former
15 current, David Hume (1711–1776), maintained that external reality is unknowable, since sense perceptions give no information whatsoever about what really exists. Hume points out that sense impressions are actually part of the contents of the mind.
20 Their presumed correspondence to external "things" cannot be verified, since it can be checked only by other sense impressions. Hume further asserts that all abstract conceptions turn out, on examination, to be generalizations from sense impressions. He
25 concludes that even such an apparently objective phenomenon as a cause-and-effect relationship between events may be no more than a subjective fabrication of the observer. Stanley Rosen notes: "Hume terminates in skepticism because he finds
30 nothing within the subject but individual impressions and ideas."

For mystics of every faith, the "experience of nothingness" is the goal of spiritual practice. Buddhist meditation techniques involve the system-
35 atic negation of all spiritual and intellectual constructs to make way for the apprehension of pure truth. St. John of the Cross similarly rejected every physical and mental symbolization of God as illusory. St. John's spiritual legacy is, as Michael Novak
40 puts it, "the constant return to inner solitude, an unbroken awareness of the emptiness at the heart of consciousness. It is a harsh refusal to allow idols to be placed in the sanctuary. It requires also a scorching gaze upon all the bureaucracies, institutions,
45 manipulators, and hucksters who employ technology and its supposed realities to bewitch and bedazzle the psyche."

Novak's interpretation points to the way these philosophical and mystical traditions prepared the
50 ground for the political nihilism of the nineteenth and twentieth centuries. The rejection of existing social institutions and their claims to authority is in the most basic sense made possible by Humean skepticism. The political nihilism of the Russian
55 intelligentsia combined this radical skepticism with a near-mystical faith in the power of a new beginning. Hence, their desire to destroy becomes a revolutionary affirmation; in the words of Stanley Rosen, "Nihilism is an attempt to overcome or repu-
60 diate the past on behalf of an unknown and unknowable, yet hoped-for, future." This fusion of skepticism and mystical re-creation can be traced in contemporary thought, for example as an element in the counterculture of the 1960s.

GO ON TO THE NEXT PAGE.

  237

78. The author's working definition of *nihilism*, as it functions in the passage, is:

    A. systematic doubt of that which one takes for granted.
    B. a mystical quest for nothingness.
    C. a form of extremist political thought.
    D. rejection of all presently established institutions.

79. The passage implies that the two strands of nihilist thought:

    A. are combined in nineteenth and twentieth century political nihilism.
    B. remained essentially separate after the eighteenth century.
    C. are necessary prerequisites for any positive, modern social thought.
    D. are derived from distinct Eastern and Western philosophical traditions.

80. In the passage, quotations from writers about nihilism are used in order to:

    I. summarize specific points made in the course of the passage.
    II. contrast points of view on the subject under discussion.
    III. make transitions between points in the discussion.

    A. I only
    B. I and II only
    C. I and III only
    D. II and III only

81. Which is a necessary assumption underlying Hume's conclusion that external reality is unknowable, as discussed in the passage?

    A. Nothing outside the mind exists.
    B. The contents of the mind consist exclusively of sense impressions.
    C. Causality is a subjective projection of the mind.
    D. Sense impressions provide our only information about external reality.

82. Novak's interpretation of St. John's spiritual legacy (lines 39–47) is important to the author's argument primarily because it:

    A. characterizes the essence of St. John's mystical doctrine.
    B. gives insight into the historical antecedents of political nihilism.
    C. draws a parallel between Christian mysticism and the Humean tradition of philosophical skepticism.
    D. suggests that St. John's teachings are influential mainly because of their sociopolitical implications.

83. The author uses all of the following techniques in developing the topic EXCEPT:

    A. discussion of individuals as representative of intellectual trends.
    B. a contrast between a common definition and his own.
    C. identification of the common elements in distinct intellectual traditions.
    D. examination of the practical consequences of a social doctrine.

GO ON TO THE NEXT PAGE.

84. In the last paragraph, the author quotes Stanley Rosen in order to make the point that modern nihilism is:

    A. impractical because of its faith in an unknowable future.
    B. more than just a movement to do away with existing institutions.
    C. a living doctrine rather than merely a part of the history of political theory.
    D. based more on the tradition of philosophical skepticism than on that of mystical affirmation.

85. Which of the following provides the best continuation for the final paragraph of the passage?

    A. Thus, the negative effects of nihilism are still being felt.
    B. Classical nihilism has thus been superseded by a new and unrelated type.
    C. The revolutionaries of that time did, after all, reject society and hope for something better.
    D. The study of nihilism, then, belongs to the past rather than to the present.

Passage II (Questions 86–91)

Agonistic behavior, or aggression, is exhibited by most of the more than three million species of animals on this planet. Animal behaviorists still
Line disagree on a comprehensive definition of the
5 term, but aggressive behavior can be loosely described as any action that harms an adversary or compels it to retreat. Aggression may serve many purposes, such as food gathering, establishing territory, and enforcing social hierarchy. In a general
10 Darwinian sense, however, the purpose of aggressive behavior is to increase the individual animal's—and thus, the species'—chance of survival.

Aggressive behavior may be directed at animals of other species, or it may be conspecific—that
15 is, directed at members of an animal's own species. One of the most common examples of conspecific aggression occurs in the establishment and maintenance of social hierarchies. In a hierarchy, social dominance is usually established according to phys-
20 ical superiority; the classic example is that of a pecking order among domestic fowl. The dominance hierarchy may be viewed as a means of social control that reduces the incidence of attack within a group. Once established, the hierarchy is rarely
25 threatened by disputes because the inferior animal immediately submits when confronted by a superior.

Two basic types of aggressive behavior are common to most species: attack and defensive threat. Each type involves a particular pattern of
30 physiological and behavioral responses, which tends not to vary regardless of the stimulus that provokes it. For example, the pattern of attack behavior in cats involves a series of movements, such as stalking, biting, seizing with the forepaws and scratching with
35 the hind legs, that changes very little regardless of the stimulus—that is, regardless of who or what the cat is attacking.

The cat's defensive threat response offers another set of closely linked physiological and
40 behavioral patterns. The cardiovascular system begins to pump blood at a faster rate, in preparation for sudden physical activity. The eyes narrow and the ears flatten against the side of the cat's head for protection, and other vulnerable areas of the body such
45 as the stomach and throat are similarly contracted. Growling or hissing noises and erect fur also signal defensive threat. As with the attack response, this pattern of responses is generated with little variation regardless of the nature of the stimulus.

50 Are these aggressive patterns of attack and defensive threat innate, genetically programmed, or are they learned? The answer seems to be a combination of both. A mouse is helpless at birth, but by its twelfth day of life can assume a defen-
55 sive threat position by backing up on its hind legs. By the time it is one month old, the mouse begins to exhibit the attack response. Nonetheless, copious evidence suggests that animals learn and practice aggressive behavior; one need look no further
60 than the sight of a kitten playing with a ball of string. All the elements of attack—stalking, pouncing, biting and shaking—are part of the game which prepares the kitten for more serious situations later in life.

86. The passage asserts that animal social hierarchies are generally stable because:

A. the behavior responses of the group are known by all its members.
B. the defensive threat posture quickly stops most conflicts.
C. inferior animals usually defer to their physical superiors.
D. the need for mutual protection from other species inhibits conspecific aggression.

GO ON TO THE NEXT PAGE.

87. According to the author, what is the most significant physiological change undergone by a cat assuming the defensive threat position?

    A. An increase in cardiovascular activity

    B. A sudden narrowing of the eyes

    C. A contraction of the abdominal muscles

    D. The author does not say which change is most significant

88. Based on the information in the passage about agonistic behavior, it is reasonable to conclude that:

    I. the purpose of agonistic behavior is to help ensure the survival of the species.

    II. agonistic behavior is both innate and learned.

    III. conspecific aggression is more frequent than interspecies aggression.

    A. I only

    B. II only

    C. I and II only

    D. I, II, and III

89. The author suggests that the question of whether agonistic behavior is genetically programmed or learned:

    A. still generates considerable controversy among animal behaviorists.

    B. was first investigated through experiments on mice.

    C. is outdated since most scientists now believe the genetic element to be most important.

    D. has been the subject of extensive clinical study.

90. Which of the following topics related to agonistic behavior is NOT explicitly addressed in the passage?

    A. The physiological changes that accompany attack behavior in cats

    B. The evolutionary purpose of aggression

    C. Conspecific aggression that occurs in dominance hierarchies

    D. The relationship between play and aggression

91. Which of the following would be most in accord with the information presented in the passage?

    A. The aggressive behavior of sharks is closely linked to their need to remain in constant motion.

    B. The inability of newborn mice to exhibit the attack response proves that aggressive behavior must be learned.

    C. Most animal species that do not exhibit aggressive behavior are prevented from doing so by environmental factors.

    D. Members of a certain species of hawk use the same method to prey on both squirrels and gophers.

GO ON TO THE NEXT PAGE.

 241

Passage III (Questions 92–99)

The Gypsies, or Romani people, are found throughout Europe, as well as in the Americas, the Middle East, and Asia. The Romani have emerged
Line as a culturally linked constellation of nomadic
5 groups, little understood by outsiders, that include, but are not limited to, the Kalderash, Machavaya, Lovari, Churari, Roanichal, Gitanoes, Kalo, Sinti, Rudari, Manush, Boyash, Ungaritza, Luri, Bashalde, Romongro, and Xoraxai. What led
10 to the original Romani diaspora remains shrouded in mystery. Historical linguists, however, have begun to trace their migratory paths, as well as to estimate when their migrations occurred.

Most scholars agree on their basic migratory
15 route, which began in Northwestern India between 800 and 950 A.D., and progressed through the upper Indus Valley, across the Himalayas, and down the Silk Road to the southern shores of the Caspian Sea. From there they
20 followed the west coast to the foothills of the Caucasus, through Armenia, and into the Byzantine Empire. Romani then entered the Balkans and drifted throughout Europe. There is considerably less consensus, however, about
25 whether there was one migration or several and what exactly was the time frame of the migration.

Linguists who support a single emigration hypothesis cite linguistic similarities between Romani and a group of Sanskrit-based languages
30 that includes Rajasthani, Hindi, Gujarati, Bengali, and Multani. According to these linguists, Romani developed in parallel with these languages until the 11th century A.D. and then diverged from the others, which continued to develop in syn-
35 chronicity. Furthermore, they point to the fact that all European Romani dialects include the same "loan words" from Dardic, Persian, Armenian, Byzantine Greek, Old Slavic, and Romanian.

40 Other scholars, however, use linguistic evidence to show that the Romani, who today fall into three major subgroups—the Domari or "Dom," Lomavren or "Lom," and Romani or "Rom"—did not separate from one original group, but were
45 rather three distinct groups who left India at three different times. These researchers look to the linguistic dissimilarities among the three branches, such as the fact that although all three branches show lexical adoption from Persian, there are no
50 specific items shared by all three branches. Further, vestiges of a third grammatical gender in Lom and Rom indicate to these linguists that these groups left India later than the Dom.

The very flexibility of the Romani language
55 ensures that historical linguists will continue to debate the migratory paths of the various Romani tribes. In one Sinto dialect, for instance, the word *svigardaj* (mother-in-law) has been constituted from *daj* (mother, of Sanskrit origin) and an adap-
60 tation of the German word *Schweiger* (*Schwieger-mutter* means mother-in-law). Among Muslim Romani in the south of Yugoslavia, the word *ledome* (frozen) can be traced to the Slav word *led* (ice) followed by the suffix *me*, which is of Greek
65 origin. While these linguistic borrowings clearly enrich the language of the Romani and provide endless fodder for speculation among academics, it also makes the difficulties of understanding between the different groups more acute, as the
70 dialects continue to diverge.

Even the origin of the name *Gypsy* is subject to linguistic debate. Some scholars claim that the word *Gypsy* refers to the dark-skinned people from the Middle East who were brought to Europe
75 before the arrival of the Romani to serve as entertainers and were loosely known as "Egyptians." When the Romani arrived, they, too, were identified as Egyptians, which was later shortened to Gypsy. Others, however, trace the origin of the
80 name to the Byzantine Empire, where Romani were falsely linked with the heretical sect of

GO ON TO THE NEXT PAGE.

Athiganoi, thus leading to the Italian *zingari*, the French *tsiganes*, the German *Zigeuner*, the Czech *cikan*, and, among others, the English word, *Gypsy*.

85 *Gypsy*.

92. According to the author, what is the major evidence that linguists cite to support the single emigration hypothesis?

    A. Similarity in dress among Romani groups in geographically diverse locations
    B. Common grammatical structures among three different branches of Gypsies
    C. Vocabulary found among all Romani that is borrowed from several foreign languages
    D. Historical records kept by the Romani indicating the path of their migration

93. The author introduces the debate over the origin of the word *Gypsy* to show that:

    A. the Romani share cultural traditions with Egyptians and Greeks.
    B. the Romani language is difficult to pronounce accurately in modern European languages.
    C. the Romani have been falsely identified as a unified group when, in fact, their members comprise three culturally and linguistically independent groups.
    D. the Romani history is incomplete and highly debated, even among scholars.

94. Which of the following would most weaken the argument that the Romani emigrated from India at three different times?

    A. Linguistic evidence that all three branches did share identical Persian words, having lost the similarity in recent centuries
    B. Variations in pronunciation of similar words among different Romani groups
    C. Historical linguistic similarity between Sanskrit-based languages and other nomadic peoples following the same migratory route as the Romani
    D. Archeological artifacts linking Byzantine-era Romani and the Athiganoi

95. According to the passage, the Romani have migrated to which of the following countries?

    I. France
    II. Armenia
    III. China

    A. I only
    B. II only
    C. I and II
    D. I, II, and III

GO ON TO THE NEXT PAGE.

96. Which of the following pieces of information, if offered as new evidence, would support the multiple emigration hypothesis described in the fourth paragraph?

    A. A Hindi text from the ninth century A.D. refers to both the Dom and the Lom.
    B. Many Persian words have three or four distinct meanings.
    C. A 13th-century Armenian folk tale mentions Gypsies.
    D. Descendants of the Romani still live in India.

97. The author of this passage would most likely look for information relevant to the arguments made in the passage in:

    A. a religious text of the *zingari*.
    B. a poem written in both Bengali and Romani.
    C. an 11th-century Romani painting.
    D. a comparison of Dom and Rom cuisines.

98. Which of the following would cast doubt on the single emigration theory?

    A. The Romani had an oral history of the migration from India that was finally committed to writing only in the 19th century.
    B. The similarities between Romani and Hindi stem from a relation between each of them and a third language that arose in the 15th century.
    C. Linguistic analysis is shown to be more useful for tracing migratory paths than for fixing the dates of migrations.
    D. Linguists supporting this theory are not involved in the linguistic debate over the origin of the word *Gypsy*.

99. Which of the following best characterizes the author's claim that the Romani are "little understood by outsiders" (line 5)?

    A. It is contradicted by the historiography of the Romani migration.
    B. It is strongly supported by objective data presented throughout the passage.
    C. It is perhaps true, but not explicitly supported by any objective data in the passage.
    D. It is refuted by the author's many references to linguistic evidence.

GO ON TO THE NEXT PAGE.

Passage IV (Questions 100–107)

The rich analyses of Fernand Braudel and his fellow *Annales* historians have made significant contributions to historical theory and research. In a
Line departure from traditional historical approaches,
5 the *Annales* historians assume (as do Marxists) that history cannot be limited to a simple recounting of conscious human actions, but must be understood in the context of forces and material conditions that underlie human behavior. Braudel was the first
10 *Annales* historian to gain widespread support for the idea that history should synthesize data from various social sciences, especially economics, in order to provide a broader view of human societies over time (although Febvre and Bloch, founders of
15 the *Annales* school, had originated this approach).

Braudel conceived of history as the dynamic interaction of three temporalities. The first of these, the *evenementielle,* involved short-lived dramatic "events," such as battles, revolutions and the
20 actions of great men, which had preoccupied traditional historians like Carlyle. *Conjonctures* was Braudel's term for larger cyclical processes that might last up to half a century. The *longue duree,* a historical wave of great length, was for Braudel the
25 most fascinating of the three temporalities. Here he focused on those aspects of everyday life that might remain relatively unchanged for centuries. What people ate, what they wore, their means and routes of travel for Braudel these things create
30 "structures" which define the limits of potential social change for hundreds of years at a time.

Braudel's concept of the *longue duree* extended the perspective of historical space as well as time. Until the *Annales* school, historians had
35 taken the juridical political unit the nation-state, duchy, or whatever as their starting point. Yet, when such enormous timespans are considered, geographical features may well have more significance for human populations than national bor-
40 ders. In his doctoral thesis, a seminal work on the Mediterranean during the reign of Philip II, Braudel treated the geohistory of the entire region as a "structure" that had exerted myriad influences on human lifeways since the first settlements on
45 the shores of the Mediterranean Sea. And so the reader is given such arcane information as the list of products that came to Spanish shores from North Africa, the seasonal routes followed by Mediterranean sheep and their shepherds, and the
50 cities where the best ship timber could be bought.

Braudel has been faulted for the imprecision of his approach. With his Rabelaisian delight in concrete detail, Braudel vastly extended the realm of relevant phenomena; but this very achievement
55 made it difficult to delimit the boundaries of observation, a task necessary to beginning any social investigation. Further, Braudel and other *Annales* historians minimize the differences among the social sciences. Nevertheless, the many
60 similarly designed studies aimed at both professional and popular audiences indicate that Braudel asked significant questions which traditional historians had overlooked.

100. The author refers to the work of Febvre and Bloch in order to:

A. illustrate the limitations of the *Annales* tradition of historical interpretation.
B. suggest the relevance of economics to historical investigation.
C. debate the need for combining various sociological approaches.
D. show that previous *Annales* historians anticipated Braudel's focus on economics.

GO ON TO THE NEXT PAGE.

101. According to the passage, all of the following are aspects of Braudel's approach to history EXCEPT that he:

    A. attempted to draw on various social sciences.

    B. studied social and economic activities that occurred across national boundaries.

    C. pointed out the link between increased economic activity and the rise of nationalism.

    D. examined seemingly unexciting aspects of everyday life.

102. In the third paragraph, the author is primarily concerned with discussing:

    A. Braudel's fascination with obscure facts.

    B. Braudel's depiction of the role of geography in human history.

    C. the geography of the Mediterranean region.

    D. the irrelevance of national borders.

103. The passage suggests that, compared to traditional historians, *Annales* historians are:

    A. more interested in other social sciences than in history.

    B. critical of the achievements of famous historical figures.

    C. skeptical of the validity of most economic research.

    D. more interested in the underlying context of human behavior.

104. Which of the following statements would be most likely to follow the last sentence of the passage?

    A. Few such studies, however, have been written by trained economists.

    B. It is time, perhaps, for a revival of the Carlylean emphasis on personalities.

    C. Many historians believe that Braudel's conception of three distinct "temporalities" is an oversimplification.

    D. Such diverse works as Gascon's study of Lyon and Barbara Tuchman's *A Distant Mirror* testify to his relevance.

105. The author is critical of Braudel's perspective for which of the following reasons?

    A. It seeks structures which underlie all forms of social activity.

    B. It assumes a greater similarity among the social sciences than actually exists.

    C. It fails to consider the relationship between short-term events and long-term social activity.

    D. It rigidly defines boundaries for social analysis.

GO ON TO THE NEXT PAGE.

106. The passage implies the Braudel would consider which of the following as exemplifying the *longue duree*?

    I.   The prominence of certain crops in the diet of a region

    II. The annexation of a province by the victor in a war

    III. A reduction in the population of an area following a disease epidemic

  A. I only

  B. III only

  C. I and II only

  D. II and III only

107. Which of the following statements is most in keeping with the principles of Braudel's work as described in the passage?

  A. All written history is the history of social elites.

  B. The most important task of historians is to define the limits of potential social change.

  C. Those who ignore history are doomed to repeat it.

  D. People's historical actions are influenced by many factors that they may be unaware of.

GO ON TO THE NEXT PAGE.

Passage V (Questions 108–113)

Although we know more about so-called
Neanderthal men than about any other early population, their exact relation to present-day human
Line beings remains unclear. Long considered sub-
5 human, Neanderthals are now known to have been
fully human. They walked erect, used fire, and
made a variety of tools. They lived partly in the
open and partly in caves. The Neanderthals are
even thought to have been the first humans to
10 bury their dead, a practice that has been interpreted as demonstrating the capacity for religious and
abstract thought.

The first monograph on Neanderthal anatomy,
published by Marcellin Boule in 1913, presented a
15 somewhat misleading picture. Boule took the
Neanderthals' low-vaulted cranium and prominent
brow ridges, their heavy musculature, and the apparent overdevelopment of certain joints as evidence of
a prehuman physical appearance. In postulating for
20 the Neanderthal such "primitive" characteristics as a
stooping, bent-kneed posture, a rolling gait, and a
forward-hanging head, Boule was a victim of the
rudimentary state of anatomical science. Modern
anthropologists recognize the Neanderthal bone
25 structure as that of a creature whose bodily orientation and capacities were very similar to those of present-day human beings. The differences in the size
and shape of the limbs, shoulder blades, and other
parts are simply adaptations that were necessary to
30 handle the Neanderthal's far more massive musculature. Current taxonomy considers the Neanderthals
to have been fully human and thus designates them
not as a separate species, *Homo neanderthalensis,*
but as a subspecies of *Homo sapiens: Homo sapiens*
35 *neanderthalensis.*

The rise of the Neanderthals occurred over
some 100,000 years—a sufficient period to account
for evolution of the specifically Neanderthal characteristics through free interbreeding over a broad
40 geographical range. Fossil evidence suggests that
the Neanderthals inhabited a vast area from Europe
through the Middle East and into Central Asia from
approximately 100,000 years ago until 35,000
years ago. Then, within a brief period of five to ten
45 thousand years, they disappeared. Modern humans,
not found in Europe prior to about 33,000 years
ago, thenceforth became the sole inhabitants of the
region. Anthropologists do not believe that the
Neanderthals evolved into modern human beings.
50 Despite the similarities between Neanderthal and
modern human anatomy, the differences are major
enough that, among a population as broad-ranging
as the Neanderthals, such an evolution could not
have taken place in a period of only ten thousand
55 years. Furthermore, no fossils of types intermediate
between Neanderthals and moderns have been
found.

A major alternative hypothesis, advanced by E.
Trinkaus and W. W. Howells, is that of localized evolu-
60 tion. Within a geographically concentrated population,
free interbreeding could have produced far more pronounced genetic effects within a shorter time. Thus
modern humans could have evolved relatively quickly,
either from Neanderthals or from some other ancestral
65 type, in isolation from the main Neanderthal population. These humans may have migrated throughout the
Neanderthal areas, where they displaced or absorbed
the original inhabitants. One hypothesis suggests that
these "modern" humans immigrated to Europe from
70 the Middle East.

No satisfactory explanation of why modern
human beings replaced the Neanderthals has yet
been found. Some have speculated that the modern
humans wiped out the Neanderthals in warfare;
75 however, there exists no archeological evidence of
a hostile encounter. It has also been suggested that
the Neanderthals failed to adapt to the onset of the
last Ice Age; yet their thick bodies should have been
heat conserving and thus well adapted to extreme
80 cold. Finally, it is possible that the improved tools
and hunting implements of the late Neanderthal
period made the powerful Neanderthal physique

GO ON TO THE NEXT PAGE.

less of an advantage than it had been previously. At the same time, the Neanderthals' need for a
85 heavy diet to sustain this physique put them at a disadvantage compared to the less massive moderns. If this was the case, then it was improvements in human culture—including some introduced by the Neanderthals themselves—that made the
90 Neanderthal obsolete.

108. Boule considered all of the following as evidence that Neanderthals were subhuman EXCEPT:

 A. posture.
 B. bone structure.
 C. cranial structure.
 D. ability to use tools.

109. The passage best supports which of the following conclusions?

 A. Neanderthals were less intelligent than early modern humans.
 B. Neanderthals were poorly adapted for survival.
 C. There was probably no contact between Neanderthals and early modern humans.
 D. Neanderthals may have had a capacity for religious and abstract thought.

110. According to the passage, the latest that any Neanderthal might have existed was:

 A. 100,000 years ago.
 B. 35,000 years ago.
 C. 33,000 years ago.
 D. 25,000 years ago.

111. By inference from the passage, the most important evidence that Neanderthals did NOT evolve into modern humans is the:

 A. major anatomical differences between Neanderthals and modern humans.
 B. brief time in which Neanderthals disappeared.
 C. difference in the geographical ranges of Neanderthals and modern humans.
 D. gap of many thousands of years between the latest Neanderthal fossils and the earliest modern human fossils.

112. All of the following are hypotheses about the disappearance of the Neanderthals EXCEPT:

 A. The Neanderthal physique became a handicap instead of an advantage.
 B. The Neanderthals failed to adapt to climatic changes.
 C. The Neanderthals evolved into modern humans.
 D. Modern humans exterminated the Neanderthals.

113. It can be inferred from the passage that the rate of evolution is directly related to the:

 A. concentration of the species population.
 B. anatomical features of the species.
 C. rate of environmental change.
 D. adaptive capabilities of the species.

GO ON TO THE NEXT PAGE.

Passage VI (Questions 114–119)

The Russia which emerged from the terrible civil war after the 1917 Revolution was far from the Bolsheviks' original ideal of a nonexploitative
Line society governed by workers and peasants. By
5 1921, the regime was weakened by widespread famine, persistent peasant revolts, a collapse of industrial production stemming from the civil war, and the consequent dispersal of the industrial working class—the Bolsheviks' original base of
10 support. To buy time for recovery, the government in 1921 introduced the New Economic Policy, which allowed private trade in farm products (previously banned) and relied on a fixed grain tax instead of forced requisitions to provide food for
15 the cities. The value of the ruble was stabilized. Trade unions were again allowed to seek higher wages and benefits, and even to strike. However, the Bolsheviks maintained a strict monopoly of power by refusing to legalize other parties.

20 After the death of the Revolution's undisputed leader, Lenin, in January 1924, disputes over the long-range direction of policy led to an open struggle among the main Bolshevik leaders. Since open debate was still possible within the Bolshevik
25 Party in this period, several groups with differing programs emerged in the course of this struggle.

The program supported by Nikolai Bukharin— a major ideological leader of the Bolsheviks with no power base of his own—called for developing agri-
30 culture through good relations with wealthy peasants, or *kulaks*. Bukharin favored gradual industrial development, or "advancing towards Socialism at a snail's pace." In foreign affairs, Bukharin's policy was to ally with non-Socialist regimes and move-
35 ments that were favorable to Russia.

A faction led by Leon Trotsky, head of the Red Army and the most respected revolutionary leader after Lenin, called for rapid industrialization and greater central planning of the economy, financed
40 by a heavy tax on the kulaks. Trotsky rejected the idea that a prosperous, humane Socialist society could be built in Russia alone (Stalin's slogan of "Socialism in One Country"), and therefore called for continued efforts to promote working-class rev-
45 olutions abroad. As time went on, he became bitterly critical of the new privileged elite emerging within both the Bolshevik Party and the Russian state.

Joseph Stalin, General Secretary of the party,
50 was initially considered a "center," conciliating figure, not clearly part of a faction. Stalin's eventual supremacy was ensured by three successive struggles within the party, and only during the last did his own program become clear.

55 First, in 1924–25, Stalin isolated Trotsky, allying for this purpose with Grigori Zinoviev and Lev Kamenev, Bolshevik leaders better known than Stalin himself whom Trotsky mistakenly considered his main rivals. Stalin maneuvered Trotsky out of
60 leadership of the Red Army, his main potential power base. Next, Stalin turned on Zinoviev and Kamenev, using his powers as head of the Party organization to remove them from Party leadership in Leningrad and Moscow, their respective power
65 bases. Trotsky, Zinoviev, and Kamenev then belatedly formed the "Joint Opposition" (1926–27). With Bukharin's help, Stalin easily outmaneuvered the Opposition: Bukharin polemicized against Trotsky, while Stalin prevented the newspapers
70 from printing Trotsky's replies, organized gangs of toughs to beat up his followers, and transferred his supporters to administrative posts in remote regions. At the end of 1927, Stalin expelled Trotsky from the Bolshevik Party and exiled him. (Later, in
75 1940, he had him murdered.) Zinoviev and Kamenev, meanwhile, recanted their views in order to remain within the Party.

The final act now began. A move by kulaks to gain higher prices by holding grain off the mar-
80 ket touched off a campaign against them by Stalin.

GO ON TO THE NEXT PAGE.

KAPLAN

Bukharin protested, but with the tradition of Party democracy now all but dead, Stalin had little trouble silencing Bukharin. Meanwhile, he began a campaign to force all peasants—not just kulaks—
85 onto state-controlled "collective farms," and a crash industrialization program during which he deprived the trade unions of all rights and cut real wages by 50 percent. Out of the factional struggle in which he emerged by 1933 as sole dictator of
90 Russia, Stalin's political program of building up heavy industry on the backs of both worker and peasant emerged with full clarity.

114. All of the following were among the factors contributing to the weakness of the Bolshevik regime in 1921 EXCEPT:

    A. the aftereffects of the civil war.
    B. low production.
    C. opposition by peasants.
    D. lack of democracy within the Party.

115. The main feature of the New Economic Policy of 1921 was:

    A. a strict economic centralization.
    B. stimulation of the economy through deliberate inflation.
    C. a limitation of trade union activity.
    D. a relaxation of economic controls.

116. An important feature of Bukharin's program was:

    A. a tax on the peasants.
    B. avoiding confrontations with the trade unions.
    C. forming alliances with friendly foreign regimes.
    D. maintaining open debate within the Party.

117. According to the passage, a similarity between Stalin and Trotsky was their attitude and policy toward:

    A. the elite of the Bolshevik Party.
    B. the importance of industrialization.
    C. democracy within the party.
    D. trade unions.

118. In his struggle with rival factions of the Party, Stalin was apparently MOST helped by:

    A. his control of the party organization.
    B. his control of the army.
    C. Trotsky's misjudgment of threats to his position.
    D. the appearance of standing above factional politics.

119. The passage supports the idea that struggles within the Bolshevik Party were primarily:

    A. reflections of struggles among important groups in the general population.
    B. the result of differences over economic policy.
    C. the result of differences over foreign policy.
    D. caused by Russian social elites outside the Party.

GO ON TO THE NEXT PAGE.

Passage VII (Questions 120–125)

One of the basic principles of ecology is that population size is to some extent a function of available food resources. Recent field experiments demonstrate that the interrelationship may be far more complex than hitherto imagined. Specifically, the browsing of certain rodents appears to trigger biochemical reactions in the plants they feed on that help regulate the size of the rodent populations. Two such examples of phytochemical regulation (regulation involving plant chemistry) have been reported so far.

Patricia Berger and her colleagues at the University of Utah have demonstrated the instrumentality of 6-methoxybenzoxazolinone (6-MBOA) in triggering reproductive behavior in the mountain vole (*Microtus montanus*), a small rodent resembling the field mouse. 6-MBOA forms in young mountain grasses in response to browsing by predators such as voles. The experimenters fed rolled oats coated with 6-MBOA to non-breeding winter populations of *Microtus*. After three weeks, the sample populations revealed a high incidence of pregnancy among the females and pronounced swelling of the testicles among the males. Control populations receiving no 6-MBOA revealed no such signs. Since the timing of reproductive effort is crucial to the short-lived vole in an environment in which the onset of vegetative growth can vary by as much as two months, the phytochemical triggering of copulatory behavior in *Microtus* represents a significant biological adaptation.

A distinct example is reported by John Bryant of the University of Alaska. In this case, plants seem to have adopted a form of phytochemical self-defense against the depredations of the snowshoe hare (*Lepus americanus*) of Canada and Alaska. Every ten years or so, for reasons that are not entirely understood, the *Lepus* population swells dramatically. The result is intense over-browsing of early and mid-successional deciduous trees and shrubs. Bryant has shown that, as if in response, four common boreal forest trees favored by *Lepus* produce adventitious shoots high in terpene and phenolic resins which effectively discourage hare browsing. He treated mature non-resinous willow twigs with resinous extracts from the adventitious shoots of other plants and placed treated and untreated bundles at hare feeding stations, weighing them at the end of each day. Bryant found that bundles containing only half the resin concentration of natural twigs were left untouched. The avoidance of these unpalatable resins, he concludes, may play a significant role in the subsequent decline in the Lepus population to its normal level.

These results suggest obvious areas for further research. For example, observational data should be reviewed to see whether the periodic population explosions among the prolific lemming (like the vole and the snowshoe hare, a small rodent in a marginal northern environment) occur during years in which there is an early onset of vegetative growth; if so, a triggering mechanism similar to that found in the vole may be involved.

GO ON TO THE NEXT PAGE.

120. The passage describes the effect of 6-MBOA on voles as a "significant biological adaptation" (lines 30–31) because it:

   A. limits reproductive behavior in times of food scarcity.

   B. leads the vole population to seek available food resources.

   C. tends to ensure the survival of the species in a situation of fluctuating food supply.

   D. maximizes the survival prospects of individual voles.

121. It can be inferred that the study of lemmings proposed by the author would probably:

   A. fully explain the interrelationship between food supply and reproductive behavior in northern rodent populations.

   B. disprove the conclusions of Berger and her colleagues.

   C. be irrelevant to the findings of Berger and her colleagues.

   D. provide evidence indicating whether the conclusions of Berger and her colleagues can be generalized.

122. The statement: "The interrelationship may be far more complex than hitherto imagined" (lines 4–5) suggests that scientists previously believed that:

   A. the amount of food available is the only food factor that affects population size.

   B. reproductive behavior is independent of environmental factors.

   C. food resources biochemically affect reproduction and the lifespan of some species.

   D. population size is not influenced by available food resources.

123. The experiments described in the passage involved all of the following EXCEPT:

   A. measuring alterations in reproductive organs after a specific compound was ingested.

   B. testing whether breeding behavior could be induced in normally nonbreeding animals by a change in diet.

   C. measuring animals' consumption of treated and untreated foods.

   D. measuring changes in the birth rate of test animals as opposed to control animals.

124. Bryant's interpretation of the results of his experiment (lines 52–55) depends on which of the following assumptions?

   A. The response of *Lepus* to resinous substances in nature may be different from its response under experimental conditions.

   B. The decennial rise in the *Lepus* population is triggered by an unknown phytochemical response.

   C. Many *Lepus* will starve to death rather than eat resinous shoots or change their diet.

   D. *Lepus* learns to search for alternative food sources once resinous shoots are encountered.

125. The experiments performed by Berger and Bryant BOTH study:

   I. the effect of diet on reproduction in rodents.

   II. a relationship between food source and population size.

   III. phytochemical phenomena in northern environments.

   A. II only

   B. III only

   C. I and II only

   D. II and III only

Passage VIII (Questions 126–130)

In examining "myths of women" in literature, Simone de Beauvoir found the images put forward by Stendhal romantic, yet feministic.
Stendhal's ideal woman was the one best able to reveal him to himself. For Stendhal, such a task required an equal. Women's emancipation was required, then, not simply in the name of liberty, but—more importantly—for the sake of individual happiness and fulfillment.

De Beauvoir wrote: "Stendhal wants his mistress intelligent, cultivated, free in spirit and behavior: an equal." Love, in Stendhal's scheme, will be more true if woman, being man's equal, is able to understand him more completely.

De Beauvoir found it rather refreshing—a kind of relief—that in Stendhal, at least, we can find a man who lived among women of flesh and blood. He rejected the mystification of women: his women were "not fury, nymph, morning star, nor siren, but human." Humanity sufficed for Stendhal, and no dream or myth could have been more entrancing.

Stendhal believes that the human, living souls of women, having rejected "the heavy sleep in which humanity is mired," may rise through passion to heroism, if they can find an objective worthy of them—an objective worthy of their spiritual and creative powers, their energies, and the ferocity and purity of total dedication. Certainly Stendhal believes such an objective exists for woman, and it is man. It is in this belief that Stendhal becomes ultimately unsatisfying to de Beauvoir. While Stendhal does grant women emotions, aspirations, and some sense of self, the only way he believes they can fully realize and fulfill their own selves is through man. It is in loving a man that the ennui of these truly living souls is driven away. Any boredom—any lack of focus, in essence, the lack of men—represents also a lack of any reason for living or dying, absolute stagnation. Meanwhile, passion—the love of a man—has an aim and that is enough justification for woman's life.

Yet de Beauvoir is still compelled by Stendhal. She finds him unique—or, at least, distinct—in going to the point of projecting himself into a female character. He does not "hover over" Lamiel, but assumes her destiny. On account of that, de Beauvoir notes, "Lamiel's outline remains somewhat speculative," but also singularly significant.

Lamiel is typical of Stendhal's women. Her creator has raised every imaginable obstacle before her: she is a poor peasant, raised by coarse, ignorant people imbued with all sorts of common prejudices. But, as de Beauvoir notes, "she clears from her path all moral barriers once she understands the full meaning of the little words: 'that's silly'. It is her freedom of mind that allows her to see through the meaninglessness and superficiality of so much social ritual, so that she may act in the world in her own fashion, responding fully to the impulses of her own curiosity and ambition, and shaping a destiny worthy of herself in a mediocre world."

In this, Lamiel conveys Stendhal's ultimate message to his readers: there is no comfortable place for great souls in society as it exists. It is in this sense that his men and women are the same: equals. Together, two who may have the chance to know each other in love, man and woman, defy time and universe—and come into absolute harmony with it. Such a couple is sufficient unto itself and realizes the absolute.

GO ON TO THE NEXT PAGE.

126. According to the passage, Stendhal believed that in order to experience self-realization, an individual requires the presence of:

 A. a muse.
 B. God.
 C. an equal.
 D. family.

127. The author suggests de Beauvoir considers Stendhal's portrait of Lamiel "somewhat speculative" (lines 49–50) because Stendhal:

 A. bases his story upon myths.
 B. sensationalizes his plot.
 C. takes on the identity of a woman.
 D. exaggerates the aspirations of his female characters.

128. The passage mentions that de Beauvoir saw the mystification of women in all of the following forms EXCEPT:

 A. nymph.
 B. morning star.
 C. fury.
 D. mistress.

129. It can be inferred from the passage that Stendhal's notion of love between a man and woman both includes and requires:

 A. faithfulness in the relationship.
 B. the mystification of woman.
 C. understanding of each other.
 D. the blessing of the union before God.

130. The author states that de Beauvoir finds Stendhal "ultimately unsatisfying" (line 31) in that Stendhal:

 A. stifles the lively spirits of women.
 B. reduces women to mere flesh and blood.
 C. defines the fulfillment of women by way of men.
 D. refuses to acknowledge the aspirations of women.

Passage IX (Questions 131–137)

The population of the United States is growing older and will continue to do so until well into the next century. For the first time in American history, elders outnumber teenagers. The U.S. Census Bureau projects that 39 million Americans will be 65 or older by the year 2010, 51 million by 2020, and 65 million by 2030. This demographic trend is due mainly to two factors: increased life expectancy, and the occurrence of a "baby boom" in the generation born immediately after World War II. People are living well beyond the average life expectancy in greater numbers than ever before, too. In fact, the number of U.S. citizens 85 years old and older is growing six times as fast as the rest of the population.

The "graying" of the United States is also due in large measure to the aging of the generation born after World War II, the "baby boomers." The baby boom peaked in 1957, with over 4.3 million births that year. More than 75 million Americans were born between 1946 and 1964, the largest generation in U.S. history. Today, millions of "boomers" are already moving into middle age; in less than two decades, they will join the ranks of America's elderly.

What will be the social, economic and political consequences of the aging of America? One likely development will involve a gradual restructuring of the family unit, moving away from the traditional nuclear family and towards an extended, multigenerational family dominated by elders, not by their adult children.

The aging of the U.S. population is also likely to have far-reaching effects on the nation's workforce. In 1989 there were approximately 3.5 workers for every person 65 and older; by the year 2030, there'll only be 2 workers for every person 65 and older. As the number of available younger workers shrinks, elderly people will become more attractive as prospective employees. Many will simply retain their existing jobs beyond the now-mandatory retirement age of 65. In fact, the phenomenon of early retirement, which has transformed the U.S. workforce over the past four decades, will probably become a thing of the past. In 1950, about 50 percent of all 65-year old men still worked; today, only 15 percent of them do. The median retirement age is currently 61. Yet recent surveys show that almost half of today's retirees would prefer to be working, and in decades to come, their counterparts will be doing just that.

Finally, the great proportional increase in the number of older Americans will have significant effects on the nation's economy in the areas of Social Security and health care. A recent government survey showed that 77 percent of elderly Americans have annual incomes of less than $20,000; only 3 percent earn more than $50,000. As their earning power declines and their need for health care increases, most elderly Americans come to depend heavily on federal and state subsidies. With the advent of Social Security in 1935, and Medicaid/Medicare in 1965, the size of those subsidies has grown steadily until by 1990, spending on the elderly accounted for 30 percent of the annual federal budget.

Considering these figures, and the fact that the elderly population will double within the next forty years, it's clear that major government policy decisions lie ahead. In the first 50 years of its existence, for example, the Social Security fund has received $55 billion more in employee/employer contributions than it has paid out in benefits to the elderly. Yet time and again the federal government has "borrowed" this surplus without repaying it in order to pay interest on the national debt.

Similarly, the Medicaid/Medicare system is threatened by the continuous upward spiral of medical costs. The cost of caring for disabled

GO ON TO THE NEXT PAGE.

elderly Americans is expected to double in the next decade alone. And millions of Americans of all ages are currently unable to afford private health insurance. In fact, the United States is prac-
85 tically unique among developed nations in lacking a national health care system. Its advocates say such a system would be far less expensive than the present state of affairs, but the medical establishment and various special interest groups have so
90 far blocked legislation aimed at creating it. Nonetheless, within the next few decades, an aging U.S. population may well demand that such a program be implemented.

131. Based on the information contained in the passage, which of the following statements about the U.S. elderly population is true?

　A.　It is largely responsible for the nation's current housing shortage.
　B.　It is expected to double within the next forty years.
　C.　It is the wealthiest segment of the U.S. population.
　D.　It represents almost 30 percent of the U.S. population.

132. According to the passage, the majority of elderly people in the United States:

　A.　currently earn less than $20,000 per year.
　B.　will suffer some sort of disability between the ages of 65 and 75.
　C.　have been unable to purchase their own homes.
　D.　continue to work at least 20 hours per week.

133. The fact that health care costs for disabled elderly Americans are expected to double in the next ten years indicates that:

　A.　the federal government will be unable to finance a national health care system.
　B.　the Medicaid/Medicare system will probably become even more expensive in the future.
　C.　money will have to be borrowed from the Social Security fund in order to finance the Medicaid/Medicare system.
　D.　"baby boomers" will be unable to receive federal health benefits as they grow older.

134. According to the U.S. Census Bureau, today's elderly population is:

　A.　larger than the current population of teenagers.
　B.　larger than the current population of "boomers."
　C.　smaller than the number of elderly people in 1950.
　D.　smaller than the number of elderly people in 1970.

135. The author speculates that, in future decades, the typical U.S. family will probably be:

　A.　youth oriented.
　B.　subsidized by Social Security.
　C.　multigenerational.
　D.　wealthier than today's family.

GO ON TO THE NEXT PAGE.

 257

136. The author suggests that, over the past three decades, many of today's elderly people:

    A. supplemented their incomes by working past the age of retirement.

    B. lost their Social Security benefits.

    C. have experienced a doubling in their cost of living.

    D. have come to depend heavily on government subsidies.

137. According to the author, the federal government has not yet instituted a program mandating health care for all U.S. citizens because:

    A. the federal deficit must first be eliminated.

    B. such a program would be too expensive.

    C. legislative lobbies have prevented it.

    D. Medicaid and Medicare have made it unnecessary.

STOP.

IF YOU FINISH BEFORE TIME HAS EXPIRED, CHECK YOUR WORK.
YOU MAY GO BACK TO ANY QUESTION IN THIS PART ONLY.

Writing Sample

DIRECTIONS: You are allotted 60 minutes to work on this part of the exam. You may work on only the Writing Sample part during that time. Should you finish early, you are permitted to check your work in this part of the exam only.

The Writing Sample test examines your writing skills. The test contains two assignments, Part 1 and Part 2, and you will have 30 minutes to complete each assignment.

You are permitted to work only on Part 1 during the first 30 minutes of the test and only on Part 2 during the second 30 minutes of the test. Should you finish writing on Part I before the time is up, you may review your work on Part 1, but do not begin writing on Part 2. Similarly, should you finish writing on Part 2 before the time is up, you are permitted to review your work on Part 2 only.

Use your time efficiently. Read the assignment carefully before you begin writing a response. Please ensure thorough comprehension of the assignment. Use the space located below each writing assignment for notation in planning your responses.

Your response to each part should be an essay composed of complete sentences and paragraphs, as this is a test of your writing skills. Your responses should be as well organized and clearly written as possible, given your time restrictions. Corrections or additions should be placed neatly between the lines of your responses.

Please note that illegible essays cannot be scored.

TURN TO THE NEXT PAGE AND BEGIN.

Part 1

Consider the following statement:

True creativity cannot be learned.

Write a unified essay in which you perform the following tasks. Explain what you think the above statement means. Describe a specific situation in which individuals *can* learn to be truly creative. Discuss what you think determines whether or not true creativity can be learned.

Part 2

Consider the following statement:

Morality can be implemented only through organized systems of justice.

Write a unified essay in which you perform the following tasks. Explain what you think the above statement means. Describe a specific situation in which morality *cannot* be implemented through organized systems of justice. Discuss what you think determines when morality is implemented through organized systems of justice.

STOP.

IF YOU FINISH BEFORE TIME HAS EXPIRED, CHECK YOUR WORK.
YOU MAY GO BACK TO ANY QUESTION IN THIS PART ONLY.

Biological Sciences Test

Time: 100 minutes
Questions 138–214

DIRECTIONS: The majority of the questions in the following Biological Sciences test are arranged in groups addressing a preceding descriptive passage. Select the single best answer to each question in the group after thorough analysis of the passage. Some discrete questions are not based on a descriptive passage. Similarly, select the best answer to these questions. If you are not certain of an answer, eliminate the answer choices known to be incorrect and select an answer from the remaining alternatives. Indicate your answer selection by blackening the corresponding oval on your answer document. A periodic table is provided below for your assistance with the passages and questions.

Periodic Table of the Elements

1 H 1.0																	2 He 4.0
3 Li 6.9	4 Be 9.0											5 B 10.8	6 C 12.0	7 N 14.0	8 O 16.0	9 F 19.0	10 Ne 20.2
11 Na 23.0	12 Mg 24.3											13 Al 27.0	14 Si 28.1	15 P 31.0	16 S 32.1	17 Cl 35.5	18 Ar 39.9
19 K 39.1	20 Ca 40.1	21 Sc 45.0	22 Ti 47.9	23 V 50.9	24 Cr 52.0	25 Mn 54.9	26 Fe 55.8	27 Co 58.9	28 Ni 58.7	29 Cu 63.5	30 Zn 65.4	31 Ga 69.7	32 Ge 72.6	33 As 74.9	34 Se 79.0	35 Br 79.9	36 Kr 83.8
37 Rb 85.5	38 Sr 87.6	39 Y 88.9	40 Zr 91.2	41 Nb 92.9	42 Mo 95.9	43 Tc (98)	44 Ru 101.1	45 Rh 102.9	46 Pd 106.4	47 Ag 107.9	48 Cd 112.4	49 In 114.8	50 Sn 118.7	51 Sb 121.8	52 Te 127.6	53 I 126.9	54 Xe 131.3
55 Cs 132.9	56 Ba 137.3	57 La* 138.9	72 Hf 178.5	73 Ta 180.9	74 W 183.9	75 Re 186.2	76 Os 190.2	77 Ir 192.2	78 Pt 195.1	79 Au 197.0	80 Hg 200.6	81 Tl 204.4	82 Pb 207.2	83 Bi 209.0	84 Po (209)	85 At (210)	86 Rn (222)
87 Fr (223)	88 Ra 226.0	89 Ac† 227.0	104 Unq (261)	105 Unp (262)	106 Unh (263)	107 Uns (262)	108 Uno (265)	109 Une (267)									

	58 Ce 140.1	59 Pr 140.9	60 Nd 144.2	61 Pm (145)	62 Sm 150.4	63 Eu 152.0	64 Gd 157.3	65 Tb 158.9	66 Dy 162.5	67 Ho 164.9	68 Er 167.3	69 Tm 168.9	70 Yb 173.0	71 Lu 175.0
*														
†	90 Th 232.0	91 Pa (231)	92 U 238.0	93 Np (237)	94 Pu (244)	95 Am (243)	96 Cm (247)	97 Bk (247)	98 Cf (251)	99 Es (252)	100 Fm (257)	101 Md (258)	102 No (259)	103 Lr (260)

GO ON TO THE NEXT PAGE.

Passage I (Questions 138–143)

Glycolysis is the sequence of reactions in the cytosol that converts glucose into two molecules of pyruvate with the concomitant generation of 2 ATP and 2 NADH. Under anaerobic conditions, NAD^+ is regenerated from NADH by the reduction of pyruvate to either lactate or ethanol. Alternatively, under aerobic conditions, NAD^+ is regenerated by the transfer of electrons from NADH to O_2 through the electron-transport chain. Glycolysis serves two main functions: it generates ATP and it provides carbon skeletons for biosynthesis.

Phosphofructokinase, which is the enzyme that catalyzes the committed step in glycolysis, is the most important control site. A high concentration of ATP inhibits phosphofructokinase. This inhibitory effect is enhanced by citrate and reversed by AMP. Thus, the rate of glycolysis depends on the cell's need for ATP, as signaled by the ATP/AMP ratio, and on the need for building blocks, as signaled by the concentration of citrate. These relationships are shown in Figure 1.

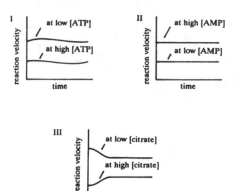

Figure 1

In liver cells, the most important regulator of phosphofructokinase activity is *fructose 2,6-bisphosphate (F-2,6-BP)*. F-2,6-BP is formed by the phosphorylation of fructose 6-phosphate in a reaction catalyzed by *phosphofructokinase 2 (PFK2)*. When blood glucose is low, a glucagon-triggered cascade leads to the phosphorylation of PFK2 and inhibition of phosphofructokinase. The control of the synthesis and degradation of F-2,6-BP is shown in Figure 2.

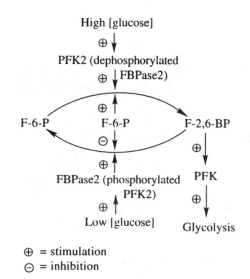

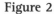

$\oplus$ = stimulation
$\ominus$ = inhibition

Figure 2

138. In an experiment with glycolytic enzymes, 10 mol of glucose produced 2 mol of ATP. This result fails to conform to the theoretical yield from 10 mol of glucose, which should produce:

   A. 1 mol of ATP.
   B. 5 mol of ATP.
   C. 10 mol of ATP.
   D. 20 mol of ATP.

GO ON TO THE NEXT PAGE.

139. One of the reactions of aerobic respiration is the addition of water to fumarate, which is shown below. This reaction is catalyzed by the enzyme fumarase, and occurs stereospecifically with water approaching on only one side of the molecule.

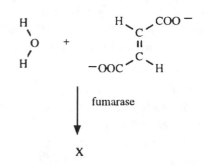

fumarase

X

The product of the reaction, X, is:

A. a racemic mixture.
B. an optically active molecule.
C. a molecule with two chiral centers.
D. an achiral molecule.

140. It can be inferred from the passage that glucagon:

A. stimulates the phosphorylation of fructose 6-phosphate.
B. stimulates F-2,6-BP synthesis.
C. inhibits phosphorylation of PFK2.
D. inhibits glycolysis.

141. Which of the following conditions would most enhance the rate of glycolysis?

A. Low concentration of F-2,6-BP
B. High ATP/AMP ratio
C. High concentration of AMP
D. High concentration of citrate

142. A high fructose-6-phosphate concentration will lead to all of the following EXCEPT:

A. increased F-2,6-BP synthesis.
B. decreased F-2,6-BP degradation.
C. stimulation of phosphofructokinase.
D. decreased ATP/AMP ratio.

143. Two bacterial colonies, A and B, are grown anaerobically on separate petri plates containing a glucose-rich medium and are found to be of equal size. The two plates are then incubated for 72 hours in an O_2-rich atmosphere. After incubation, Colony A exhibited growth, and an assay of the medium revealed that most of the glucose in the plate had been consumed; Colony B had nearly disappeared. These results suggest that Colonies A and B most likely contain:

A. facultative aerobes and obligate aerobes, respectively.
B. facultative aerobes and obligate anaerobes, respectively.
C. obligate aerobes and obligate anaerobes, respectively.
D. obligate anaerobes and facultative aerobes, respectively.

GO ON TO THE NEXT PAGE.

Passage II (Questions 144–149)

There are four phases of the *human immunodeficiency virus (HIV)* life cycle. In *binding and entry,* the virus binds to the CD4 receptor on CD4+ T-cells via the viral glycoprotein, *gp120.* The binding results in the fusion of the viral and cellular membranes, followed by the entrance of the viral core into the cell. After entry, *synthesis and integration* occurs, during which viral RNA is transcribed into double-stranded DNA by reverse transcriptase. Viral DNA enters the nucleus and integrates into the host genome. Following integration, *expression* of viral genes occurs. Finally, during *assembly and release,* viral structural proteins are synthesized and assemble into particles containing the viral enzymes and two copies of the viral RNA. The particles bud from the cell.

One of the most puzzling cytopathic effects of HIV is the depletion of T-cells, despite the fact that relatively few cells are actually infected. Four models that attempt to account for this effect are summarized below:

Hypothesis 1
HIV particles that fail to integrate into the CD4+ T-cell genome produce a toxic factor that functionally impairs T-cells and eventually leads to cell death.

Hypothesis 2
HIV integration promotes the synthesis of terminal maturation factors in CD4+ T-cells, increasing their susceptibility to the body's normal cell-destruction process.

Hypothesis 3
Viral glycoproteins (gp120 and gp41) expressed on the surface of HIV-infected T-cells fuse with CD4 receptors on healthy cells, forming a non-functional cell mass (syncytia formation).

Hypothesis 4
gp120 molecules are released into circulation by infected T-cells and bind to the CD4 receptors on healthy T-cells, making the latter subject to an autoimmune attack by anti-gp120 antibodies.

144. A researcher wanting to study the process by which viral mRNA is transcribed in an HIV-infected CD4+ T-cell would add all of the following reagents to her cell culture EXCEPT:

   A. radiolabeled thymine.
   B. radiolabeled guanine.
   C. radiolabeled uracil.
   D. radiolabeled adenine.

145. If Hypothesis 1 were true, which of the following pairs of processes would HIV have to undergo before a toxic factor could be produced?

   A. Binding and entry; synthesis and integration
   B. Reverse transcription and host cell death
   C. Binding and entry
   D. Reverse transcription; synthesis and integration

146. Which of the following supports Hypothesis 3?

   A. Some CD4+ T-cell lines do not form syncytia, but are susceptible to the cytopathic effects of HIV.
   B. Syncytia formation is transient in some CD4+ T-cell lines.
   C. gp120 and gp41 bind almost irreversibly to CD4 receptor molecules in vitro.
   D. Syncytia formation does not lead to cell death in some CD4+ T-cell lines.

GO ON TO THE NEXT PAGE.

147. Hypothesis 4 is based on the assumption that:

   A. healthy CD4+ T-cells are not normally subject to autoimmune attacks.
   B. healthy CD4+ T-cells will produce anti-gp120 cells in response to exposure to the HIV virus.
   C. healthy CD4+ T-cells normally synthesize gp120.
   D. proteins travel through the body by way of the immune system.

148. If Hypothesis 3 were true, which of the following cellular organelles would be responsible for directing the newly synthesized gp120 and gp41 molecules toward the plasma membrane, on which they would eventually be expressed?

   A. Centrioles
   B. Golgi complex
   C. Mitochondria
   D. Lysosomes

149. HIV infection is detected by the presence of anti-HIV antibodies in the blood. This indicates that during infection:

   A. helper T-cells are still able to activate cytotoxic T-cell proliferation.
   B. B-lymphocytes are still able to produce antibodies in response to the foreign antigens of HIV.
   C. anti-HIV antibodies are effective against the virus.
   D. HIV has not infected host macrophages.

GO ON TO THE NEXT PAGE.

Passage III (Questions 150–154)

A chemist investigated the reactivity of four organic compounds; their melting and boiling points are given in Table 1. The compounds were treated with an oxidizing agent and a reducing agent. Their ability to react with Br_2 and HBr was also investigated.

Table 2 records the molecular formulas of the reaction products from these experiments.

Table 1

Compound	I	II	III	IV
	$CH_3CH=CHCH_3$	$CH_3CH_2CH=CH_2$	$CH_3C \equiv CCH_3$	$CH_3CH_2C=CH$
Melting point, °C	−106/−139	−195	−24	−122
Boiling point, °C	+1/+4	−6	+27	+9

Table 2

Compound	I	II	III	IV
H_2/Pd	C_4H^{10}	C_4H_{10}	C_4H_{10}	C_4H_{10}
Br_2	$C_4H_8Br_2$	$C_4H_8Br_2$	$C_4H_6Br_4$	$C_4H_6Br_4$
HBr	C_4H_9Br	C_4H_9Br	$C_4H_8Br_2$	$C_4H_8Br_2$
Cold, dilute $KMnO_4$	$C_4H_{10}O_2$	$C_4H_{10}O_2$		
Hot, basic $KMnO_4$/H^+	$2C_2H_4O_2$	$C3H6O_2 + CO_2$		

GO ON TO THE NEXT PAGE.

150. Compound I has two melting points because it can exist as either of two:

   A. anomers.
   B. enantiomers.
   C. conformational isomers.
   D. geometric isomers.

151. What is the name of the product formed when Compound I is reacted with hot, basic $KMnO_4$?

   A. Acetic acid
   B. 2,3-Butanediol
   C. Ethanal
   D. Ethylene glycol

152. The reaction of Compound IV with HBr primarily differs from Compound II in that it proceeds through which of the following intermediates?

   A. A secondary carbocation
   B. A vinylic anion
   C. A vinylic cation
   D. A tertiary carbocation

153. Hydrogenation and bromination of Compound I occur, respectively, via the mechanisms of:

   A. *syn* addition and *anti* addition.
   B. *anti* addition and *syn* addition.
   C. nucleophilic addition and electrophilic addition.
   D. electrophilic addition and nucleophilic addition.

154. Why do Compound I and Compound II form the same product in the reaction with HBr?

   A. Both have equally stable double bonds
   B. Both have equally reactive double bonds
   C. Both obey Markovnikov's rule
   D. Neither obeys Markovnikov's rule

GO ON TO THE NEXT PAGE.

Passage IV (Questions 155–160)

An epidemiologist was called in to investigate an outbreak of illness following a sewage leak into a city's water supply. Blood tests of the affected individuals revealed the presence of an unknown infectious agent, which the epidemiologist determined to be either viral or bacterial. Further examination determined that the infectious agent was bacterial, and when the results were more closely analyzed, it appeared that more than one strain of bacteria was infecting the patients. Four different strains of bacteria, labeled Microbe Q, Microbe R, Microbe S, and Microbe T, were eventually isolated.

Four different types of nutrient plates were prepared, each containing only four amino acids, and the microbes were inoculated onto the plates to determine the essential amino acids of each strain. Those amino acids that an organism cannot synthesize are said to be *essential* to that organism.

Plate 1: cysteine, phenylalanine, serine, threonine

Plate 2: cysteine, phenylalanine, proline, tryptophan

Plate 3: cysteine, proline, threonine, tryptophan

Plate 4: phenylalanine, serine, threonine, tryptophan

The results are shown in Table 1.

Table 1

Microbe

	Q	R	S	T
Plate 1	+	+	−	+
Plate 2	−	+	+	+
Plate 3	+	−	−	−
Plate 4	−	−	−	+

+ = growth; − = no growth

After the microbes were isolated, it was determined that Microbe R and Microbe S were not pathogenic. Potential antibiotics against Microbe Q and Microbe T were then selected, and the microbes were inoculated onto their respective growth media. Antibiotic discs X, Y, and Z were then placed on each nutrient plate. After 24 hours of incubation (enough time to allow growth), the plates were re-examined. The shaded areas of Figure 1 represent regions of good bacterial growth.

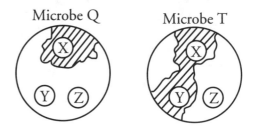

Figure 1

GO ON TO THE NEXT PAGE.

155. Which of the following techniques would have been *most* effective in helping the epidemiologist determine that the infectious agent was bacterial?

    A. Hybridize the infectious agent with radiolabeled probes specific for the genes encoding viral structural proteins; only viral genes would hybridize.

    B. Analyze a patient's serum in a spectrophotometer to measure its absorption wavelength; the photosynthetic pigments found in all bacteria would distinguish them from viruses, which lack such pigments.

    C. Stain the infectious agent for the presence of RNA; only bacteria would stain positive.

    D. Stain the infectious agent for the presence of protein; only bacteria would stain positive.

156. Which of the following structures would NOT have been detected when the epidemiologist determined Microbe R's structural composition?

    A. Nuclear membrane
    B. DNA
    C. Cell wall
    D. Ribosomes

157. According to Table 1, which of the following amino acids is essential to Microbe Q?

    A. Serine
    B. Threonine
    C. Phenylalanine
    D. Proline

158. According to Table 1, which of the four nutrient media could the epidemiologist have used when determining the effectiveness of the antibiotic discs against the pathogenic microbes?

    A. The medium from Plate 1
    B. The medium from Plate 2
    C. The medium from Plate 3
    D. The medium from Plate 4

159. Based on the information in Figure 1, which of the following antibiotics would be *most* effective in treating patients infected with both Microbe Q and Microbe T?

    A. Antibiotic X
    B. Antibiotic Y
    C. Antibiotic Z
    D. Antibiotic Y and Antibiotic Z are equally effective

GO ON TO THE NEXT PAGE.

160. Which of the following would be the easiest method to isolate Microbe Q from Microbe T when they coexist in the same patient?

A. Centrifuge a serum sample from a patient infected with both bacteria; the two strains should layer at different levels and could thus be isolated.

B. Take a blood sample from a patient infected with both bacteria. Put some blood on a nutrient plate containing only phenylalanine, and some on another plate containing only cysteine. Incubate and isolate what grows.

C. Take a blood sample from a patient infected with both bacteria. Put some on a nutrient plate with all the amino acids except cysteine, and some on another plate with all the amino acids except phenylalanine. Incubate and isolate what grows.

D. There is no way to isolate the two bacteria, since all bacteria are similar in their structure and nutritional requirements.

GO ON TO THE NEXT PAGE.

161. The hormone calcitonin acts as a regulator of serum Ca^{2+} levels by promoting the incorporation of Ca^{2+} into bone. Which of the following hormones is antagonistic to calcitonin?

A. Parathyroid hormone
B. Prolactin
C. ACTH
D. Thyroxine

162. In a healthy individual, which of the following blood vessels has the highest partial pressure of carbon dioxide?

A. Pulmonary arteries
B. Pulmonary veins
C. Aorta
D. Coronary arteries

163. Which of the following structures is NOT derived from embryonic ectoderm?

A. Eye lens
B. Pituitary gland
C. Digestive tract
D. Adrenal medulla

164. Transfusion with which of the following blood types would cause severe agglutination in a patient with type B blood, Rh positive?

A. Type B blood, Rh negative
B. Type A blood, Rh positive
C. Type O blood, Rh positive
D. Type O blood, Rh negative

165. The graph below plots the transmembrane diffusion rates for Compound A and Compound B as a function of their extracellular concentrations. Given that both compounds are approximately the same size, and there are no facilitated diffusion sites, it would most likely be inferred that:

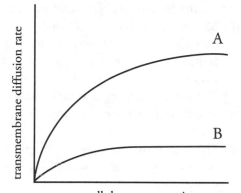

A. Compound A is polar and Compound B is nonpolar.
B. Compound A is nonpolar and Compound B is polar.
C. Compound A is polar and Compound B is polar.
D. Compound A is nonpolar and Compound B is nonpolar.

GO ON TO THE NEXT PAGE.

 275

Passage V (Questions 166–170)

A student working in a laboratory accidentally touches a hot plate with his right hand. An involuntary (reflex) action that operates through a polysynaptic reflex arc involving two synapses causes him to immediately withdraw his hand. This withdrawal is mediated by the following sequence of events:

1) Skin receptors sense "hot" pain.
2) Stimulation of these receptors leads to the transduction of an impulse along a sensory neuron.
3) The sensory neuron synapses with an interneuron in the dorsal horn of the spinal cord.
4) The interneuron synapses with a motor neuron in the ventral horn of the spinal cord.
5) The motor neuron relays the impulse to the muscles in his right arm.
6) The arm muscles react in antagonistic pairs: the biceps (flexor muscle) contract and the triceps (extensor muscle) relax.

The sensation of pain is also conveyed to the sensory cortex; however, this is slower than conduction to the motor neuron because the impulse must travel along thin myelinated fibers and cross several synapses.

Research has elucidated the chemical and molecular events that produce a reflex contraction. The link between a nerve terminal and the sarcolemma of a muscle fiber is known as a neuromuscular junction; the space between the two is a synapse. The nerve terminal is characterized by the presence of numerous mitochondria and synaptic vesicles containing the neurotransmitter acetylcholine. Transmission of an impulse to the terminal triggers the release of acetylcholine into the synapse via exocytosis. The acetylcholine diffuses across the synapse and then binds to receptors on the muscle sarcolemma. These receptors form the extracellular part of ligand-gated ion channels. Receptor binding causes a change in the conformation of the channels, causing them to open, allowing a rapid influx of Na^+ into the sarcoplasm. This produces an action potential. The action potential is conducted along the sarcolemma and the T system into the muscle fiber, triggering the release of Ca^{2+} into the sarcoplasm and thereby stimulating muscle contraction.

166. Calcium ions stimulate muscle contraction by:

   A. binding to the sarcolemma.
   B. binding to troponin.
   C. causing the formation of permanent actin-myosin cross-bridges.
   D. binding to actin.

167. Which of the following provides the most plausible explanation for the presence of numerous mitochondria in the nerve terminals?

   A. All cells have mitochondria.
   B. Neurons are aerobic cells.
   C. The diffusion of acetylcholine across a synapse requires ATP.
   D. The exocytosis of synaptic vesicles requires ATP.

GO ON TO THE NEXT PAGE.

168. If the student's receptors for the sensation of "hot" pain had been severed, then the student would have:

    A. felt no pain, and his hand would have remained on the hot plate.
    B. felt no pain, but would have immediately removed his hand from the hot plate.
    C. felt pain, but would have been unable to remove his hand from the hot plate.
    D. felt pain, but would have slowly removed his hand from the hot plate.

169. Which of the following best explains why the withdrawal of a limb from a burning hot plate occurs faster than the withdrawal of a limb from an uncomfortably warm tub of water?

    A. Intense heat causes a greater amount of acetylcholine to be released into the neuromuscular junction, producing an action potential of greater magnitude.
    B. Intense heat directly stimulates the sensory areas of the brain that respond to temperature, allowing the information to be processed more rapidly.
    C. Intense heat stimulates the secretion of epinephrine from the neuromuscular junction, triggering the "fight-or-flight" responses and decreasing reaction time.
    D. Intense heat stimulates a simple reflex involving only two synapses, allowing the information to be processed more rapidly.

170. When a strong stimulus such as burning heat is applied to a limb, the limb's withdrawal is accompanied by a concomitant extension of the opposite limb; this is known as the crossed extensor reflex. This implies that as the student withdraws his right hand from the hotplate:

    A. his right biceps relax and his right triceps contract.
    B. his right biceps contract and his right triceps contract.
    C. his left biceps relax and his left triceps contract.
    D. his left biceps contract and his right biceps relax.

GO ON TO THE NEXT PAGE.

Passage VI (Questions 171–175)

Alkanes, in the presence of light, react with halogens to produce alkyl halides. The reactions result in the substitution of halogen atoms for hydrogen atoms on the carbon skeleton. The reactions involve free radical intermediates as illustrated in this general mechanism:

$$\text{Initiation:} \quad X_2 \xrightarrow{\text{light}} 2X \bullet \quad (1)$$

$$\text{Propagation:} \quad RH + X \bullet \rightarrow R \bullet + HX \quad (2)$$
$$X_2 + R \bullet \rightarrow RX + X \bullet \quad (3)$$

(R = alkyl chain, X = F, Cl, Br, I)

The reactivity of an alkane depends on the types of hydrogens that are available to be substituted. Differences in the bond strengths, and in the energies of the transition states, make tertiary hydrogens most reactive, followed by secondary and then primary hydrogens. For instance, in substitution by bromine, tertiary hydrogens are five times more reactive than primary ones.

The order of reactivity of the halogens is:

$$F > Cl > Br > I$$

171. The chlorination of butane is accompanied by which of the following?

    I.   The formation of chiral products
    II. No observed change in optical rotation
    III. The formation of achiral products

A. I only
B. III only
C. II and III only
D. I, II, and III

172. Reaction of alkanes containing equal numbers of primary and tertiary hydrogens with fluorine produces approximately equal amounts of each possible product. By contrast, reaction with bromine produces five times as much tertiary product as primary. Which of the following statements is most strongly supported by these facts and the passage?

A. The reactivity of the halogens is inversely related to their selectivity between hydrogens in free-radical substitutions.
B. Bromine is a more efficient halogenating reagent for all classes of alkanes than fluorine.
C. Fluorine is less reactive with respect to substitution of tertiary hydrogens in alkanes than bromine.
D. Fluorine forms stronger bonds to primary carbons than bromine does.

173. Light of low intensity is sufficient to cause the alkanes and halogens to react because:

A. the reactions have low activation energies.
B. only a small, catalytic amount of X radicals must be produced in Step 1.
C. the bonds in the halogen molecules are weak.
D. alkanes are very reactive molecules.

GO ON TO THE NEXT PAGE.

174. Which of the following represents a chain termination step?

A. $Br^\bullet + Br_2 \rightarrow Br_2 + Br^\bullet$

B. $Br^\bullet + R^\bullet \rightarrow RBr$

C. $RH + Br_2 \rightarrow RBr + HBr$

D. $Br_2 + R^\bullet \rightarrow RBr + Br^\bullet$

175. What is the IUPAC name of the product formed when the most reactive hydrogen of 2-methylpropane is substituted by a bromine atom?

A. 2-bromomethylpropane

B. 2-bromobutane

C. 1-bromo-2-methylpropane

D. 2-bromo-2-methylpropane

GO ON TO THE NEXT PAGE.

Passage VII (Questions 176–181)

Current theories of carcinogenesis are based on the concept of cellular and viral *oncogenes*. It is believed that the genome of any eukaryotic cell contains DNA segments, called *proto-oncogenes,* that normally code for cell growth-related proteins such as transcription factors, growth factors, growth-factor receptors, and tyrosine kinases (enzymes thought to regulate cell division). These cellular proto-oncogenes can be transformed into tumorigenic oncogenes (*c-onc*) by a number of mechanisms.

A common mechanism by which a cellular proto-oncogene is transformed into a *c-onc* is point mutation, which leads to formation of a defective protein. For example, one well-studied cellular proto-oncogene codes for the *ras* protein. *Ras* proteins have GTPase activity, and their activity is regulated by the presence of GTP or GDP. In the wild-type protein, growth-factor receptors with tyrosine kinase activity stimulate *ras* to exchange GDP with GTP through an indirect process involving intermediate proteins. *Ras* then activates a cytosolic kinase (also an oncogene) *c-raf. c-raf* then activates *MAP kinase-kinase,* which in turn activates *MAP-kinase. MAP-kinase* appears capable of phosphorylating transcription factors in the nucleus. After the appropriate genes have been transcribed, *ras* GTPase activity hydrolyzes GTP, converting *ras* to its inactive form. Mutant *ras* proteins are unable to hydrolyze GTP, and therefore remain in the active GTP-bound form.

Alternatively, a proto-oncogene may become an oncogene through a mutation that causes it to produce an excess of a normal protein. Such a mutation may place the gene under the control of a stronger promoter via either chromosomal translocation, or by the integration of a provirus with a strong promoter in the immediate proximity of the proto-oncogene. An excess of a normal protein may also be caused by gene amplification of the proto-oncogene.

Another mechanism of carcinogenesis that also depends on oncogenes is viral carcinogenesis, which is caused by transforming viruses. Transforming viruses, which occur widely in the avian and animal kingdoms, are retroviruses whose genomes contain oncogenes (called viral oncogenes, or *v-onc*) derived from their former eukaryotic hosts. Such viruses can later cause other host cells to become tumorigenic.

176. Which of the following activities would you expect to increase in a tumorigenic cell?

    I.   mRNA synthesis
    II. Ribosomal assembly
    III. Cell division

A. I only
B. I and II only
C. II and III only
D. I, II, and III

177. A *c-onc* activated by point mutation differs from the proto-oncogene from which it was derived by:

A. a single base-pair.
B. two base-pairs.
C. a triplet insertion.
D. a triplet deletion.

GO ON TO THE NEXT PAGE.

178. Based on the information in the passage, cellular proto-oncogenes can become tumorigenic oncogenes by all of the following mechanisms EXCEPT:

    A. a mutation that results in the synthesis of a faulty protein.

    B. a chromosomal translocation that produces an excess of a protein.

    C. binding of complementary nucleic acid sequences to proto-oncogene transcripts.

    D. a mutation that causes gene amplification of the proto-oncogene.

179. Comparison of a *v-onc* sequence with a corresponding *c-onc* sequence reveals that the organization of the viral gene corresponds to the mRNA of the *c-onc* gene, rather than to its own genomic organization. Which of the following best accounts for this observation?

    A. The *v-onc* gene contains only *c-onc* introns.

    B. The *v-onc* gene has a greater level of expression than the corresponding *c-onc* gene.

    C. The *v-onc* gene was captured from a host cell in the form of RNA during a retroviral infection.

    D. Since retroviral DNA is incorporated into the cellular genome, the alternating exons and introns in the *v-onc* gene are spliced by cellular enzymes.

180. Which of the following processes function in an analogous way to *ras* activity?

    A. Formation of antibody-antigen complexes during an immune response

    B. Sodium-potassium pump in neurons

    C. Krebs cycle in mitochondria

    D. Second messenger system involving cAMP

181. The incorporation of a strong promoter near a proto-oncogene may lead to cancer because the stronger promoter most likely:

    A. increases the rate of translation.

    B. increases the rate of transcription.

    C. increases the rate of translocation.

    D. increases the rate of point mutations.

GO ON TO THE NEXT PAGE.

Passage VIII (Questions 182–187)

Radioimmunoassay (RIA) is a technique used for measuring hormone concentrations in blood serum based on highly specific antigen-antibody interactions. To carry out an RIA for a particular human hormone, an antibody to that hormone is prepared by immunizing mice or rabbits with an extract from the human endocrine gland that produces the hormone. A measured quantity of this antibody is then mixed with a known concentration of isotopically labeled hormone and the blood sample to be assayed, which contains an unknown concentration of unlabeled hormone. RIA is based on the principle that as long as there is too little antibody to bind both the labeled hormone and unlabeled hormone completely, then the unlabeled and the labeled hormone will compete for antibody-binding sites. Thus, as the concentration of unlabeled hormone in the sample increases, the percentage of antibody-bound radiolabeled hormone decreases.

Hormone concentrations can be calculated by comparing the radioactivity counts obtained from the original RIA to a standard curve, such as the one shown in Figure 1. To generate a standard curve for a particular hormone, RIAs are performed on a series of solutions containing different known concentrations of unlabeled hormone. After the radioactivity of each solution is measured, these concentrations are then plotted against the percentage of antibody-bound radiolabeled hormone.

For most hormones, the form that circulates in the blood (the active form) is different from that extracted from the tissues and used to prepare the antibodies and standard curve used for RIAs (the precursor form), though typically, the two forms are very similar in structure and chemistry.

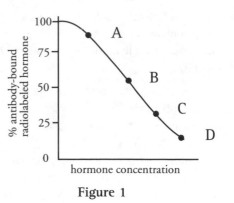

Figure 1

182. According to the passage, an antibody to a particular human hormone is prepared by immunizing laboratory animals with an extract of the human hormone. Which of the following best explains why this technique works?

A. The lab animal's immune system recognizes the human hormone as "foreign," or antigenic, and produces antibodies in response to its presence.

B. Human gland cells must first be injected into a host organism, such as a mouse or rabbit, before they can produce the antibodies.

C. Human hormones will elicit antibody production in mice and rabbits, but not in other animals, such as rats and chimpanzees.

D. Immunization with human hormone, prior to actual exposure to the hormone, protects the lab animal from infection upon second exposure to the hormone.

GO ON TO THE NEXT PAGE.

KAPLAN

183. An RIA for antidiuretic hormone (ADH) performed on a healthy person yielded a concentration of 3 pg/mL. If an RIA were performed on a patient suffering from severe blood loss, which of the following ADH concentrations would the RIA most likely yield?

    A. 0.5 pg/mL
    B. 2 pg/mL
    C. 3 pg/mL
    D. 5 pg/mL

184. If Figure 1 were the standard curve for FSH, which point on the graph would most likely represent FSH concentration in a woman before pregnancy and in her sixteenth week of pregnancy, respectively?

    A. Point A and Point D
    B. Point B and Point D
    C. Point C and Point D
    D. Point B and Point A

185. RIA is based on the principle that radiolabeled and unlabeled hormone will compete for binding sites on the antibody. Which of the following conditions would NOT compromise the validity of an RIA?

    A. The antibody binds the radiolabeled hormone with a greater affinity than the unlabeled hormone.
    B. The antibody binds the radiolabeled hormone and the unlabeled hormone with equal affinity.
    C. There is enough antibody in the solution to completely bind with the radiolabeled and the unlabeled hormone.
    D. The radiolabeled hormone binds to a site on the antibody other than the antigen-binding site, inducing a conformational change that inhibits the binding of unlabeled hormone.

186. If Figure 1 were the standard curve for insulin, which points on the graph would most likely represent the serum insulin concentration calculated from the RIA performed before and 1 hour after glucose infusion, respectively?

    A. Point B and Point A
    B. Point B and Point D
    C. Point C and Point C
    D. Point C and Point A

187. Suppose that a researcher who wanted to measure the concentration of a particular *active* hormone unwittingly used its *precursor* form to develop the antibodies and generate the standard curve used for the RIA. If the researcher then performed an RIA on a sample of unlabeled active hormone contaminated with unlabeled precursor hormone, how would this affect the RIA?

    A. The standard curve generated for the precursor form would be inaccurate and therefore could not be used to calculate unknown concentrations of that form.
    B. The percentage of antibody-bound radiolabeled hormone would be greater than normal, because there would be twice as much unlabeled hormone for the radiolabeled hormone to compete with.
    C. The calculated concentration of the active hormone would be greater than its actual concentration, because the antibody would bind to both the active hormone and its precursor form.
    D. The calculated concentration of the active hormone would be less than its actual concentration, because the antibody would bind to both the active hormone and its precursor form.

GO ON TO THE NEXT PAGE.

Questions 188 through 192 are NOT based on a descriptive passage.

188. Marine and freshwater fish have different problems in maintaining their internal salt and water balances. Osmosis causes freshwater fish to gain water and marine fish to lose water. Based on this information, which of the following must be true?

A. Marine fish live in an environment hypertonic to their body fluids.
B. Marine fish live an environment hypotonic to their body fluids.
C. Freshwater fish live in an environment hypertonic to their body fluids.
D. Freshwater fish live in an environment isotonic to their body fluids.

189. Myoglobin, which is an oxygen-carrying protein found in muscle tissue, consists of a single polypeptide chain with an attached heme group. In contrast, hemoglobin consists of four heme-carrying polypeptide subunits. Which of the following best accounts for the difference in shape between the hemoglobin and myoglobin oxygen-dissociation curves?

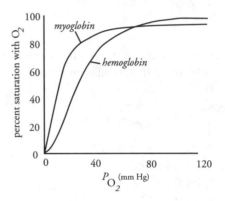

A. Bohr effect
B. Cooperative binding of oxygen to myoglobin
C. Difference in P_{O_2} between blood and muscle
D. Cooperative binding of oxygen to hemoglobin

GO ON TO THE NEXT PAGE.

190. Which of the following is not a meta-directing group in electrophilic aromatic substitution?

A. $-\overset{\overset{\displaystyle O}{\|}}{C}-OH$

B. $-NH_2$

C. $-\overset{\overset{\displaystyle O}{\|}}{C}-R$

D. $-SO_3H$

191. An amino acid is subjected to electrophoresis at pH 8.5 and is observed to migrate to the anode. The isoelectric point of this amino acid:

A.   is less than 8.5.
B.   is more than 8.5.
C.   is equal to 8.5.
D.   cannot be determined without more information.

192. It is hypothesized that the binding of testosterone to corticosteroid receptors in the hypothalamus of a developing male fetus accounts for the sexual differentiation of the human brain. This binding causes the hypothalamus to switch from cyclic production of gonadotropin-releasing factors (which is characteristic of females) to acyclic production. This switch, therefore, is likely to affect the release patterns of:

A.   LH.
B.   FSH.
C.   both LH and FSH.
D.   neither LH nor FSH.

GO ON TO THE NEXT PAGE.

Passage IX (Questions 193–198)

Cystic fibrosis (CF) is the most common autosomal recessive disease in the Caucasian population. The disease affects 1 in 2,500 newborns, and ranges in degree of severity even within the same family. In some cases, individuals do not survive past the age of five, while in others, adults live full lives through careful management.

It has been determined that CF is caused by a mutation of chromosome 7. In 75 percent of all CF cases, the mutation involves a deletion of three base pairs in a DNA sequence that codes for a transmembrane chloride channel. As a result of the deletion, the chloride channel is unable to operate efficiently.

CF is characterized by sticky, viscous, mucus secretions that impair the normal physiological functions of many organs, most especially the pancreas and lungs. Patients usually suffer from diarrhea, pancreatic exocrine insufficiency, and chronic obstructive pulmonary disease. Breathing is often difficult, and carbon dioxide tends to remain in the blood of CF patients longer than in that of healthy individuals. The diarrhea and pancreatic troubles are treated with enzyme supplementation; the respiratory ailments prove more trying in their treatment. Patients must undergo intense, daily respiratory therapy, and take heavy doses of antibiotics in order to maintain adequate ventilation. One such antibiotic is *cephalosporin C*, which is effective against penicillin-resistant bacteria. Despite the rigorous treatments, individuals with CF usually die as a result of pneumonia or bacterial infections secondary to the respiratory aspects of the disease.

193. One of the most common bacteria to infect patients with CF is *Staphylococcus*. If a sample from a CF patient were cultured, how would *Staphylococcus* appear when stained and viewed under a microscope?

  A. Helical
  B. Sickle-shaped
  C. Rodlike
  D. Spherical

194. According to the passage, pancreatic insufficiency in CF patients can be effectively treated with enzyme supplementation. Which of the following substances is LEAST likely to be found in such a supplement?

  A. Lipase
  B. Trypsin
  C. Enterokinase
  D. Chymotrypsinogen

195. What is the probability that a child of two carriers of the CF gene will be affected with CF?

  A. 0%
  B. 25%
  C. 50%
  D. 66%

GO ON TO THE NEXT PAGE.

196. The discovery that the sweat of children with CF contained excessive salt led to the measurement of sodium and chloride in sweat as a means of diagnosing CF. This suggests that, as compared to the chloride channel coded for by the normal gene, the channel coded by the CF gene:

   A. transports less chloride from surrounding epithelial cells into the sweat ducts.
   B. transports less sodium from surrounding epithelial cells into the sweat ducts.
   C. transports more sodium but less chloride from surrounding epithelial cells into the sweat ducts.
   D. is unable to transport chloride out of the sweat ducts and into surrounding epithelial cells.

197. CF patients suffer from pancreatic exocrine insufficiency as a result of obstruction of the pancreatic ducts leading into the small intestine. Which of the following CF symptoms is most likely caused by this insufficiency?

   A. Pulmonary obstruction
   B. Fat malabsorption
   C. Carbohydrate malabsorption
   D. Susceptibility to penicillin-resistant bacteria

198. Based on the information in the passage, compared to healthy individuals, CF patients most likely have a blood pH that:

   A. is more acidic.
   B. is more basic.
   C. is the same.
   D. wildly fluctuates.

GO ON TO THE NEXT PAGE.

Passage X (Questions 199–203)

Ketones are known to readily react with halogens in the presence of acid or base to form alpha-halogenated products. The overall reaction is shown below:

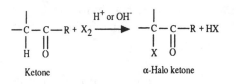

Reaction 1

In basic solution (Figure 1), the hydroxide ion removes a proton from the alpha carbon, yielding a carbanion intermediate (Step 1). Finally, the alpha-halogenated ketone is formed by the addition of a positively polarized bromide to the carbanion (Step 2):

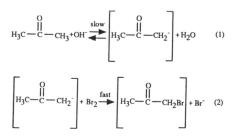

Figure 1

Alpha halogenation under acidic conditions (Figure 2) initially involves protonation of the carbonyl oxygen, resulting in the formation of an enol (Step 2). This molecule then undergoes electrophilic addition to yield another intermediate that can then be deprotonated to form the α-halo ketone (Step 4).

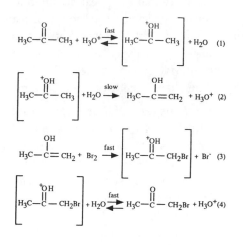

Figure 2

199. What is the function of the hydrogen and hydroxide ions in the acidic and basic solutions, respectively?

   A. They both act as catalysts.
   B. They are both reactants.
   C. The hydrogen ion is a reactant, while the hydroxide ion acts as a catalyst.
   D. The hydrogen ion acts as a catalyst, while the hydroxide ion is a reactant.

200. In Figure 2, the first two steps are characteristic of isomerization between which of the following?

   I.   Tautomers
   II. Enantiomers
   III. Geometric isomers

   A. I only
   B. III only
   C. I and II only
   D. I, II, and III

GO ON TO THE NEXT PAGE.

201. Alpha halogenation of acetone in basic solution usually results in multiple halogenations on the alpha carbon (known as the Haloform reaction). This reaction occurs because:

  A. introduction of the first halogen makes the remaining α-hydrogens more acidic and therefore easily removed by the base.
  B. the base is very strong and will easily abstract protons.
  C. α-halo ketones are highly unstable and susceptible to further reaction.
  D. the first halogen stabilizes any carbocations that are formed.

202. From the mechanism drawn in Figure 1, the overall rate of reaction for alpha halogenation is dependent on the concentration of which of the following?

  I. CH_3COCH_3
  II. Br_2
  III. OH^-

  A. I only
  B. II only
  C. I and III only
  D. I, II, and III

203. What would be the likely product if acetone was reacted with methylmagnesium bromide and then water?

  A. Butanone
  B. *tert*-Butyl alcohol
  C. *tert*-Butyl bromide
  D. Isopropyl methyl ether

GO ON TO THE NEXT PAGE.

Passage XI (Questions 204–209)

Acetylcholine (AC), a vital neurotransmitter of the autonomic nervous system, is released by the presynaptic knob of a neuron in response to an action potential. Once acetylcholine has interacted with the receptors of the postsynaptic membrane, it is quickly inactivated by *acetylcholinesterase* (ACE), the principal enzymatic component of the synaptic cleft.

The active site of ACE consists of two separate regions. The *binding region* contains a carboxylate group, which is responsible for attachment to the quaternary nitrogen atom of acetylcholine. The *catalytic region*, which is responsible for the esterase activity, contains serine (Ser), histidine (His), and tyrosine (Tyr) residues.

Figures 1–8 show how the changes in the active site of ACE are coupled with the breakdown of acetylcholine.

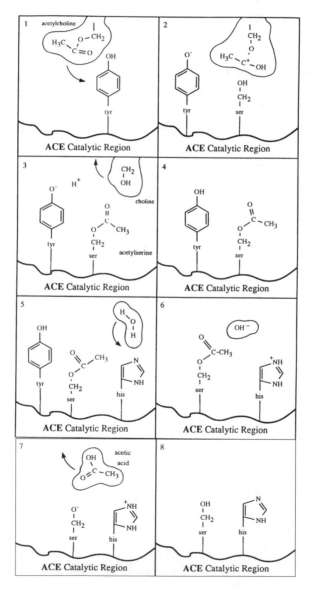

GO ON TO THE NEXT PAGE.

KAPLAN

204. It can be inferred from the passage that ACE acts to:

    A. prevent AC from being reabsorbed by the presynaptic knob.
    B. prevent AC from being released by the presynaptic knob.
    C. restore the excitability of the postsynaptic membrane.
    D. restore the excitability of the presynaptic knob.

205. Assuming that the carboxylate group in the binding region of ACE is not protonated, what type of interaction is likely to occur between this group and the quaternary nitrogen of acetylcholine?

    A. Hydrogen bonding
    B. Electrostatic interaction
    C. Hydrophobic interaction
    D. London forces

206. In Figure 5, the nitrogen in the imidazole ring becomes protonated because it:

    A. acts as a Lewis base by accepting a lone pair of electrons.
    B. acts as a Lewis acid by donating a lone pair of electrons.
    C. acts as a Lewis acid by accepting a lone pair of electrons.
    D. acts as a Lewis base by donating a lone pair of electrons.

207. In what way does protonation of AC by the tyrosine residue enhance the activity of ACE?

    A. It makes choline a better leaving group, thereby making the reaction of AC with the serine residue more complete.
    B. It makes AC more susceptible to nucleophilic attack, thereby making the reaction of AC with the serine residue more complete.
    C. It makes choline a better leaving group, thereby increasing the rate of the reaction with the serine residue.
    D. It makes AC more susceptible to nucleophilic attack, thereby increasing the rate of the reaction with the serine residue.

208. Based on the passage, which of the following is true?

    A. Acetylserine is the product of S_N1.
    B. Acetylserine is the product of S_N2.
    C. OH^- is a better leaving group than CH_3^-.
    D. $SerCH_2O^-$ is a better leaving group than choline.

209. The process of acetic acid formation in Figures 6 and 7 is an example of which of the following reactions?

    A. Basic hydrolysis of an ester
    B. Acidic cleavage of an ether
    C. Oxidation of an alcohol
    D. Decarboxylation of a carboxylic acid

GO ON TO THE NEXT PAGE.

210. Destruction of which of the following organelles would most inhibit intracellular protein digestion?

   A. Lysosomes
   B. Peroxisomes
   C. Rough endoplasmic reticulum
   D. Ribosomes

211. A researcher is trying to determine the contents of a viral genome. Upon chemical analysis, the nucleic acid is found to contain 27 percent cytosine, 27 percent adenine, 23 percent uracil, and 23 percent guanine. Based on this data, the viral genome most likely consists of:

   A. single-stranded DNA.
   B. double-stranded DNA.
   C. single-stranded RNA.
   D. double-stranded RNA.

212. Which of the following would form the most stable carbocation?

   A. $(CH_3)_2CHBr$ dissolved in toluene
   B. $(CH_3CH_2)_3COH$ dissolved in acetone
   C. $(CH_3)_3COH$ dissolved in H_2SO_4
   D. CH_3CH_2I dissolved in diethyl ether

213. Which of the following graphs best corresponds to the optimal pH for pepsin activity?

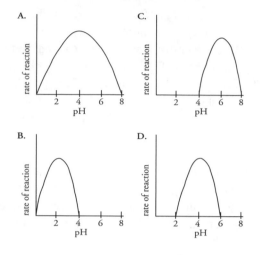

214. Mammalian fetal circulation is similar to amphibian adult circulation in that:

   A. gas exchange occurs only in the lungs.
   B. gas exchange occurs only in the placenta.
   C. the heart has only three chambers prior to birth.
   D. there is a mixing of oxygenated and deoxygenated blood within the heart.

STOP.

IF YOU FINISH BEFORE TIME HAS EXPIRED, CHECK YOUR WORK.
YOU MAY GO BACK TO ANY QUESTION IN THIS PART ONLY.

Answer Key

Full-Length Practice MCAT

PHYSICAL SCIENCES

1.	C	9.	A	17.	B	25.	B	33.	C	41.	D	49.	C	57.	B
2.	D	10.	B	18.	D	26.	D	34.	B	42.	D	50.	B	58.	D
3.	B	11.	D	19.	A	27.	D	35.	B	43.	A	51.	D	59.	C
4.	C	12.	B	20.	C	28.	C	36.	A	44.	D	52.	B	60.	B
5.	A	13.	B	21.	B	29.	A	37.	A	45.	C	53.	C	61.	A
6.	B	14.	C	22.	A	30.	D	38.	B	46.	A	54.	A	62.	C
7.	C	15.	C	23.	B	31.	B	39.	B	47.	A	55.	A	63.	D
8.	D	16.	A	24.	C	32.	A	40.	A	48.	B	56.	A	64.	C

65.	D	73.	D
66.	D	74.	B
67.	A	75.	C
68.	C	76.	A
69.	D	77.	C
70.	C		
71.	B		
72.	D		

VERBAL REASONING

78.	A	84.	B	90.	A	96.	A	102.	B	108.	D	114.	D	120.	C
79.	A	85.	C	91.	D	97.	B	103.	D	109.	D	115.	D	121.	D
80.	C	86.	C	92.	C	98.	B	104.	D	110.	D	116.	C	122.	A
81.	D	87.	D	93.	D	99.	B	105.	B	111.	A	117.	B	123.	D
82.	B	88.	C	94.	A	100.	D	106.	A	112.	C	118.	A	124.	C
83.	D	89.	D	95.	C	101.	C	107.	D	113.	A	119.	B	125.	D

126.	C	132.	A
127.	C	133.	B
128.	D	134.	A
129.	C	135.	C
130.	C	136.	D
131.	B	137.	C

BIOLOGICAL SCIENCES

138.	D	146.	C	154.	C	162.	A	170.	C	178.	C	186.	B	194.	C
139.	B	147.	A	155.	A	163.	C	171.	D	179.	C	187.	C	195.	B
140.	D	148.	B	156.	A	164.	B	172.	A	180.	D	188.	A	196.	D
141.	C	149.	B	157.	B	165.	B	173.	B	181.	B	189.	D	197.	B
142.	D	150.	D	158.	A	166.	B	174.	B	182.	A	190.	B	198.	A
143.	B	151.	A	159.	C	167.	D	175.	D	183.	D	191.	A	199.	D
144.	A	152.	C	160.	C	168.	A	176.	D	184.	D	192.	C	200.	A
145.	C	153.	A	161.	A	169.	D	177.	A	185.	B	193.	D	201.	A

202.	C	210.	A
203.	B	211.	C
204.	C	212.	C
205.	B	213.	B
206.	D	214.	D
207.	D		
208.	B		
209.	A		

Score Conversion Chart

Full-Length Practice MCAT

Physical Science		Verbal Reasoning		Biological Science	
Raw Score*	Estimated Scaled Score*	Raw Score*	Estimated Scaled Score*	Raw Score*	Estimated Scaled Score*
0	1	0–24	1	0–10	1
1–14	2	25–27	2	11–21	2
15–20	3	28–30	3	22–25	3
21–26	4	31–33	4	26–30	4
27–32	5	34–36	5	31–35	5
33–38	6	37–40	6	36–40	6
39–42	7	41–43	7	41–43	7
43–47	8	44–47	8	44–47	8
48–51	9	48–49	9	48–52	9
52–55	10	50–51	10	53–55	10
56–59	11	52–53	11	56–60	11
60–62	12	54–55	12	61–62	12
63–66	13	56–57	13	63–66	13
67–74	14	58–59	14	67–71	14
75–77	15	60	15	72–77	15

* This score coversion chart has been derived from a large representative sample of Kaplan students around the country. It will provide you with a score based on your performance compared to others who have taken this exam. Because the exam has been designed to closely match the MCAT content and format specifications, and because so many MCAT test takers prepare with Kaplan, this chart provides a rough estimate of your performance against the population who will sit for the MCAT. No test or score conversion chart can exactly predict actual test-day performance.

Answers and Explanations

Physical Sciences

Passage I (Questions 1–5)

1. C

To answer this question, you need to use Wien's law, which is given in the passage. It states that $\lambda = 2.9 \times 10^6/T$, where λ is the most intense wavelength emitted in nm and T is the temperature in kelvins. Since the temperature of the Sun's photosphere is 5,800 K, the most intense wavelength emitted is given by $\lambda = 2.9 \times 10^6/5,800 = 500$ nm, which is choice C.

2. D

When an electron makes a transition from a higher energy state to a lower energy state, a photon is emitted with energy equal to the difference between the energies of the two states. The table in the passage provides energies for photon transitions from energy state $n - 2$ to various higher energy states in hydrogen. The absolute energy difference between states $n = 4$ and $n = 3$ is equal to the difference between their energies relative to the $n = 2$ state. Therefore, the energy of the photon emitted in the transition from $n = 4$ to $n = 3$ is $4.08 \times 10^{-19} - 3.02 \times 10^{-19} = 1.06 \times 10^{-19} \approx 10^{-19}$ J.

The energy of a photon E is given by $E = hc/\lambda$, where h is Planck's constant, c is the speed of light in a vacuum, and λ is the photon's wavelength. Rearranging to solve for λ gives $\lambda = hc/E$. Using $E = 10^{-19}$ J from above, we find:

$$\lambda = (6.6 \times 10^{-34})(3 \times 10^8)/(10^{-19}) \text{ m.}$$

Rounding to the nearest integer gives $\lambda = 20 \times 10^{-34+8+19}$ m $= 2 \times 10^{-6}$ m. Since 1 nm $= 10^{-9}$ m, $\lambda = 2,000$ nm, which is choice D.

3. B

The binding energy of an electron is by definition the energy required to detach an electron from an atom in its ground state. Hydrogen's ground state is the $n = 1$ state. When the atom is ionized, the electron is separated from the atom and makes a transition to the highest energy state, the $n = \infty$ state. This is not a distinct energy state, but rather it defines the minimum energy that must be transferred to the electron to free it from the atom. Hence, the energy difference between the $n = \infty$ and the $n = 1$ state is the binding energy of the electron in the hydrogen atom, and choice B is correct.

Choices A, C, and D can all be ruled out based on the data presented in the passage which indicates that the energy increases as n increases. This implies that the energy of the $n = 2$ state is greater than that of the $n = 1$ state by some finite, positive amount E_{12}. Furthermore, according to the table, the energy of the $n = \infty$ state is 5.44×10^{-19} J greater than the energy of the $n = 2$ state. Since the energy difference between $n = \infty$ and $n = 1$ is the sum of these two finite, positive quantities ($E_{12} + 5.44 \times 10^{-19}$ J), it must also be finite and positive. Therefore, choice A is wrong. Choice C is wrong because a zero frequency photon would correspond to zero energy, as shown by the formula $E = hf$, but, as discussed above, the energy absorbed must be positive. Choice D is also wrong because the sum $E_{12} + 5.44 \times 10^{-19}$ J is clearly greater than

5.44×10^{-19} J, the energy absorbed in the $n = 2$ to $n = \infty$ transition.

4. C

This question asks for the frequency f of light given its wavelength λ. If you didn't remember the relationship between the two, you could have figured it out from the formula $hf = hc/\lambda$ given in the passage. Dividing both sides by h, we obtain $f = c/\lambda$, where c is the speed of light in a vacuum. Plugging in $\lambda = 550$ nm, we obtain

$$f = \frac{3 \times 10^8 \text{m/s}}{550 \text{ nm}} = 5 \times 10^{14} \text{Hz}$$

which most closely corresponds to choice C.

5. A

This question asks you to apply Wien's law to the case of a star changing its size and temperature. Wien's law, $\lambda = 2.9 \times 10^6/T$, indicates that the wavelength of the peak intensity only depends on temperature. Therefore, if the star's temperature doesn't change when it doubles in size, the wavelength of the peak intensity of the star's radiation will not change. Choice A is therefore the correct answer, and choices B and C are wrong. Since the shape of the spectrum, like the location of the peak, is also a function of temperature choice D is wrong as well.

Passage II (Questions 6–12)

6. B

When the half-reactions are written as reductions—as they are here—the cell voltage is determined by the equation

$$E_{cell} = E_{cathode} - E_{anode}$$

(Remember that E_{cell} must be greater than zero for the reaction to be spontaneous.) The cell voltage is therefore 2.05 V:

$$1.69 \text{ V} - (-0.36 \text{ V}) = 2.05 \text{ V}$$

Since the potentials of cells connected in series are additive, a 20 V battery needs ten 2.05 V cells, choice B. Choice A is a 10 V battery, choice C is a 30 V battery, and choice D is a 40 V battery.

7. C

Oxidation—the loss of electrons—occurs at the anode. When both half-reactions are written as reductions, the following equation is used to determine the cell potential:

$$E_{cell} = E_{cathode} - E_{anode}$$

(Again, remember that E_{cell} must be greater than zero for the reaction to be spontaneous.) The cell potential is positive when the reduction potential of the second reaction in Table 1 is subtracted from the first reaction, making the first reaction the cathode and the second reaction the anode. Since oxidation occurs at the anode, the reaction must proceed to the left, making choice C the correct answer. Choice A and choice B are wrong because the first reaction is the cathode reaction, not the anode reaction. Choice D is wrong because the second reaction proceeds to the left, not to the right.

8. D

Oxidation occurs when a species' oxidation number increases; reduction occurs when a species' oxidation number decreases. Also discussed earlier, oxidation occurs at the anode and reduction occurs at the cathode. From the answer choices, it can be seen that lead oxide and lead are the only species that have to be investigated. In

Reaction 1, Pb^{4+}, in lead oxide, is going to Pb^{2+}, in lead sulfate. Since lead's oxidation number has decreased, it has been reduced. Choice A, choice B, and choice C can, therefore, all be eliminated, leaving choice D as the correct answer. Choice D is correct because lead is being reduced at the anode—where oxidation occurs—from Pb to Pb^{2+}.

9. A

The battery is being recharged, so Reaction 1 is proceeding to the left. Since aqueous sulfuric acid, H_2SO_4, is one of the products of recharging, the concentration of H^+ will increase, making choice A the correct answer. Choice B is wrong because $PbSO_4(s)$ is serving as a reactant during recharging, and is therefore consumed during the reaction. Choice C is wrong because water is also a reactant during recharging. Choice D is wrong because the amount of lead oxide increases, not decreases as the battery is being recharged.

10. B

As can be seen in Reaction 1, when the lead-acid battery is being discharged, sulfuric acid, a reactant, is being consumed. Since it is stated in the passage that sulfuric acid is the electrolyte, the density will decrease as the discharge progresses, so the density at point A is less than that at point B. Choice A is wrong because at point A there is less electrolyte present, not more. Choice C is wrong because the density decreases as the discharge progresses. Choice D is wrong because there is a direct relationship between the density of the electrolyte and the state of discharge.

11. D

Remembering that a $k\Omega$ is $10^3\ \Omega$ and using the relationship that $V = IR$, a current of 0.1 A times a resistance of 10,000 Ω gives a voltage of 1000 V. You might have chosen choice B if you did not convert kiloohms to ohms. Choices A and D represent other conversion errors.

12. B

The reason that the battery "goes dead" with decreasing temperature is that the viscosity of the electrolyte increases. At higher viscosities the ions are moving much slower, which leads to an increase in resistance and a decrease in the power output. Roman numeral I states that the resistance of the electrolyte has decreased. This is not true, the resistance of the electrolyte increases with decreasing temperature. Since choice A, choice C, and choice D all contain Roman numeral I, they can be eliminated, leaving choice B as the correct answer.

Passage III (Questions 13–17)

13. B

The question stem states that the voltage source, which according to the passage has negligible internal resistance, is replaced by a battery with a small, but significant internal resistance. A battery with significant internal resistance can be modeled as a voltage source connected in series with a resistor. Hence, the new circuit is the same as the one in Figure 1, except for the addition of a second resistor (call its resistance R_{int}) in series with the original resistor (call its resistance R_0). To determine how this additional resistance affects the circuit, use Ohm's law $V = IR$, where V is the voltage, I is the current, and R is the resistance. Solving for I gives $I = V/R$. Thus, in the original circuit, the voltage source supplies a voltage V and the ammeter measures a current $I_{original} = V/R_0$. In the new circuit, the total resistance is given by the addition rule for resistors in series, $R_{total} = R_0 + R_{int}$. Therefore, the current measured by the ammeter in the new circuit will be $I_{new} = V/(R_0 + R_{int})$, which is clearly smaller than Ioriginal since its denominator is larger. So choice B is correct, and choice A is wrong.

Choices C and D are wrong because the resistance of a resistor is a property that does not change with the addition of other resistors to the circuit. The resistance of a resistor remains constant when the voltage across it or the current through it changes.

14. C

Like charges repel each other and opposite charges attract each other. Since electrons have negative charge, they will move away from a negative terminal and move towards a positive terminal. This corresponds to the counterclockwise direction. So choices A and B can be ruled out.

By convention, current flows in the direction that positive charge would flow. This means that in the circuit in Figure 1, the current flows in the clockwise direction, from the positive terminal to the negative terminal, and choice C is the correct answer. If you couldn't figure out the direction of current flow or the direction that the electrons travel, but you knew they were opposite directions, you could have eliminated choices B and D.

15. C

Ammeters, like all components of electric circuits, have some internal resistance. Therefore, adding an ammeter to the circuit is like adding another resistor in series. If the ammeter has a large resistance, then the current flowing through the resistor will be significantly reduced when it is added to the circuit. If it has a small resistance, the current will be only slightly affected; so choice C is correct.

Choice A is wrong since insulated wires are wires surrounded by a nonconducting material, which prevents unintended contact with the current. Insulating the wires won't directly affect the current through the resistor and won't affect the way that the ammeter works. Choice B is wrong

as well: The current in the wire to the right of the resistor is the same as the current to the left of the resistor, so an ammeter will function identically at either location. In both cases, the ammeter is in series with the resistor. You can eliminate choice D because an ammeter that can detect current in either direction might be useful. But whether it can or not is unrelated to the ammeter's effect on the current flowing through the resistor.

16. A

When the electrons collide with the atoms of the resistor, the vibration of the atoms increase, and the atoms' kinetic energy, which is the energy of motion, increases as well. By definition, the temperature of a gas, liquid, or solid is a measure of the average kinetic energy of the atoms that make up the substance. Thus, the increase in the kinetic energy of the atoms is directly related to the increase in temperature, and choice A is correct.

Since temperature is related to the average kinetic energy and not the potential energy, choices B and D are wrong. As for choice C, the passage states that the atoms vibrate as a result of the collisions. A moving electron hits an atom which is basically stationary and starts it in motion. This means that the electron transfers some of its kinetic energy to the atom. So the electron's kinetic energy actually decreases as a result of the collisions, and choice C is wrong.

17. B

The energy delivered to a piece of toast must be equal to the energy dissipated by the toaster's resistor. The rate of energy dissipation, or the energy released per unit time, is known as the power. Mathematically, this can be expressed as $P = E/t$, where P is the power, and E is the energy released in time t. The passage gives the relation $P = I^2R$, where P is the power, I is the current, and R is the resistance of the resistor. Equating the two expressions for power and solving for E, gives $E = I^2Rt$. Now we substitute the values given in the question stem into the last equation for the energy and obtain $E = (4 \times 10^{-3}\ A)^2(10 \times 10^3\ \Omega)$ $(1\ s) = 0.16\ J$, which is choice B.

As is often the case with questions involving calculations, the wrong answer choices are the results of math errors. For example, you would have obtained choice D if you forgot to square the current.

Passage IV (Questions 18–23)

10. D

If the pH of blood increases to 7.6, it becomes more alkaline, and the pH of blood must be kept at approximately pH 7.4. Since it is stated in the second sentence of the last paragraph that blood pH can be adjusted rapidly by changes in the rate of CO_2 exhalation, choice A and choice B can be eliminated. In order to bring the pH of blood back to its normal value of 7.4, it must become more acidic; it becomes more acidic by increasing the concentration of H^+. Reaction 1 has H^+ as a product, and according to Le Châtelier's principle, you should know that a reaction will proceed in a direction that will consume an added reactant or product. In other words, the concentration of a product can be increased by increasing the concentration of a reactant. If the concentration of carbon dioxide is allowed to increase, it will react to produce more H^+, resulting in a lowering of the pH. The concentration of carbon dioxide will increase if it is not exhaled, making choice D the correct response.

19. A

Carbonic acid, H_2CO_3, is the intermediate formed when carbon dioxide and water combine, making choice A the correct response. You should be able to recognize that when the products of Reaction 1 combine, carbonic acid will result. Choice B is incorrect because it is just not a logical intermediate: water and carbon dioxide would not react to form H^+ and CO_3^{2-}. Choices C and D can be eliminated because they both contain carbon dioxide, which is one of the two reactants.

20. C

You should know that the smaller the pK_a the stronger the acid. Looking at Table 1, it can be seen that the histidine side chains buffer has a stronger conjugate acid than both the organic phosphates buffer and the ammonium buffer. Choice C is therefore the correct response. Choice A is wrong because the pK_a of the histidine side chains buffer is not equal to the organic phosphates buffer. Choice B is wrong because it is the reverse of what it should be. Choice D is wrong because, again, the pK_a of the histidine side chains buffer is not equal to the organic phosphates buffer.

21. B

In Region I the following reaction takes place:

$$H_3PO_4(aq) + OH^-(aq) \rightarrow H_2PO_4^-(aq) + H_2O$$

As OH^- is added, $H_2PO_4^-$ is formed and a buffer is realized. So, in this region, there is a point where the concentration of H_3PO_4 will equal that of $H_2PO_4^-$. In Region II there is a point where exactly enough base has been added to react with all of the H_3PO_4; this point is called an equivalence point. In Region III the following reaction takes place:

$$H_2PO_4^-(aq) + OH^-(aq) \rightarrow HPO_4^{2-}(aq) + H_2O$$

Again, this system constitutes a buffer, and there is a point in this region where—after enough base has been added—the concentration of $H_2PO_4^-$ will equal that of HPO_4^{2-}. Choice B is therefore the correct response. In Region IV there is another equivalence point when exactly enough base has been added to react with all of the $H_2PO_4^-$. In Region V the following reaction takes place:

$$HPO_4^{2-}(aq) + OH^-(aq) \rightarrow PO_4^{3-}(aq) + H_2O$$

This system is, of course, a buffer as well.

22. A

When a weak acid is reacted with a strong base, the equivalence point will be in the basic region. Consider the titration of equimolar solutions of acetic acid and NaOH. Before the equivalence point, the following reaction takes place:

$$HC_2H_3O_2(aq) + OH^-(aq) \rightarrow H_2O + C_2H_3O_2^-(aq)$$

At the equivalence point, only $C_2H_3O_2^-$ exists. When $C_2H_3O_2^-$ undergoes hydrolysis (i.e., reacts with water), hydroxide ions are formed according to the following equilibrium:

$$C_2H_3O_2^-(aq) + H_2O \rightleftharpoons HC_2H_3O_2(aq) + OH^-(aq)$$

The numerical value of the equilibrium constant along with the initial concentration of acetate is all that is needed to determine the hydroxide ion concentration. When equimolar solutions of a strong acid and a strong base are titrated, the equivalence point will be neutral. It is neutral because neither of the ions present at the equivalence point can undergo hydrolysis. Choice A is therefore the correct response. Choice B would be correct if a weak base was titrated with a strong acid.

23. B

As the passage states, the immediate buffering effect of bicarbonate is controlled by changes in the breathing rate. When acidosis occurs, the concentration of H^+ is too high. As discussed earlier, Le Châtelier's principle applies: In order to decrease the concentration of H^+, the concentration of carbon dioxide must decrease. If the breathing rate increases, more carbon dioxide is exhaled and its concentration in the blood decreases. Since the effect of this rapid breathing is to remove carbon dioxide from the body, the ultimate effect is to decrease the total CO_2/HCO_3^- concentration in the blood. Therefore choice B is correct. Choice A is wrong because the ratio of CO_2 to HCO_3^- would decrease, not increase. Choices C and D are wrong because the breathing rate would increase, not decrease.

Discrete Questions

24. C

Since rotation about a point is at issue, an understanding of torques is necessary to solve the problem. The torque τ, or rotational force on a rigid body resting on a pivot point, is given by $\tau = rF$, when a force F acts at a distance r from the pivot in a direction perpendicular to the axis of rotation. Balance is achieved when the net torque is zero, i.e., the clockwise torque equals the counterclockwise torque.

Draw a little sketch of the telephone handset, balanced horizontally on a pivot point. The weight of the mouthpiece is (100 grams)g, where g is the acceleration due to gravity. Call the distance between the point where this force acts and the pivot r_m. Similarly, the weight of the earpiece is (150 grams)g and acts a distance r_e from the pivot. To achieve balance, the opposing torques must be equal to each other, so (100 grams)gr_m = (150 grams)gr_e. Solving for r_m and canceling out g gives $r_m = (3/2)r_e$. So the mouthpiece must be (3/2) times farther from the pivot than the earpiece, and choice C is correct.

25. B

The relationship between ΔG, ΔH, ΔS, and temperature is

$$\Delta G = \Delta H - T\Delta S$$

For a reaction to be spontaneous, ΔG must be less than zero. If a reaction is not spontaneous at any temperature, ΔH must be positive and ΔS must be negative. No matter what the temperature, ΔG will always be positive and the reaction will be nonspontaneous. Choice B is therefore the correct response. Choice A is for a reaction that would be spontaneous if the temperature was sufficiently high. Choice C is for a reaction that is spontaneous at ALL temperatures. Choice D is for a reaction that would be spontaneous if the temperature was sufficiently low.

26. D

To achieve boiling, intermolecular forces holding the liquid together have to be overcome so that the molecules of the substance can enter the vapor phase. Boiling points of substances, therefore, often reflect the strength of the intermolecular forces operating among the molecules. Choice D is correct because the intermolecular hydrogen-oxygen bonds in water are stronger than the intermolecular hydrogen-sulfur bonds in hydrogen sulfide. When hydrogen is bonded to a strongly electronegative element such as nitrogen, oxygen, or fluorine, very strong intermolecular forces exist. These forces are called hydrogen bonds. Choice A is wrong because, although it is true that intramolecular oxygen-hydrogen bonds are stronger than intramolecular sulfur-hydrogen bonds, it is not the reason that water boils at a higher temperature than hydrogen sul-

fide. Choice B is wrong because if the enthalpy of vaporization of water is less than that of hydrogen sulfide, less energy is required to evaporate a given quantity of water at a constant temperature than for hydrogen sulfide. This is not what happens: The heat of vaporization of water is greater than that of hydrogen sulfide, so water boils at a higher temperature. Choice C is wrong because it is the ability of water to hydrogen bond that makes it boil at a higher temperature.

27. D

A semipermeable membrane allows the movement of solvent molecules, but not solute molecules. This means that water molecules can move through the semipermeable membrane and that glucose molecules cannot. Choice A, choice B, and choice C can all be eliminated, leaving choice D as the correct response. You should be aware that osmosis is the net movement of solvent molecules through a semipermeable membrane from a pure solvent or a dilute solution to a more concentrated solution. In this case, solution A, which is 5 percent glucose, is more concentrated than solution B, which is only 1 percent glucose. So, there will be a movement from the more dilute solution, solution B, to one of higher concentration, which is solution A.

28. C

Normality is defined as the number of equivalents of solute per liter of solution. An equivalent of an acid is the amount of acid required to give one mole of H^+. Phosphoric acid, which contains three moles of protons per mole of acid, therefore contains three equivalents per mole. A one-molar solution of phosphoric acid is said to be 3 normal. The solution in question contains 49 grams of phosphoric acid, and the molar mass of phosphoric acid is 98. Since 49 is half of 98, the amount of phosphoric acid in this sample is half of the 3 equivalents in each mole of the acid. So there are 1.5 equivalents of phosphoric acid in this solution. We know the total volume of the solution is 2000 milliliters, or 2 liters. So this solution contains 1.5 equivalents of acid per 2 liters. This comes to 0.75 equivalents per liter, which is a 0.75 N solution.

Passage V (Questions 29–33)

29. A

The passage mentions that metals have partially filled valence bands. This means that there are low energy unoccupied atomic orbitals in metals through which electrons may move freely. Therefore, the valence band for metals is the conduction band, and consequently, there is no band gap. Metals such as iron are good conductors of electricity because of these unoccupied low energy orbitals. (All of this information is contained in the passage and requires little or no background knowledge.) Choice B is incorrect because metals, unlike semiconductors, do not have a band gap. Choice C is wrong because iron's 3d orbital is not filled; it has only 6 electrons, not 10. Choice D is true of many solids including metals, semiconductors, and insulators, but it does not answer the question and so is incorrect.

30. D

Statement I says that heat could be expected to reduce the frequency of collisions between moving electrons. This is not true: Heat increases the kinetic energy of electrons, thereby increasing, not decreasing, the frequency of collisions. Choice A and choice C can be eliminated. Statement II says that heat breaks covalent bonds. This is true: Sufficient energy—in this case supplied by heat—will break covalent bonds. The passage doesn't tell you explicitly that heat breaks covalent bonds in semiconductors, but it

is implied in the description of the semiconductive properties of silicon. In the first sentence of the second paragraph, you are told that silicon forms tetrahedral covalent bonds, and that when heated, it will conduct. Since silicon is sp^3 hybridized—forming a filled valence band—bonds must be broken in order to promote electrons to the conduction band. Choice B can therefore be eliminated, making choice D the correct response. The truth of Statement III should then be obvious: In order for the freed electrons to "jump" to the higher energy band gap, they must gain energy. Heat supplies the energy and permits this to happen.

31. B

The passage states that phosphorus atoms increase the conductivity of silicon because phosphorus provides the crystal with unbonded electrons, while boron atoms produce holes in the bonding structure. From the Periodic Table, it can be seen that boron has three valence electrons, silicon has four, and phosphorus has five. Since the bonds in the silicon crystal are tetrahedral, a phosphorus atom surrounded by silicon atoms will be able to form covalent bonds with only four of its valence electrons, leaving the fifth one unbonded. Boron has only three valence electrons, so a boron atom surrounded by silicon atoms will only be able to form three covalent bonds, leaving a hole in the bonding structure of silicon. It is the presence of these unbonded electrons and holes that enhances the conductivity of phosphorus. Choice B is therefore the correct answer. Choice A is wrong because the difference in electronegativity between boron, phosphorus, and silicon is quite small. Choice C is wrong for two reasons: Phosphorus isn't a semimetal, and even if these two elements were both semimetals and good semiconductors, this in itself wouldn't explain the enhancement of silicon's conductivity produced by doping silicon with some of these elements. Choice D is wrong because, like choice

C, it wouldn't explain the phenomenon the question asks about even if it were true.

32. A

Since the band gap is 1.1 eV, an applied voltage in excess of 1.1 V would give the electrons enough energy to cross the band gap and populate the conduction band. (You should know that an electron volt is equal to the energy required to move an electron through a potential difference of one volt.) Choice A is therefore the correct response. Choice B is wrong because pure, undoped silicon doesn't have any holes. The passage states that holes are produced when the silicon is doped with boron choice C is wrong because there is no information in the passage that suggests that the band gap is affected by an external potential. Choice D is wrong because the electrons do have enough energy to overcome the band gap and would move into the conduction band.

33. C

The passage provides almost all the necessary information to answer this question. The only piece of background information needed is that electrons flow from the negative terminal to the positive terminal. The passage states that phosphorus-doped silicon has more electrons than pure silicon and that boron-doped silicon has fewer electrons than pure silicon. In addition, it is stated that electrons flow more easily from a side with excess electrons—the phosphorus-doped silicon—to a side with fewer electrons—the boron-doped silicon. So, if the semiconductor orientation were switched, electron flow would not be as easy as the original configuration.

Passage VI (Questions 34–38)

34. B

This question is a straightforward application of the equation given in the passage, $E = 1240/\lambda$. In this equation, E is the energy in electron-volts of a photon having a wavelength λ in nanometers. Note that this formula is a variant of the more familiar equation $E = hc/\lambda$. Plugging $\lambda = 632.8$ nm, we obtain $E = 1240/632.8 \approx 2.0$ eV, which is closest to choice B. It is a good idea to save time by estimating because the answer choices are relatively far apart.

35. B

To answer this question, you have to refer to the passage to find the description of the condition called a population inversion. The passage states that a population inversion exists when the percentage of neon atoms with electrons in the 20.66 eV energy level is greater than the percentage of neon atoms with electrons in lower levels. The distinctive characteristic of this distribution is that the percentage of atoms with electrons in a higher energy level is greater than the percentage of atoms with electrons in lower levels. The only choice that is consistent with this is choice B.

36. A

To solve this problem, apply the law of conservation of energy to atomic systems. In the absence of dissipative forces, the total energy of a system, which is the sum of the kinetic and potential energies, is conserved. In the case of atoms, the potential energy is the energy stored when the electron moves to a higher energy state by absorbing a photon.

In the collision between the helium and neon atoms, the helium atom loses 20.61 eV of potential energy because its electron returns to the ground state and the neon atom gains 20.66 eV of potential energy. Since energy is conserved, the helium atom must have lost some kinetic energy as well. The neon atom cannot gain more energy than the helium atom loses. Therefore, the minimum amount of kinetic energy that the helium atom must lose is equal to the difference between the two potential energies. This is equal to 20.66 – 20.61 = 0.05 eV, which is choice A. If the helium atom loses only this amount of kinetic energy, then the neon atom's kinetic energy will not change during the collision. If the helium atom loses more than 0.05 eV, then the neon atom's kinetic energy will increase.

37. A

The power of the laser is 6.2×10^{15} eV/s, which means that the laser produces 6.2×10^{15} eV of energy each second. This energy takes the form of photon energy. To solve for the number of photons produced per second, figure out how many photons correspond to an energy of 6.2×10^{15} eV. The formula given in the passage states that the energy (in eV) of one photon is given by $E = 1,240/\lambda$, where λ is the photon's wavelength in nm. Hence, the energy of n photons must given by $n(1,240/\lambda)$. Setting this expression equal to 6.2×10^{15} eV and solving for n, we obtain $n = \lambda(6.2 \times 10^{15}/1,240)$. The question stem states that for this laser, $\lambda = 200$ nm. Substituting in, we calculate $n = 200(6.2 \times 10^{15}/1,240) = 1.0 \times 10^{15}$, which is choice A.

38. B

To answer this question, you have to figure out the difference between stimulated and spontaneous emission. The passage states that a photon is emitted in a random direction when an atom spontaneously decays. This process is called spontaneous emission. It also states that a photon can stimulate an electron transition in an atom. The photon that is emitted in this process, called stimulated emission, travels in the same direction as the stimulating photon. Therefore, spontaneous emission produces photons that travel in random directions, whereas stimulated emission produces photons that travel in the same direction as the stimulating photon. A coherent beam of light consists of photons travelling in the same direction.

Choices A and C are wrong because, as stated in the third paragraph, the photon produced by spontaneous emission causes stimulated emission by inducing the *same* electron transition in another excited atom. Since the electron transition is the same, the photon energy released by the transition is the same, and the photon wavelengths must be the same because energy and wavelength are related by the formula $E = 1240/\lambda$.

Choice D is incorrect because stimulated emission is necessary to obtain a large number of photons traveling in the same direction.

Passage VII (Questions 39–44)

39. B

The passage states that after death, the ^{14}C in a skeleton that beta decays is not replaced by new ^{14}C. Consequently, as time passes, the amount of ^{14}C in the skeleton decreases.

The half-life quantifies the rate of this decrease. The half-life of an isotope is the length of time it takes for half of the atoms in a sample of that isotope to decay. A skeleton starts out with 8 g of ^{14}C, and the half-life of ^{14}C is 5,730 years. Therefore, after 5,730 years, 8 g of ^{14}C will decay to 4 g. After another 5,730 years, 4 g will decay to 2 g, and after yet another 5,730 years, 2 g will decay to 1 g, which is the amount present in the prehistoric skeleton. Hence, the prehistoric skeleton must be 3(5,730) = 17,190 years old, and choice B is correct.

40. A

The number of atoms decaying per unit time is directly proportional to the number of atoms present. To see this, recall that the definition of half-life is the time required for half of a sample to decay. The half-life is a constant for a given material regardless of the sample size. Therefore, if the initial amount of material is greater, then a larger amount of material will decay during each half-life. If the production rate of ^{14}C increases, then there will be more ^{14}C present. Hence, the number of ^{14}C atoms decaying per unit time will increase. So choice A is correct and choice B is incorrect.

The second paragraph describes how a balance between ^{14}C production and decay is reached, so that the total amount of ^{14}C on Earth approaches a constant. If ^{14}C production is increased, then the weight of ^{14}C on Earth will initially increase. However, as this ^{14}C begins to decay, the total amount of ^{14}C will approach a new constant as a new balance is reached between the production and decay processes. Hence, choice C is wrong.

If the production of ^{14}C increases, then a larger fraction of the carbon on Earth will be ^{14}C, and living organisms will ingest a larger fraction of ^{14}C. Therefore, the percentage of ^{14}C in living organisms will increase, and choice D is wrong.

41. D

Carbon dating uses the fact that ^{14}C is unstable and decays over time, while ^{12}C is stable and does not decay. Let's say the ratio of ^{14}C to ^{12}C in an organism is known at the moment of death. By measuring the ratio of ^{14}C to ^{12}C in a fossil, the age of the fossil can be determined because the ^{14}C in the dead organism decays over time in a quantifiable way.

Although it is not explicitly stated in the passage, choice D is an assumption of carbon dating. It correctly states that the half-life of ^{14}C does not depend upon conditions external to the ^{14}C nucleus. This means that the half-life does not depend on the weather, the amount of ^{14}C present, etc. Because the half-life is a constant with respect to conditions external to the nucleus, it can be used to measure elapsed time accurately. Since measuring time is the goal of carbon dating, choice D is a necessary assumption.

Choice A is wrong because ingestion is an event that is external to the nucleus. Choice C is wrong because the type of molecule in which ^{14}C is incorporated is also a condition external to the nucleus. Choice B is wrong because we know from biology that some carbon leaves the body as waste. This does not affect carbon dating, however, because what matters is the ratio of ^{14}C to ^{12}C left in the body, not the specific amount of ^{14}C left in the body.

42. D

The age of the galaxy is much greater than that of fossils on the Earth. Therefore, in determining the age of the galaxy, it makes sense to use an isotope with a longer half-life than ^{14}C, which is used in determining the age of Earth fossils. This is because ^{14}C will decay to undetectable quantities more quickly than an isotope with a longer half-life, like ^{232}Th. Hence, choice D is correct, and choice A is incorrect.

Choice B is wrong because there is no reason to think that ^{14}C is more abundant in stars. And if it were true, ^{14}C *would* be more suitable for this application because the larger abundance would be easier to measure. Choice C is wrong because the instability of ^{14}C, and ^{232}Th for that matter, is precisely what makes them useful as dating tools.

43. A

To answer this question, you have to balance a nuclear reaction. The question stem suggests the reaction

$$^{14}_{7}\text{N} + ^{1}_{0}\text{n} \rightarrow ^{14}_{6}\text{C} + ^{a}_{b}?,$$

which has a nitrogen nucleus and a neutron on the left side and a carbon nucleus and the unknown particle on the right.

Two things must be balanced in a nuclear reaction: the charge of the nucleus (which corresponds to the number of protons), and the number of nucleons (which is the number of protons plus the number of neutrons). Balancing nuclear charge, we obtain $7 + 0 = 6 + b$, which implies $b = 1$. Balancing the number of nucleons, we obtain $14 + 1 = 14 + a$, which implies $a = 1$. Thus, the unknown particle is a nucleon with a charge of +1. The only particle that fits both criteria is the proton, choice A. Choice B is wrong because an electron is not a nucleon and it has a charge of −1. Choice C is wrong because a helium nucleus has 4 nucleons and a charge of +2. Choice D is wrong because a neutron has a charge of 0.

44. D

Kinetic energy, the energy of motion, equals $(1/2)mv^2$, where m is the mass of the object and v is its speed. The electron emitted when a ^{14}C nucleus decays is emitted with some initial speed and thus has kinetic energy. After it enters lead and is stopped, the electron's speed is zero so its kinetic energy is also zero. In other words, all the electron's kinetic energy is gone. Since energy is conserved, 100 percent of the electron's kinetic energy must have been transferred somewhere, and in this case, it is transferred to the lead. Hence, choice D is correct.

Passage VIII (Questions 45–49)

45. C

This question is testing your knowledge of phase diagrams. You should know that Region I—the lower temperature region—is where the solid state exists, Region II—the higher temperature and pressure region—is where the liquid phase exists, and that Region III—the higher temperature and lower pressure region—is where the vapor phase exists. Choice C is correct because at this temperature and pressure the liquid phase exists. Choice A and choice B are wrong because the vapor phase exists at these points. Choice D is wrong because the solid phases exists at this point.

46. A

Calcium chloride, by forming solid hydrates with water, is often used as a desiccant, or drying agent. It is used in this experiment because the presence of water might prevent the arsine gas from igniting. Choice B is wrong because calcium chloride is not basic, rendering it ineffective in removing HCl. Choice C is wrong because—as seen in Figure 1—calcium chloride and zinc ion do not have any contact. Choice D is wrong because arsine gas is the analyte, removing it would defeat the purpose of the test.

47. A

It is stated in the last sentence of the first paragraph that yellow arsenic is unstable. Since it is less stable than gray arsenic, meaning that it is at a higher potential energy, more energy will be released when it converts to As_4O_6. Choice B is wrong because gray arsenic, being more stable than the yellow, will release less energy. Choices C and D are wrong because, as just discussed, they release different amounts of energy.

48. B

The solubility of one compound in another is usually governed by the rule that "like dissolves like." Water and ammonia, both being polar, are quite soluble in each other. Arsine has a similar geometry to that of ammonia, but the electronegativity of arsenic is substantially less than that of nitrogen, and remember: ammonia can hydrogen bond with water, arsine cannot. In fact, the electronegativity of arsenic is very close to that of hydrogen. Because of arsenic's electronegativity, arsine has a small dipole moment, rendering it insoluble in polar solvents such as water. While choices A, C, and D are true statements, each are less important factors in influencing the solubility of compounds, especially in the case of arsine.

49. C

Because there are three sulfides in orpiment and the molecule has no charge overall, the total negative charge of the sulfides, minus six, must be balanced by the positive charges of the arsenics. The two arsenics, therefore, have a collective charge of plus six, and each arsenic has a charge of plus three.

Discrete Questions

50. B

Ammonia has a central nitrogen atom, bonded to three hydrogen atoms. According to the valence-shell electron-pair repulsion theory, or VSEPR theory, a central atom surrounded by three bonded pairs of electrons and one lone pair of electrons has a pyramidal geometry. Choice A is wrong because a trigonal planar molecule has the central atom surrounded by three bonding pairs of electrons and no lone pairs, such as BF_3. Choice C is wrong because a tetrahedral molecule has the central atom surrounded by four bonding

pairs of electrons and no lone pairs, such as CH_4. Choice D is wrong because a trigonal bipyramidal shape has the central atom surrounded by five bonding electron pairs and no lone pairs, such as PF_5.

51. D

Archimedes' principle states that the buoyant force exerted by a fluid on a submerged object is equal to the weight of the fluid displaced. In this case, the submerged object is the research module and the fluid is ocean water. Mathematically, the buoyant force is given by $F = m_wg$, where m_w is the mass of the water and g is the acceleration due to gravity. Since we are not given the mass of the water displaced, we express it as $m_w = \rho_wV_w$, where ρ_w is the density of the water and V_w is the volume of the water displaced. But the volume of the water displaced is identical to the volume of the submerged module, V_0. Hence, $m_w = \rho_wV_w = \rho_wV_0$, and $F = m_wg = \rho_wV_0g$. Since the answer choices are far apart, we round off the values given in the question and calculate:

$$F = \rho_wV_0g \approx (1{,}000 \text{ kg/m}^3)(150 \text{ m}^3)(10 \text{ m/s}^2) = 1.5 \times 10^6 \text{ N},$$

which is choice D. Note that no conversions are necessary since all the values are given in SI units.

52. B

To solve this problem, apply Hooke's law $F = kx$, where F is the force applied to the spring, x is the distance the spring stretches, and k is the spring constant. The forces applied in this case are weights. Since weight is proportional to mass, the distance the spring stretches is also proportional to the mass of the object attached to the spring.

The spring starts out with a length of 64 cm. When the 0.5 kg mass is attached, it stretches 8 percent longer, or 64(0.08) = 5.12 cm. Since the distance stretched and the mass attached are proportional, the ratio of the distance stretched to the mass attached is $(5.12 \text{ cm})/(0.5 \text{ kg}) \approx 5/(0.5) = 10$ cm/kg. In other words, each kilogram attached to the spring stretches it 10 cm. Thus, when the 0.4 kg mass is attached, the spring is stretched a distance $(0.4 \text{ kg})(10 \text{ cm/kg}) = 4$ cm. Therefore, the total length of the spring is its original length plus the distance it stretches, or 64 + 4 = 68 cm. This is choice B.

53. C

The electrostatic force between two charged particles is given by $F = kq_1q_2/r^2$, where k is a constant, q_1 and q_2 are the charges on the particles, and r is the distance between the two charges. Since the force is proportional to each of the charges, halving the charge on one of the particles will also halve the force, and choice C is correct. Halving the charge on both particles will reduce the force by one fourth, so choice B is wrong. Since the force is inversely proportional to the square of the distance, doubling the distance will reduce the force by one fourth, and choice A is wrong. Watch out for choice D. It is wrong because the presence of a third charge will not change the force of attraction between the first and second charges. The third charge, however, will change the net force on the first and second charges because it interacts with each separately.

54. A

When heat is absorbed during a reaction, ΔH is positive; when heat is released, ΔH is negative. The melting of ice requires absorption of heat to disrupt the attractions between molecules, so the change in enthalpy is positive, and you can eliminate choice B and choice D. Now, entropy is the measurement of the disorder in a system; the change in entropy is expressed as ΔS. When the

disorder of a system increases, ΔS is positive; when disorder decreases, ΔS is negative. When ice melts, the individual molecules of water become freer to move around, so there is an increase in disorder and ΔS is positive. Therefore, choice C is wrong and choice A is correct.

Passage IX (Questions 55–59)

55. A

The velocity of the softball is a vector, which means that it has both a magnitude and direction. At Point A, the velocity vector points up and to the right, because the softball is traveling in this direction. At Point C, however, the velocity vector points down and to the right. Since the velocity's direction has changed, it is not the same at Points A and C, and choice A is correct.

You should know that the gravitational potential energy of the softball is given by $U = mgy$, where m is the mass, g is the acceleration due to gravity, and y is the height above the earth. Since Points A and C are at the same height y, the gravitational potential is the same and choice C is incorrect.

The passage says to ignore air resistance, so the total mechanical energy, which is the kinetic plus potential energy, is conserved in this system. Since the gravitational potential is the same at Points A and C, the kinetic energy $(1/2)mv^2$ must be the same as well. Because the mass m does not change, the speed v must be the same at both points also, and choice B is wrong.

Since air resistance is negligible, the only force present is that of gravity, which acts in the vertical direction. Consequently, there is no horizontal force on the softball, which means there can be no horizontal acceleration. Therefore, the horizontal component of the velocity must remain the same throughout the softball's flight, and choice D is wrong.

56. A

Newton's second law $F = ma$ states that a force produces an acceleration in the same direction as the force. In the absence of a force, there is no acceleration. In this situation, the only force present is the force of gravity, which is the same at all times during the softball's flight. Near the earth's surface, the gravitational force is directed downward and its magnitude is given by $F = mg$, where m is the softball's mass and g is the acceleration due to gravity. Putting the gravitational force into Newton's second law, we obtain $ma = mg$. Canceling the masses, we obtain $a = g$. In other words, the acceleration of the softball is the same as the acceleration due to gravity.

Figure 1 shows that the unit vector j points upwards, which means that $-j$ points downwards. Because j is a unit vector, its magnitude is 1. Since the softball accelerates downward with a magnitude of g, the acceleration is symbolically given by $g(-j) = -gj$. Thus, choice A is correct. Choice C is incorrect because it has the wrong magnitude. Choices B and D are wrong because they both include an acceleration in the horizontal direction $-i$.

57. B

You should know that the change in momentum of a body is equal to the impulse applied to that body. The magnitude of the momentum of a body is given by mv, where m is its mass and v is its speed. In this situation an impulse is applied to the softball to launch it from the cannon. Before the impulse the speed of the softball is zero, so we can write $J = \Delta(mv) = mv_0 - m(0) = mv_0$, where J is the impulse. Solving for v_0, we obtain $v_0 = J/m$. Since m is inversely proportional to v_0, doubling the mass will halve v_0, so choice B is correct.

58. D

Figure 2 shows that the curve is symmetric around $t = t_b$. Since the axes of graphs are always linear unless otherwise stated, the time elapsed at Point C is twice the time elapsed at Point B. There are no horizontal forces because air resistance is negligible. Therefore, the horizontal speed is the constant v_0 throughout the softball's flight. The horizontal distance traveled is then given by $x = v_0 t$, where t is the time elapsed. Since the time elapsed at Point C is twice the time elapsed at Point B, the horizontal distance traveled at Point C is twice the horizontal distance traveled at Point B, and choice D is correct.

59. C

The softball starts off at rest and acquires a speed v_0 as it is launched from the cannon. The work-energy theorem states that the work done equals the change in the kinetic energy. Since the softball acquires a kinetic energy equal to $(1/2)mv_0^2$, the automatic pitcher must have done work on it. The pitcher uses air pressure, which builds up behind a disk, to do the work when the disk is released. The angle of the barrel to the horizontal will not affect this mechanism, and the softball will still be ejected with the same kinetic energy. Hence, the work done by the pitcher does not change.

Although it is true that the softball's maximum height increases and that the distance it lands from the cannon decreases, the work done by the pitcher does not change, so choices A and B are wrong. Although it is also true that gravity is a conservative force, it is irrelevant because the question asks about the work done by the pitcher, not the work done by gravity. Hence, choice D is incorrect as well.

Passage X (Questions 60-65)

60. B

To solve this problem, apply the formula given in the passage which quantifies the positions of the intensity maxima. The formula is $d\sin\theta = n\lambda$, where d is the distance between the slits, θ is the angle, and λ is the wavelength. The note in the passage says that $\sin\theta \approx \theta$ when θ is small. You have to know that this approximation is only valid when θ is measured in radians. Making this approximation, we obtain $d\theta = n\lambda$, and solving for θ we obtain $\theta = n\lambda /d$. Note that the distance units of λ and d can be anything as long as they are the same. n is given in the question stem, and λ and d are given in Figure 1. Substituting, we obtain

$$\theta = \frac{3(500\times10^{-9}m)}{(5\times10^{-4}m)} = 3\times10^{-3} \; radians,$$

which is choice B.

61. A

If a quantity is quantized, it means that there is a fundamental unit of that quantity which cannot be further divided. For example, charge is quantized, so charges only appear in nature as multiples of the fundamental charge e. There is not a continuous range of values for the possible charge on an object. Similarly, light energy is quantized. The fundamental unit of light energy is called a photon. The photon, because it cannot be subdivided, is similar to other elementary particles. Thus, quantization implies particle-like characteristics, and choice A is correct.

The passage states that the wave theory, not the particle theory, predicts that light will exhibit interference, so choice B is incorrect. The Doppler effect refers to the change in frequency observed when a wave source or detector is in motion. That the Doppler effect occurs with light as well as sound waves indicates that light has wave, not particle, characteristics and choice C is wrong. Neither particles nor waves can travel faster than the speed of light, so the fact that particles cannot travel faster than light does not support or weaken the particle theory, and choice D is wrong.

62. C

The easiest way to solve the problem is to check the units of each of the answers, a process called dimensional analysis. Since wavelength is measured in meters, the correct answer will be in meters as well. First, note that h has the units of J•s, and v, a speed, has the units of m/s. Then, choice C has the units of $hv/E = (J•s)(m/s)/J = m$, so it is correct. The other choices are incorrect. Choice A has the units of $E = (J•s)(m/s)(J) = J^2m$. Choice B has the units of

$$\frac{hE}{v} = \frac{(J•s)(J)}{(m/s)} = \frac{(J•s)(kg•m^2/s^2)}{(m/s)} = (J•kg)m.$$

Choice D has the units of $E/hv = J/[(J•s)(m/s)] = m^{-1}$.

Another way to solve the problem is to recall that the photon energy E is given by $E = hc/\lambda$, where c is the speed of light, and λ is the photon's wavelength. Solving for λ, we obtain $\lambda = hc/E$. To find the "wavelength" of an electron, replace the speed of light c with the speed of the electron v, and obtain $\lambda = hv/E$, where E is now the energy of the electron. Again, this is choice C.

63. D

You should know that the speed of light is different in different media. The formula associated with this concept is $n = c/v$, where n is the index of refraction of a given medium, c is the speed of light in a vacuum, and v is the speed of light in the given medium. Hence, if the index of refraction and the speed of light in a vacuum are known, we can solve for the speed of light in the medium. Thus, choice D is correct.

We would need the air's index of refraction, along with the variables in choice A, to calculate the water's index of refraction using Snell's law. Even if we could calculate the water's index of refraction, we would need the speed of light in a vacuum to calculate the speed of light in water, so choice A is wrong. Similarly, the variables in choice B allow the calculation of the index of refraction, but the speed of light is still required, so choice B is wrong. Choice C is incorrect because while density might play an indirect role in the index of refraction, the density is not sufficient information to determine the index of refraction.

64. C

You should know that the speed v of a wave is given by $v = f\lambda$, where f is the frequency of the wave, and λ is its wavelength. This makes sense, since λ is the distance traveled by the wave in one cycle, and frequency is the inverse of the period, which is the time it takes for one wave to cycle. Now solve the relation in the question stem $k = 2\pi/\lambda$ for λ to obtain $\lambda = 2\pi/k$. Also solve $\omega = 2\pi f$ for f to obtain $f = \omega/2\pi$. Substituting these expressions into the speed equation, we obtain $v = f\lambda = (\omega/2\pi)(2\pi/k) = \omega/k$, which is choice C. Choice A, while a correct relation, is not the right answer because it does not express v in terms of ω and k. Choices B and D can be eliminated on the basis of dimensional analysis because they do not have the units of speed, m/s. k has units of m^{-1} and ω has units of s^{-1}, so choice B is nonsensical and choice D has units of $1/(ms)$.

65. D

A particle of light is known as a photon. You should know the formula $E = hf$, which states that the energy E of a photon is equal to Planck's constant h times the frequency f of the light. The photon energy is thus proportional to the frequency of the light. Since the photon energy is a property of a particle and frequency is a property of a wave, this relationship successfully connects the particle and wave descriptions of light, and choice D is correct.

Choice A is incorrect because the number of particles passing by per unit time is related to the intensity of the light, not its frequency. Choice B is wrong because photons have zero mass. Choice C is wrong because photons are thought of as point-like particles without size.

Passage XI (Questions 66-72)

66. D

You should know that helium, a noble gas, is very unreactive and would almost certainly not react with any of the species in the furnace. Because the helium does not react with any of the species that participate in the equilibrium, the equilibrium is unaffected by the addition of helium. Even though it increases the total pressure inside the system, the partial pressures of the reacting gases are unchanged (Dalton's law) and therefore they keep on behaving as if the helium weren't present. The correct selection is therefore choice D.

67. A

The entropy of a reaction is a measure of the disorder of the system. The sign of the value of the entropy indicates whether the products of a reaction are more or less disordered than the reactants. A reaction that experiences an increase in disorder in going from reactants to products would have a positive ΔS for the reaction. Similarly, a reaction that decreases its disorder would have a negative ΔS for the reaction. In this reaction, 1 mole of carbon dioxide, a gas, reacts with 1 mole of solid carbon to give two moles of carbon monoxide gas. Since there are more moles of gas in the products than in the reactants, there is an increase in entropy, meaning that the sign of the change is positive.

68. C

The carbon dioxide molecule has a central carbon bonded to two oxygen atoms: carbon shares two electrons with each oxygen, and each oxygen shares two electrons with carbon. As a result of this sharing pattern, two double bonds are formed. You should know that a double bond consists of one sigma bond and one pi bond. Since there are two double bonds, there are two pi bonds, making choice C the correct choice.

69. D

You should know the relationship $\Delta G = \Delta H - T\Delta S$. ΔS for this reaction is positive, because there are more moles of gaseous products than reactants, but there is no information about the sign of ΔH. Since ΔH cannot be determined, neither can ΔG. Choice A is wrong (that is, the statement is certainly true) because, as was just stated, the entropy change is positive. Choice B is wrong because, according to Le Châtelier's principle, a decrease in pressure will favor the side of the reaction with more moles of gas. In this case, it is the products side, and the equilibrium is said to have shifted to the right. Choice C is wrong because, again, according to Le Châtelier's principle, addition of a product will shift the equilibrium to the left, that is, the reactants side.

70. C

The first thing that should be done is to determine which choices have the proper number of valence electrons. Carbon monoxide must have a total of 10 electrons: six from the oxygen and four from the carbon. Choice B and choice D can be eliminated because they both have 12 electrons. In

choice A, the carbon has one pair of unbonded electrons, plus four more electrons in the double bond. This gives the carbon a total of only six electrons in its valence shell, so the carbon doesn't have a complete octet, and choice A must be wrong. Choice C shows the correct Lewis structure for carbon monoxide: each atom has a complete octet, and there is a total of ten electrons.

71. B

P_e, as the table explains, is the expected pressure at each temperature if no reaction had taken place. When the carbon dioxide is introduced into the furnace chamber, it is at a pressure of 1 atmosphere and a temperature of 298 K. Above 298 K, P_e is greater than 1 atmosphere because, at constant volume, the pressure increases as the temperature increases. Since P_e is the pressure if no reaction had taken place, any change in the number of moles of gas present does not have to be considered. Since the pressure of a gas is directly proportional to its temperature in Kelvins, the ratio of the *expected* pressure to the original pressure of 1 atmosphere must be equal to the ratio of the temperature of the trial to the original temperature of 298 K. The equation is as follows:

$$P_e /(1 \text{ atm}) = T/298$$

Solving for P_e yields answer choice B.

72. D

Since carbon has a molar mass of 12 grams, a tenth of a mole would be 1.2 grams, and the 0.6 grams stated in the question is one twentieth of a mole. The equation given in the passage shows that for every one mole of carbon consumed, two moles of CO are produced. So, if one twentieth of a mole of carbon is consumed, two twentieths, or one tenth, of a mole of CO will be produced. One tenth of the molar mass of CO, 28 grams, is 2.8 grams.

Discrete Questions

73. D

The question is about refraction, which is the process that bends light as it travels from one medium into another. Snell's law $n_1\sin\theta_1 = n_2\sin\theta_2$ describes this process, where n_1 and n_2 are the indices of refraction of the two media, and θ_1 and θ_2 are the angles that the light rays make with the normal to the interface between the two media. This law predicts that light traveling into a medium with a higher index of refraction will be refracted towards the normal. Light traveling into a medium with a lower index of refraction will be refracted away from the normal. In the question, the light is refracted away from the normal, so the new medium must have an index of refraction lower than air. The vacuum has the lowest index of refraction possible, $n = 1$, so choice D is correct.

Steel is opaque, so light will not travel through it at all. The steel surface will absorb or reflect light, not refract it, so choice C is wrong. Water and glass both have indices of refraction that are higher than air, so both choices A and B are wrong. Note that even if you did not remember whether higher indices cause refraction towards or away from the normal, you could have eliminated choices A and B because they both would bend the light in the same direction, and both cannot be right.

74. B

The K_{sp}, or solubility product constant, is found by multiplying together the concentrations of the dissociated ions, each raised to a power equal to the number of ions in one formula unit of the salt. When a mole of the salt, X_mY_n, dissolves, m moles of X^{n+} ions and n moles of Y^{m-} ions enter solution. So, the coefficient of X is m, and the coefficient of Y is n. The expression is as follows:

$$K_{sp} = [X^{n+}]^m[Y^{m-}]^n$$

Choice A is wrong because it has the coefficients reversed. Choice C and choice D can be eliminated because the K_{sp} is not a fraction.

75.

A resonance hybrid is a molecule that cannot be represented by just one Lewis structure; the molecule is said to be a composite of the possible structures. Choice A is wrong because all the atoms have a complete octet—hydrogen having its two electrons—and only one Lewis structure is possible:

$$H\!-\!C\!\equiv\!\ddot{N}$$

Choice B is wrong because it too has only one structure:

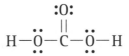

Choice C is correct because it does exist as a resonance hybrid:

$$:\!\ddot{O}\!-\!N\!=\!\ddot{O} \longleftrightarrow \ddot{O}\!=\!N\!-\!\ddot{O}\!:^-$$

Keep in mind that the nitrite ion does not exist as one or the other of the above resonance structures but is a composite of them, having a structure somewhere in-between the two. Choice D is wrong because it has only one Lewis structure as well:

$$:\!\ddot{C}l\!-\!\ddot{O}\!:^-$$

76. A

A comparison of trials 1 and 2 in the table shows that if the concentration of R is held constant and the concentration of species Q is doubled, the reaction rate also doubles. So, the rate of the reaction is proportional to the concentration of Q, and, thus, the reaction is first order for Q. Now, if the reaction is *third* order overall, then it must be *second* order for R. Now that we know that the reaction is second order for R, we can proceed to figure out what concentration of R would result in the observed rate for trial 3. Looking at the table, you can see that the concentration of Q in trial 3 is equal to the concentration of Q in trial 2. Therefore, the difference in rate between trial 2 and trial 3 must be due entirely to the change in the concentration of R. Now, the rate in trial 3 is 4 times the rate in trial 2. But, since the reaction is second order with respect to R, the rate will be quadrupled simply by *doubling* the concentration of R. So, the concentration of R in trial 3 must be double its concentration in trial 2, and, therefore, the concentration of R in trial 3 is 2.00. Thus, choice A is correct.

77. C

To answer the question, apply the formula for the thermal expansion of a solid. This formula is given by $\Delta L = \alpha L \Delta T$, where ΔL is the change in length, L is the original length, ΔT is the change in temperature, and α is some constant which depends on the type of material. This formula makes sense intuitively: As the length increases, there is more material available to expand, and as the temperature increases, the more vigorously the material expands.

Compared with the first iron bar, the second iron bar is twice as long, so $L_2 = 2L_1$, and is raised twice as much in temperature, so $\Delta T_2 = 2\Delta T_1$. Note that α is the same for both bars because they are made of the same material. Therefore, the ratio of the first bar's length change to the second bar's length change is

$$\frac{\Delta L_1}{\Delta L_2} = \frac{\alpha L_1 \Delta T_1}{\alpha L_2 \Delta T_2} = \frac{\alpha L_1 \Delta T_1}{\alpha (2L_1)(2\Delta T_1)} = \frac{\alpha L_1 \Delta T_1}{4(\alpha L_1 \Delta T_1)} = \frac{1}{4},$$

so choice C is correct.

KAPLAN

Verbal Reasoning

Passage I (Questions 78–85)

78. A

This question asks you for the author's working definition of *nihilism*. Remember that the author's definition is not the same as the usual definition of nihilism, a form of extremist political thought, so C is not correct. The definition that reflects the author's own thinking is provided in the second and third sentences of paragraph one. The author says there that nihilism is a complex intellectual stance whose essence is systematic negation of perceptual orders and assumptions. Choice B defines the essence of mysticism, not nihilism. Choice D is too narrow, being an aspect of political nihilism derived purely from skepticism.

79. A

The correct answer is a restatement of the first sentence of paragraph four, which says that the two traditions prepared the ground for the political nihilism of the nineteenth and twentieth centuries. If skepticism and mysticism paved the way for modern political nihilism, then they must be combined in modern political nihilism. Choice B contradicts the whole thrust of the last paragraph of the passage. Choice C goes too far in saying that the two strands of nihilist thought are necessary prerequisites of any positive modern social thought. The second sentence of paragraph one says that nihilism forms the basis for many positive assertions of modern thought, but this doesn't mean that it must form the basis for all of them. Choice D is out because mysticism appears in both Eastern and Western philosophical traditions.

80. C

Statement I is true. There are three quotations used in the passage, two by Stanley Rosen in the second and fourth paragraphs, and one by Novak in paragraph three. Rosen's first quote, at the end of paragraph two, summarizes Hume's argument, and Rosen's second quote sums up what the author wants to say about the political nihilism of the Russian intelligentsia. Statement I will therefore be part of the correct answer; this eliminates choice D. Statement II is false because the author never presents any contrasting points of view in the entire passage. This rules out choice B. Statement III, on the other hand, is true. In the opening sentence of paragraph four, the author refers to the quote from Novak in the previous paragraph in order to make the transition from the discussion of mysticism to the larger point about how skepticism and mysticism paved the way for nihilism. Since Statements I and III are true, choice C is correct.

81. D

This question centers on Hume's conclusion in paragraph two that external reality is unknowable. Hume argued that there is no way to verify whether our sense impressions actually correspond to external reality because all we have to check one of our sense impressions is other sense impressions. He assumed, therefore, that we have no source of information about external reality other than sense impressions—choice D. Hume never concluded, at least as far as we know, that "nothing outside the mind exists"; he just said that we couldn't know what was outside the mind. This rules out choice A. Choice B twists Hume's belief that sense impressions are actually part of the

 315

contents of the mind; Hume didn't say that sense impressions were all that we have upstairs. Choice C is a distortion of Hume's conclusion that causality may be a subjective projection of the mind.

82. B

In the beginning of the last paragraph, the author says that Novak's quote "points to the way [the] philosophical and mystical traditions prepared the ground for the political nihilism of the 19th and 20th centuries." Correct choice B paraphrases this statement. Although Novak does characterize St. John's doctrine, this is not why his interpretation is important to the author's argument, so A is wrong. Novak does not draw a parallel between Humean skepticism and Christian mysticism, which rules out choice C, nor does he say that St. John's teachings were influential, so D is wrong as well.

83. D

You have to pick the choice that is a technique not used by the author to develop his thesis. The best approach to this type of question is simply to go through the choices one by one. The author discusses David Hume as a representative of skepticism and St. John of the Cross as a representative of mysticism, so choice A is not the answer. B is out, too; the author contrasts the common definition of nihilism with his own definition in the first three sentences of the passage. It is also in the first paragraph that the author states that skepticism and mysticism are "united by their categorical rejection of the known"; this identification of the common element in the two traditions is choice C. Eliminating these three choices leaves us with choice D as the correct answer. The author never examines the practical consequences of any social doctrine, let alone those of nihilism.

84. B

The author uses Rosen's quote to support his own thesis that the Russian political nihilists combined radical skepticism and the rejection of existing institutions with a faith in the power of a new beginning: "their desire to destroy becomes a revolutionary affirmation." The quote confirms that nihilism is more than just the desire to reject or destroy society. Neither the author nor Rosen suggests that the nihilists were impractical, so A is wrong. C can't be correct because the author never speaks of nihilism as a doctrine that is currently "alive." Choice D suggests that the fusion of the skeptical and mystical traditions in nihilism is weighed more heavily towards skepticism than towards mysticism, but the author never says anything to this effect, so it can be eliminated as well.

85. C

You are looking for a choice that follows logically from the flow of the author's argument. So you can bet that the right answer will somehow refer to the counterculture movement of the 1960s that is mentioned in the passage's final sentence. Choice A suggests that the negative effects of nihilism are still being felt, but the author never hints that any form of nihilism had a negative effect on anything. The nihilistic element of the counterculture movement is not new and different from classical nihilism, so B is wrong. Choice C would conclude the passage by commenting further on the nihilism of the 1960s revolutionaries—this is more like what you're looking for. A quick look at choice D confirms that choice C is the best answer. Since the author has obviously been studying nihilism, he isn't going to say that the study of nihilism belongs to the past but not the present.

Passage II (Questions 86–91)

86. C

The reason for the stability of these hierarchies is revealed in the final sentence of paragraph two; hierarchies are rarely threatened by disputes because the inferior animal immediately submits when confronted by a superior. Correct choice C paraphrases this assertion. Choice A doesn't make any sense; even if the behavior responses of the group (whatever those behavior responses are supposed to be) are known by all of the members, this won't automatically make the hierarchy stable. The author never says that the defensive-threat posture stops most conflicts (choice B) or that conspecific aggression is inhibited by the nccd for protection from other species (choice D).

87. D

The defensive threat response is discussed primarily in paragraph four. An increase in cardiovascular activity (choice A), narrowing of the eyes (choice B), and stomach muscle contraction (choice C) are all mentioned in the paragraph as being part of the defensive threat response. However, the author never says that one of these is more significant than the others, so choice D is correct.

88. C

The entire passage is about agonistic, or aggressive, behavior, so you need to rely on your memory of the topics of different paragraphs if you want to go back and verify the statements in this Roman numeral question. Statement I is taken practically verbatim from the final sentence of paragraph one. Since the statement is true, you can eliminate choice B. Statement II paraphrases the entire final paragraph, so it is true as well, and choice A has to be ruled out. Statement III, on the other hand, is not supported by anything in the passage; all you know from the second paragraph is that both conspecific and interspecies aggression exist. Choice C is the correct answer.

89. D

This question centers on the nature-versus-nurture argument discussed in the final paragraph. Keep the author's conclusion—that aggressive patterns are both innate and learned—in mind when you're looking for the right choice. It allows you to rule out choice C immediately,

since it is clear that scientists have not resolved the question in favor of genetics. The only thing the passage says is controversial is the definition of aggression, so choice A is wrong. Choice B is out because the author never says that the experiments on mice were the first investigations done to answer the nature-nurture question. This leaves choice D as the only possible correct answer, and it seems reasonable to infer from the author's remark, "copious evidence suggests that animals learn and practice aggressive behavior," that there has been a lot of study devoted to this subject.

90. A

Scan the choices and eliminate the ones that look familiar. Choice B, the evolutionary purpose of aggression, is explicitly addressed in the final sentence of paragraph one. Conspecific aggression occurring in dominance hierarchies, choice C, is discussed in paragraph two. The relationship between play and aggression, choice D, is mentioned in the final two sentences of the passage. Choice A seems to be the winner by the process of elimination. Indeed, the physiological changes that accompany aggressive behavior were discussed in detail only with respect to defensive threat response and not with respect to attack behavior in cats.

91. D

You already know a considerable amount from the passage about aggressive behavior in animals; you just have to decide which new assertion fits in with what you already know. The author doesn't say anything about a link between aggressive behavior and breathing (the reason a shark has to stay in motion), so choice A is out. The inability of newborn mice to exhibit the attack response is *not* proof that aggressive behavior must be learned, as choice B claims. On the contrary, mice attack after only a month, too short a time to have learned this behavior, which is why the author cites this as evidence that aggressive behavior is partially genetic. Choice C is wrong because the author never discusses animal species that don't exhibit aggressive behavior. That leaves choice D, which says that certain hawks use the same means of attack on both squirrels and gophers. This fits right in with the facts of the passage, since the second sentence of paragraph three states that the physiological and behavioral patterns that make up aggressive behavior change very little regardless of the stimuli that provoke them (the stimuli here being the squirrels and the gophers).

Passage III (Questions 92–99)

92. C

The evidence for the single emigration hypothesis will be found in paragraph three. The passage mentions linguistic similarities with Sanskrit-based languages and "loan words" from several other languages. By looking to the passage first in this explicit text question, you will easily be able to identify the relevant information to pick choice C as the correct answer. Choice A is never mentioned in the passage. Choice B is half-right, half-wrong, because it brings in the idea of there being three branches of Gypsies, a concept espoused by the multiple-emigration folks. Choice D not only is irrelevant, but also misconstrues details from the passage: The Romani kept NO historical records.

93. D

This question asks you why a piece of information was included in the passage. Why was the word *Gypsy* discussed at some length? Examples are generally included to further illustrate a main point, which in this case is that the history of the Romani people is little understood by outsiders. Choice A takes details outside their context, details used to explain the origin of the word *Gypsy*, rather than the other way around. Choice

B involves information that was never mentioned in the passage. Choice C distorts information from paragraph four, one of the hypotheses about Romani migratory patterns, and takes it as truth. Even if the detail were uncontested, however, it still would not relate to why the word *Gypsy* was highlighted in the last paragraph. Choice D gives us exactly the explanation we are seeking.

94. A

This logic question asks you to weaken the argument that the Romani emigrated from India at three different times. To weaken the argument, you will want to contest evidence or remove assumptions that would be crucial to the argument's integrity. On a difficult question like this, look carefully at the paragraph where the argument is presented, paragraph four. You can eliminate choice D immediately, as it involves a faulty use of detail from a different paragraph. Choice C is outside the scope: We don't care about other nomadic groups, only the Romani. Introducing this extraneous information just distracts us from the issue; it does nothing to the argument. Choice B fails because it offers evidence that would seem to support the argument, rather than weaken it. Choice A is correct because it undermines evidence that was used to support the multiple-emigration hypothesis.

95. C

This question requires you to locate the relevant details within the passage. Paragraph two discusses what is known about the Romani migration, and there Armenia is explicitly mentioned, eliminating choice A. The phrase "throughout Europe" (line 24) clearly implies that the Romani also migrated to France, so choice B is also out. China is never mentioned in the passage at all, so choice C is the correct answer.

96. A

The word "support" means that the answer should strengthen the argument. The fourth paragraph deals with the fundamental dissimilarities among the three branches of Romani. Choice A is a good choice because the ninth century is when the Romani began to leave India, according to paragraph two. If the two branches were distinct that early, it supports the idea that the Romani were already distinct groups that far back, and less likely to be migrating as a single group. Choice B is irrelevant; differences in meaning within Persian has no bearing on Romani. The 13th-century date mentioned in choice C is too late to be relevant to the migrations, which are dated in the ninth, tenth, and eleventh centuries in paragraphs two and three. Nothing in the passage suggests that all Romani left India in the migrations, so choice D adds nothing.

97. B

The passage deals entirely with linguistic evidence. Choice B refers to the Romani language and Bengali, one of the languages listed as "Sanskrit-based." So this would be a likely source of further data on the relationships between these language groups. The *zingari*, choice A, are mentioned once, in paragraph 6, in the context of the possible origin of the word *Gypsy*—not in reference to the competing migration theories. Nor does the passage suggest that religious beliefs or differences are relevant. The passage never discusses evidence from painting or cuisine, so choices C and D are out.

98. B

To answer this question you should research paragraph three, which reviews the evidence supporting the single migration theory. There the similarities between Romani and Sanskrit languages such as Hindi are cited as evidence that these languages developed in synchronicity until the late 11th century and then diverged during the single migration. The correct answer, choice B, throws this evidence into doubt, thus weakening the single-migration theory. The other choices would have no effect on the argument as presented in the third paragraph.

99. B

The entire passage refers to the many ways outsiders disagree with each other over the history and origins of the Romani, so choice B is correct. Choices A and D are contrary to all the evidence given; clearly the author wouldn't make such a statement only to contradict it with the ensuing argument. Choice C is wrong because the many linguistic debates discussed—everything from the competing migration theories to the debate over the origin of the word *Gypsy*—clearly support the statement.

Passage IV (Questions 100–107)

100. D

The reason that the author refers to Febvre and Bloch is explained in the parentheses at the end of paragraph one. The author states that Febvre and Bloch had anticipated Braudel by originating the historical approach that emphasized economics. Choice A is out because the limitations of the *Annales* approach are not discussed until the end of the passage. The relevance of economics to history has already been suggested by the time the author mentions Febvre and Bloch, so choice B is wrong. Choice C is incorrect because the need for combining various sociological approaches is not debated in the first paragraph or anywhere else.

101. C

Nationalism is never mentioned in the passage. All the other choices are aspects of Braudel's approach to history. Choice A is mentioned in paragraph one. Paragraph three explains that Braudel ignored national boundaries in favor of geographical features in his work on the Mediterranean (choice B). In the same paragraph, you find out that unchanging aspects of everyday life (choice D) were what the French historian studied most closely.

102. B

The right answer has to cover the entire paragraph; beware of choices that are just details from the paragraph in question (in this case the third paragraph), like choice C. The author only mentions the geography of the Mediterranean in the context of discussing his real subject: Braudel's depiction of the role of geography in human history (choice B) when a long view of history is taken. You can eliminate choice A because Braudel's use of obscure facts does not mean that he was "fascinated" with them. D is out because the author never says that national borders are irrelevant; they were just less significant to Braudel than geographical boundaries.

103. D

The author states in paragraph one that unlike conventional historians, the *Annales* historians emphasized understanding history in the context of the forces and material conditions underlying human behavior. Choice D paraphrases this. Annales historians are interested in synthesizing data from social sciences in order to do history, but they are not more interested in other social sciences than in history, so choice A is wrong. Braudel incorporated the study of great figures into his framework of the three temporalities, so there is no reason to think *Annales* historians would be critical of the achievements of histori-cal figures (choice B). Choice C is incorrect because the author states in paragraph one that the *Annales* historians advocate using economic data in historical research.

104. D

The author ends the paragraph by affirming the value and influence of Braudel's approach; he cites the number of similarly designed studies as evidence. The next sentence will most likely refer to these studies in some way and be similarly upbeat about Braudel's work. Choice D fits the bill. Choice A, on the other hand, is wrong because it contradicts the positive tone the last sentence of the passage established. Choice B is incorrect because it does not continue the thought from the last sentence and is inconsistent with the main ideas of the passage as a whole. Choice C is wrong because it too is negative in tone when a positive sentence is appropriate.

105. B

The author voices the possible criticisms of Braudel in the last paragraph. One of them is that he minimized the differences among the social sciences. The author is never critical of Braudel's "structures," so choice A is out. The relationship between short-term events and long-term social activity is not mentioned by the author at all, so C is wrong, and choice D can be eliminated because Braudel is criticized for having no boundaries for social analysis, not for having rigid boundaries.

106. A

The *longue duree* are the aspects of daily life—what people eat, what they wear, how they travel—that remain unchanged for centuries. Statement I, then, is certainly an example of what Braudel would consider the *longue duree*. Statement II, however, falls into the category of *evenementielle*, the short-lived dramatic events of a region, and the reduction in the population of a region (Statement III) from a disease might last a half-century or so, placing it into the category of *conjonctures*. Since Statement I is the only one that exemplifies *longue duree,* choice A is correct.

107. D

The author suggests in the first paragraph that one fundamental principle of Braudel's work is that history must be understood in the context of forces and material conditions that underlying human behavior. So the assertion that historical actions are influenced by forces which individuals may be unaware of is perfectly consistent with Braudel's principles. Choice A, on the other hand, is wrong because neither written history nor social elites are mentioned in the passage. Choice B is incorrect because defining the limits of potential social change in the *longue duree* was but one aspect of Braudel's work and certainly not the historian's most important task. Finally, choice C is a cliché and neither particularly relevant to nor descriptive of Braudel's analysis.

Passage V (Questions 108–113)

108. D

The characteristics which Boule took as evidence that the Neanderthals were subhuman are listed in paragraph three. Choice D is correct because Boule never cites the use of tools as evidence of subhuman development.

109. D

Choice A can be eliminated because the intelligence of the Neanderthals is never compared to that of humans. Choice B may have been true of the Neanderthals, but only after the onset of the Ice Age, so there must be a better answer. Choice C is incorrect because explanations of the disappearance of the Neanderthals posit that modern

humans wiped them out or displaced or absorbed them. Choice D is the correct answer; the author states in paragraph one that the Neanderthals' burial of their dead is regarded as an indication that they had capacity for religious and abstract thought.

110. D

According to the third paragraph, Neanderthals inhabited a vast area from 100,000 to 35,000 years ago and then disappeared within a period of five to ten thousand years. If they actually took the whole 10,000 years to disappear, that means the latest any Neanderthal could have existed was 25,000 years ago (choice D).

111. A

The evidence that the Neanderthals did not evolve into modern humans is laid out in the second half of paragraph three. The author says that the anatomical differences between Neanderthals and modern humans (choice A) are major enough that evolution could not have taken place in a span of ten thousand years. Choice B is a close wrong answer choice, since the brief time frame of 10,000 years *is* part of the reason that scientists think humans did not evolve from Neanderthals. But the time frame isn't evidence enough; presumably, if Neanderthals and humans were close enough anatomically, 10,000 years would have been enough time for evolution to take place. It's the anatomical differences that seem to make the whole thing impossible. Choices C and D aren't mentioned in the passage at all.

112. C

The hypotheses about the disappearance of the Neanderthals are all in paragraph five. Of the choices listed, only choice C is not put forward in this paragraph as a possible explanation. Even if humans did evolve from an isolated group of Neanderthals, as Trinkaus and Howells suggest, knowing this would not shed light on the mystery of the disappearance of the entire population of Neanderthals.

113. A

According to the fourth paragraph, interbreeding in a concentrated population can produce more pronounced genetic effects in a shorter period of time than interbreeding in a sparser population would. From this it can be inferred that the rate of evolution is directly related to the concentration of the species population (choice A). Changes in the anatomical features of a species (choice B) may be a way to measure the rate of evolution, but anatomical features do not directly affect the rate of evolution. The rate of environmental change (choice C) and the adaptive capabilities of a species (choice D) may both affect a species' survival, but they too do not speed evolution up in the way that concentrating the population can.

Passage VI (Questions 114–119)

114. D

This is an All Except question, so you have to pick out the choice that did not contribute to the weakness of the Bolshevik regime. The author discusses the problems facing the Bolshevik regime in 1921 in the first paragraph. These problems included a collapse of industrial production stemming from the civil war (choices A and B), and persistent peasant revolts (choice C). A lack of democracy (choice D), however, did not hurt the Bolsheviks; rather, they were able to monopolize power by refusing to legalize other political parties.

115. D

The author describes the details of the New Economic Policy at the end of paragraph one. The author lists the permission of private trade—which was previously banned—as one feature of the policy. Forced requisitions were eliminated and trade unions were allowed to be active again. In other words, the New Economic Policy relaxed economic controls—choice D. Economic centralization (choice A) and deliberate inflation (choice B) can be ruled out because they are not mentioned in the first paragraph. Choice C directly contradicts the fact that trade unions were once again allowed to fight for higher wages and benefits and to strike.

116. C

The features of Bukharin's program are listed in paragraph three. At the end of the paragraph, the author states that one of Bukharin's policies was to form alliances with nonsocialist foreign regimes that were favorable to Russia. Choice A is one of Trotsky's policies, not Bukharin's. Avoiding confrontations with the trade unions (choice B) was presumably the idea behind the New Economic Policy's lifting of restrictions; this wasn't Bukharin's policy either. Choice D was not a feature of anyone's program.

117. B

Details of Trotsky's and Stalin's policies and attitudes can be found in paragraphs four and seven. Trotsky called for rapid industrialization and Stalin sought to build up heavy industry, so it's clear that industrialization was important to both of them. Choice A is incorrect; the author states that Trotsky was critical of the elite, but Stalin's attitude toward them is left unstated. Similarly, you don't know how either of them felt about democracy within the party (choice C) or how Trotsky felt about trade unions (choice D).

118. A

You can throw out choices B and D right away—Trotsky had control of the Red Army, not Stalin, and there is no reason to think that Stalin's initially neutral appearance helped him at all once he began to maneuver. Trotsky's misjudgment of threats (choice C) enabled Stalin to force him out of Red Army leadership, but control of the party helped Stalin much more. He was able to use his powers to remove Zinoviev and Kamenev from Party leadership and to expel Trotsky from the Party and have him murdered.

119. B

You know from the second paragraph that disputes over the long-range direction of policy led to the struggles within the Bolshevik party. This rules out choices A and D, and all you have to figure out is whether the policy was foreign or economic policy. Since foreign policy is mentioned only once in the passage, the differences were clearly over economic policy (choice B).

Passage VII (Questions 120–125)

120. C

The biological adaptation to which the sentence is referring is the "phytochemical triggering of copulatory behavior" in voles—that is, the chemical MBOA in young mountain grasses causes voles to reproduce at just the right time, when there is a lot of grass for voles to feed on. This is important because the amount of available grass varies considerably. 6-MBOA, then, ensures the survival of voles in a situation of fluctuating food supply (choice B). 6-MBOA doesn't limit reproduction; it encourages reproduction, so choice A is wrong. Use your common sense to eliminate choice B: seeking available food resources comes pretty naturally to animals. D is wrong because a biological adaptation maxi-

mizes the survival of the entire species, not just individual voles.

121. D

The author recommends research on the reproductive behavior of lemmings because lemmings are similar in kind and in habitat to voles. Knowing whether lemmings have a reproductive trigger mechanism similar to that of voles would allow us to determine whether Berger's findings about voles are true of other species as well. This idea is captured by choice D. Choices B and C contradict this notion entirely. Choice A goes way too far: there is no way one study of lemmings could tell us all there is to know about the interrelationship between food supply and reproductive behavior in northern rodent populations.

122. A

Ecologists have long thought, according to the first sentence of the paragraph, that population size is a function of available food (this rules out choice D). They just didn't realize that the interrelationship of food and population size was so complex. In other words, they thought that the amount of available food was the only food factor that affected population (answer choice A); they didn't know about food that biochemically encouraged or discouraged reproduction (which eliminates choice C). We don't know what scientists formerly thought about the link between environmental factors and reproductive behavior, so B is not an option.

123. D

In this All Except question, you have to identify the choice that is not an element of either experiment. Choice A is mentioned in the middle of paragraph two as part of the mountain vole experiment. Choice B was part of that experiment as well, as indicated at the beginning of paragraph two. Measuring consumption of treated and untreated foods (choice C) was the method used in the experiment on hares. Choice D is the one choice that was not an element of either experiment discussed in the passage. The passage does discuss the use of a control group in the 6-MBOA experiment, but this experiment was not measuring changes in the birth rate of the animals, so D is the correct answer.

124. C

This question asks for the assumption upon which Bryant's interpretation rests. Bryant concluded from his experiment that avoidance of unpalatable resins in the natural food source of *Lepus* may play a role in the decline in the *Lepus* population. He is assuming that hares will not eat anything at all, and thus starve to death, if they find resin on their food. The gist of this is captured in choice C. Certainly choice A is not an underlying assumption. Bryant's experiment would be worthless if the hares' behavior in the experiment didn't give us an idea of how they behaved in nature. Choice B is out because Bryant's experiment does not investigate the reasons for the decennial rise in hare population. Choice D makes no sense because if the hares learned to look for new sources of food once they couldn't eat the resinous shoots, their population wouldn't decrease.

125. D

You must consider what was or was not part of both studies. Statement I is not true because the effect of diet on reproduction is part of Berger's study only. Both studies investigate the relationship between food source and population size, so Statement II is true. Statement III is clearly true as well, so choice D is the answer.

Passage VIII (Questions 126–130)

126. C

In the first paragraph, the author says that in Stendhal's view, the ideal woman is one that reveals a man to himself, and in order to do so she must be his equal. Self-realization can be attained, then, through an equal (choice C). Muses (choice A), God (choice B), and family (choice D) are not mentioned in the passage.

127. C

Go back to the sentence in question and read the surrounding sentences. Stendhal projected himself into Lamiel, his female character, de Beauvoir notes; he "assumed Lamiel's destiny." This is why Lamiel is "somewhat speculative"; Stendhal takes on the identity of a woman (choice C), which means he had to rely on speculation. Choice A is wrong because we know from the third paragraph of the passage that Stendhal rejected myth, rejected the mystification of women. Nothing in the passage indicates that Stendhal sensationalized his plots (choice B) or exaggerated the aspirations of his female characters (choice D).

128. D

According to the third paragraph, de Beauvoir rejected the mystification of women in "fury, nymph, morning star . . . siren." The choice not included here is D, "mistress."

129. C

The answer appears both in the second paragraph—"love will be more true if woman, being man's equal, is able to understand him more completely"—and in the last paragraph—"two who may have the chance to know each other in love defy time." The key is clearly understanding of each other (choice C). There is no mention in the passage of faithfulness or of blessing of the union, which means choices A and D are wrong. Stendhal rejected the mystification of women, so B is wrong as well.

130. C

The line reference leads you to the middle of paragraph four; read the surrounding lines. Stendhal's belief that the fulfillment of women is dependent upon total dedication to men is what disappoints de Beauvoir. Choice A is wrong because Stendhal does believe that women can use their spiritual and creative powers if they have a worthy objective (paragraph four). Similarly, Stendhal does acknowledge the aspirations of women, as seen in his character Lamiel (contrary to choice D). Choice B is incorrect because de Beauvoir was happy that Stendhal "lived among women of flesh and blood."

Passage IX (Questions 131–137)

131. B

The answer to this question is a direct quote from the first sentence of paragraph six: the elderly population will double in the next forty years. No current housing shortage (choice A) is discussed in the passage, nor does the author ever state that the elderly represent 30 percent of the United States population, choice D. Choice C contradicts the second sentence in paragraph five, which notes that only 3 percent of today's elderly Americans make more than $50,000 a year.

132. A

The second sentence in paragraph five states that according to government figures, 77 percent of elderly Americans earn less than $20,000 per year (choice A). None of the other choices is a fact drawn from the passage.

133. B

Since the first sentence of paragraph seven says that the Medicaid/Medicare system is already threatened by the continuous upward spiral of medical costs, you can infer that the projected doubling of the cost of care for disabled elderly Americans will represent a further drain on the system. In other words, Medicaid and Medicare will probably become even more expensive in the future, so choice B is correct. Choice A is never implied. In fact, it seems that a national health care system might be less expensive than the current system. Choice C distorts paragraph six's reference to the fact that the government has borrowed against the Social Security system to pay interest on the national debt. Choice D is too pessimistic. The author says that aging "boomers" may well demand that national health care be provided.

134. A

The second sentence of paragraph one says that elders now outnumber teenagers for the first time in American history (choice A). Since the boomers are the largest generation in U.S. history, numbering 75 million, choice B is highly unlikely. Finally, the author never actually states how many elderly people there are in the current U.S. population, but the current number must surely be greater than the number in 1950, choice C, or in 1970, choice D.

135. C

Speculation on the nature of the family of the future is in paragraph three. The second sentence of that paragraph states that one likely development will be a gradual restructuring towards a extended multigenerational family, making choice C correct.

 325

136. D

Since you don't know where the answer will come from in the passage, you have to go through the choices one by one. A contradicts the statement from the middle of paragraph four that only 15 percent of 65-year-old-men still work. There is no evidence that any elderly people have lost their Social Security benefits, so B is out. Choice C distorts the second sentence of the final paragraph, which says that the cost of caring for disabled elderly Americans is expected to double in the next decade alone. Choice D, therefore, must be the correct answer; in fact, the author does say at the end of paragraph six that elderly Americans have come to depend on government subsidies.

137. C

The last question in this set is based on the last paragraph of the passage. As the author says, the medical establishment and various special interest groups have so far blocked legislation aimed at creating a national health care system. The institution of a national health care system is never tied in the passage to the elimination of the Federal deficit, so choice A is wrong. B contradicts the suggestion in the passage that a national health care program may be less expensive than the current system. C is wrong because it is the problems with Medicare/Medicaid that may make a national health care program necessary.

Writing Sample

THE THREE TASKS

Task One
Analyze a given statement. Define and explore its deeper meaning and describe the implications of the statement.

Task Two
Describe an example that contrasts with the statement as you developed it in the first task.

Task Three
Derive and articulate a method of deciding when the statement should be applied and when it shouldn't.

Characteristics of Holistic Scores

Score: 6

- Fulfills all three tasks
- Offers an in-depth consideration of the statement
- Employs ideas that demonstrate subtle, careful thought
- Organizes ideas with coherence and unity
- Shows a sophisticated use of language that clearly articulates ideas

Score: 5

- Fulfills all three tasks
- Offers a well-developed consideration of the statement
- Employs ideas that demonstrate some in-depth thought
- Organizes ideas effectively, though less so than a Level 6 essay
- Shows above-average command of word choice and sentence structure

Score: 4

- Addresses all three tasks
- Offers a consideration of the statement that is adequate but limited
- Employs ideas that are logical but not complex
- Organizes ideas with coherence but may contain digression(s)
- Shows overall control of word choice and sentence structure

Score: 3

- Overlooks or misinterprets one or more of the three tasks
- Offers a barely adequate consideration of the statement
- Employs ideas that may be partially logical, but may also be superficial
- Shows a fundamental control of word choice and sentence structure
- May present problems in clear communication

Score: 2

- Significantly overlooks or misinterprets one or more of the three tasks
- Offers a flawed consideration of the statement
- Organizes ideas with a lack of unity and/or coherence
- May show repeated mistakes in grammar, punctuation, etcetera
- Contains language that may be hard to understand

Score: 1

- Exhibits significant problems in grammar, punctuation, usage, and/or spelling
- Presents ideas in a confusing and/or disjointed manner
- May completely disregard the given statement

SAMPLE RESPONSE TO STIMULUS 1

"True creativity cannot be learned."

As individuals, all human beings have within them creative abilities. There is some quality in every person to imagine and then create that cannot be completely described or explained. These abilities cannot be learned, as they already exist in each and every one of us.

Some of us, however, may find that we have difficulty accessing our creativity. In this way, creativity <u>can</u> be "learned." Everyone, whether privileged or disadvantaged, can, with help, unlock creative capacities in themselves. Take, for example, the process of learning to draw. So often, people are "taught" to be "creative" by being told that they must function like someone else. In a typical art class, students are shown models of "good" drawings, given a paper and pencil, and told to produce an equivalent work of art. Then their attempts are criticized, and the novice artists become frustrated and discouraged, losing all sense of their own abilities. This technique serves only to kill whatever natural creative impulses the students might have. Another technique, outlined in the book <u>Drawing on the Right Side of the Brain</u>, has students begin with exercises that create a supportive environment. In one exercise, students look at an object while they draw it, never lifting pencil from paper, and never looking at what they're doing. In another, students reproduce a drawing which has been turned upside down. In both cases, the point is to draw students' attention away from how "real" the drawing looks and put their attention on what the object they're drawing actually looks like. Thus, students are encouraged to do what they, as individuals, can do.

Creativity requires innovation, and innovation requires risk-taking. No one will take a risk when the result may be severe criticism and humiliation. The quality of creativity rests on positive self-esteem. In the case of those learning to draw, an approach that doesn't seek to criticize what they do seems to work better than one that compares their work to "successful art." So being in a supportive and non-judgmental atmosphere in which they are totally accepted is the way to encourage people to take the risk of trying to do something they have never done before and thus unlock their creative capacities.

ANALYSIS OF SAMPLE RESPONSE TO STIMULUS 1

Holistic Score: 4

Task 1

As individuals, all human beings have within them creative abilities. There is some quality in every person to imagine and then create that cannot be completely described or explained. These abilities cannot be learned, as they already exist in each and every one of us.

Task 2

Some of us, however, may find that we have difficulty accessing our creativity. In this way, creativity <u>can</u> be "learned." Everyone, whether privileged or disadvantaged, can, with help, unlock creative capacities in themselves. Take, for example, the process of learning to draw. So often, people are "taught" to be "creative" by being told that they must function like someone else. In a typical art class, students are shown models of "good" drawings, given a paper and pencil, and told to produce an equivalent work of art. Then their attempts are criticized, and the novice artists become frustrated and discouraged, losing all sense of their own abilities. This technique serves only to kill whatever natural creative impulses the students might have. Another technique, outlined in the book <u>Drawing on the Right Side of the Brain</u>, has students begin with exercises that create a supportive environment. In one exercise, students look at an object while they draw it, never lifting pencil from paper, and never looking at what they're doing. In another, students reproduce a drawing which has been turned upside down. In both cases, the point is to draw students' attention away from how "real" the drawing looks and put their attention on what the object they're drawing actually looks like. Thus, students are encouraged to do what they, as individuals, can do.

This changes the focus of your argument from "Can creativity be learned?" to the simpler question of, "What's the best way to teach it?"

good details

Task 3

Creativity requires innovation, and innovation requires risk-taking. No one will take a risk when the result may be severe criticism and humiliation. The quality of creativity rests on positive self-esteem. In the case of those learning to draw, an approach that doesn't seek to criticize what they do seems to work better than one that compares their work to "successful art." So being in a supportive and non-judgmental atmosphere in which they are totally accepted is the way to encourage people to take the risk of trying to do something they have never done before and thus unlock their creative capacities.

Your essay addresses all three tasks clearly, but you tend to oversimplify by not focusing specifically on whether or not creativity can be learned. This weakness is shown in particular by your sketchy treatment of Task 1. Your main point appears to be that "true creativity" is an inherent ability, but you don't explain this thoroughly. Thus, your example in paragraph 2 leaves us wondering: Is drawing a picture without looking at the paper "truly creative" in the way the statement means? And in paragraph 3 we wonder: Is self-esteem all we need to become truly creative?

Biological Sciences

Passage I (Questions 138–143)

138. D

The complete catabolism of a mole of glucose yields a net of 36 moles of ATP. The glycolytic portion of this pathway, however, yields only a net of 2 moles of ATP. Therefore, if 10 moles of glucose were to undergo glycolysis, then the total ATP produced would be 10 times the amount formed from the glycolysis of one mole, so 10 × 2 moles of ATP = 20 moles of ATP. Therefore, choice D is correct and choice A, choice B, and choice C are wrong.

139. B

If the reaction was not stereospecific, water could add to the double bond of fumarate to form two enantiomers:

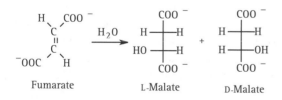

Fumarate → L-Malate + D-Malate

However, the question stem states that the reaction is stereospecific. Therefore, fumarate, which is a *trans* isomer, will react differently to its *cis* counterpart, forming a stereochemically different product. As a result, only one enantiomer will be formed, which is an optically active molecule. A racemic mixture consists of an equal quantity of enantiomers. This would only be produced if the reaction was not stereospecific. Therefore, choice A is wrong. Choice C is wrong because only one chiral center is produced in the reaction. An

achiral molecule is one which doesn't contain any chiral centers, or if it does, it possesses an internal plane of symmetry. Since the product has a chiral center and no internal plane of symmetry, choice D is wrong.

140. D

According to the passage and Figure 2, a low blood glucose concentration stimulates a glucagon-triggered cascade that leads to the phosphorylation of PFK2 to form the enzyme FBPase 2 which degrades F-2,6-BP into fructose 6-phosphate, inhibiting phosphofructokinase activity in the process. Since phosphofructokinase catalyzes the committed step in glycolysis, its inhibition will in turn inhibit glycolysis. Choice D is thus correct, since glucagon inhibits glycolysis.

Choice A and choice B are wrong, since glucagon does not stimulate the production of F-2,6-BP, it promotes its degradation. Choice C is wrong, since according to Figure 2, the phosphorylation of PFK2 occurs when blood glucose levels are low. Glucagon, therefore, promotes the phosphorylation of PFK2.

141. C

According to Figure 1, a high AMP concentration results in a greater glycolytic reaction velocity than a low AMP concentration. Therefore, choice C enhances the rate of glycolysis, and is thus correct.

Choice A is wrong because a low concentration of fructose 2,6-bisphosphate inhibits phosphofructokinase activity, which leads to an inhibition of glycolysis. Choice B is wrong since a high

ATP to AMP ratio corresponds to a high ATP concentration or a low AMP concentration, and since Graphs I and II tell you that a high ATP concentration and a low AMP concentration reduces the rate of glycolysis, choice B can be eliminated. Choice D is wrong since, as seen in Graph III, a high citrate concentration reduces the rate of glycolysis.

142. D

A high fructose-6-phosphate concentration will lead to increased phosphofructokinase activity and enhanced glycolysis, so there will be more ATP. Greater ATP concentration will raise the ATP/AMP ratio, so choice D is correct, since the ATP/AMP ratio will not decrease with high concentrations of fructose 6-phosphate.

Choice A and choice B can be eliminated, since according to Figure 2, fructose 6-phosphate stimulates the synthesis of F-2,6-BP and inhibits its degradation. Choice C can also be discarded, since high concentrations of F-2,6-BP stimulate phosphofructokinase.

143. B

Colony A survived under both anaerobic and aerobic conditions, and demonstrated considerable growth and glucose consumption under aerobic conditions. This implies that the Colony A bacteria are facultative aerobes. That Colony B practically disappeared when incubated under aerobic conditions implies that Colony B bacteria must be obligate anaerobes. Thus, Colonies A and B are, respectively, facultative aerobes and obligate anaerobes, so choice B is correct and choice A, choice C, and choice D are all incorrect. You should have eliminated choice A and choice C right away, since the fact that the bacteria from both colonies existed for some time under anaerobic conditions implies that neither of them could be obligate aerobes, since obligate aerobes require molecular oxygen for existence.

Passage II (Questions 144–149)

144. A

The transcription of viral mRNA in an HIV-infected CD4+ T-cell requires the same reagents as does the transcription of eukaryotic mRNA in a healthy CD4+ T-cell: RNA polymerase, ribose, phosphate, and adenine, cytosine, guanine, and uracil. Unlike DNA, RNA doesn't contain thymine. So, if the researcher wanted to study mRNA synthesis (transcription) then she would add radiolabeled adenine, guanine, cytosine, and uracil, but not radiolabeled thymine, since it wouldn't be incorporated into the mRNA transcripts.

145. C

Hypothesis 1 is based on the premise that HIV fails to integrate. These unintegrated viruses produce a factor that results in CD4+ T-cell death. So if Hypothesis 1 is true, integration doesn't occur. However, for HIV to be capable of producing a toxic factor that causes the death of its host CD4+ T-cell, it must be inside the host cell, implying that binding and entry do occur. So, choice C is correct.

You can immediately eliminate choice A and choice D, since they both include integration. Reverse transcription is the process by which DNA is synthesized from an RNA template with the enzyme reverse transcriptase. There's not enough information in the description of Hypothesis 1 to determine whether or not reverse transcription must occur before the toxic factor can be produced. Furthermore, it would be virtually impossible for HIV to produce a toxic factor after it had already induced the death of its host cell. Thus, choice B is wrong.

146. C

According to Hypothesis 3, HIV-infected cells express the viral proteins gp120 and gp41 on their surfaces, and that these proteins bind to the

KAPLAN

CD4 receptors on healthy T-cells, yielding a mass of immune-impaired cells known as syncytia. The net result is an effective depletion of T-cell activity. If gp120 and gp41 bound almost irreversibly to CD4 receptors, then syncytia formation would account for the depletion of T-cells associated with HIV infection. Therefore, choice C supports Hypothesis 3 and is correct.

Choice A is wrong, because it contradicts Hypothesis 3 by saying that some CD4+ T-cell lines do not form syncytia yet are still susceptible to depletion due to HIV infection. Hypothesis 3 states that syncytia formation is the cause of the T-cell depletion. Choice B does not support Hypothesis 3, either. If syncytia formation were transient, then these T-cells would be only temporarily nonfunctional, and the supply of T-cells would not be depleted. Choice D neither supports nor contradicts Hypothesis 3. Although syncytia formation does lead to cell death, the cell death is not necessary for syncytia formation to render the T-cells nonfunctional.

147. A

According to Hypothesis 4, gp120 molecules are released by HIV-infected CD4+ T-cells and bind to healthy CD4+ T-cells. According to the passage, gp120 binds to the CD4 receptor molecules expressed on the surface of other T-cells. Since CD4 receptor molecules are a normal part of CD4+ T-cell structure, they are recognized by the immune system as "self." However, CD4 receptor molecules bound to gp120 molecules are recognized as "foreign," since the gp120 molecules are not normally present in the body. In response to the presence of gp120, the immune system produces anti-gp120 antibodies, thereby attacking its own CD4+ T-cells. This is known as an autoimmune response. Therefore, Hypothesis 4 only makes sense if healthy CD4+ cells are not normally subject to autoimmune attacks, and so choice A is correct.

Choice B is wrong because the B-cells are the antibody-producing components of the immune system. Choice C is wrong because healthy CD4+ T-cells do not synthesize gp120 molecules. Choice D is wrong because it would be impossible for gp120 to travel through the body by way of the immune system, since the immune system is not a system in the traditional sense of the word. The immune system refers to a group of nonspecific and specific defense mechanisms mediated by specialized cells, such as B-cells, T-cells, and macrophages, that travel through the body via the circulatory system.

148. B

The Golgi complex (Golgi apparatus) is the organelle responsible for the packaging and distribution of newly synthesized proteins, including viral proteins, such as gp120 and gp41. Choice A is wrong because centrioles are cylindrical structures whose role, if any, in animal cell mitosis is unclear to date. Choice C is wrong because mitochondria are the sites of cellular respiration in eukaryotic cells. Choice D is wrong because lysosomes are responsible for the digestion of various cellular and extracellular metabolites as well as the degradation of unwanted toxins.

149. B

According to the question stem, the test for the presence of HIV is the detection of anti-HIV antibodies circulating in the blood. HIV depletes the body's supply of T-cells, which are crucial for the proliferation and activity of the B-cells that produce the anti-HIV antibodies detected in the blood. This means that at some point during HIV infection, there are enough healthy T-cells in circulation to allow for the production of anti-HIV antibodies by B-cells, and so choice B is correct.

Though choice A is most likely a true statement, it is wrong because cytotoxic T-cells are not the cells responsible for the presence of anti-HIV antibodies in the blood of an HIV-infected person. Choice C is wrong because, even if it were true, it still wouldn't account for the presence of circulating anti-HIV antibodies. Choice D is wrong, since the presence of anti-HIV antibodies would not imply that macrophages have not been infected. Macrophages are phagocytic mononuclear white cells that serve accessory roles in cellular immunity; they are not directly involved in antibody production. By the way, macrophages have been shown to harbor HIV in vivo, yet they are relatively resistant to HIV cytopathic effects, most likely due to their low level of CD4 expression. Some studies have suggested that these cells may be the basis of the neurological abnormalities seen in some AIDS patients.

Passage III (Questions 150–154)

150. D

In Compound I, there is no rotation of substituents attached to the double bond. Therefore, the methyl substituents can be located on the same side of the double bond (*cis*) or on opposite sides (*trans*):

H₃C   CH₃   H   CH₃
cis-2-Butene   *trans*-2-Butene
H   H   H₃C   H

The *cis/trans* arrangement of substituents around a double bond is known as geometric isomerism, making choice D the correct response. *Cis* and *trans* isomers have different physical properties, attributed to a difference in their dipole moments and symmetry. Choice A is wrong since anomers are cyclic forms of carbohydrates that differ in the configuration about the anomeric carbon (usually carbon 1). Enantiomers are chiral molecules that are non-superimposable mirror images of each other. In addition, they have identical chemical and physical properties (except the ability to rotate plane-polarized light).

Compound I is achiral and its isomers have different physical properties, so choice B is wrong. Conformational isomers arise by the rotation around a single bond, not a double bond. At normal temperatures, these isomers cannot be isolated, therefore choice C is also wrong.

151. A

In hot basic potassium permanganate, non-terminal alkenes will be oxidatively cleaved to form 2 molecules of carboxylic acid. Compound I is symmetrical, so cleavage and subsequent oxidation will result in the formation of two molecules of acetic acid:

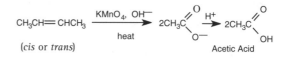

The molecular formula of acetic acid is $C_2H_4O_2$ and since two molecules are formed, the overall result is $2C_2H_4O_2$ which corresponds exactly with Table 2. Choice B and Choice D are incorrect because these molecules are diols and are formed when alkenes are treated with cold dilute potassium permanganate. Choice C is wrong because the molecular formula doesn't match that in the table. Also, aldehydes will not form under these conditions.

152. C

The addition of HBr to Compound II follows Markovnikov's rule: H⁺ adds to the least substituted, double bonded carbon first to form a carbocation intermediate–$CH_3CH_2CH^+CH_3$. Br⁻ then adds to this molecule to form 2-bromobutane:

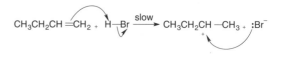

HBr adds to Compound IV in much the same way as Compound II. H⁺ adds to the least substituted carbon, but this time the intermediate $CH_3CH_2C^+=CH_2$ is formed. This is called a vinylic cation—an intermediate in which the positive charge is adjacent to a double bond. Therefore, choice C is the correct answer. After the vinylic cation is formed, Br⁻ adds to form $CH_3CH_2CBr=CH_2$:

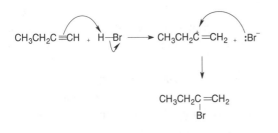

The double bond can then add another molecule of HBr to form a *gem*-dihalide—$CH_3CH_2CBr_2CH_3$. Choice A and choice D are incorrect because carbocations are formed when HBr adds to alkenes, not alkynes. Choice B is wrong since the positive charge on the vinylic intermediate means that it is a cation not an anion.

153. A

Catalytic hydrogenation of alkenes is always a syn process, because the alkene molecules collide with the surface of the solid catalyst bearing hydrogen in such a way that only one side of the double bond is left exposed to attack by hydrogen:

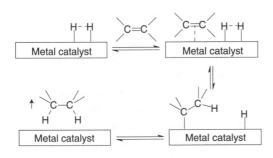

On the other hand, the addition of bromine to an alkene occurs through an anti addition mecha-

nism. A cyclic bromonium ion is initially formed; bromide then adds to the molecule 180° to the first bromine, i.e., on the opposite face of the molecule. Hence, the hydrogenation and bromination of Compound I are respectively, syn and anti addition; Choice A is therefore the correct response. Choice B is incorrect because this states that the opposite occurs. Choice C is wrong because hydrogenation does not occur through nucleophilic addition. Choice D is wrong because bromination is classified as electrophilic addition, not nucleophilic addition.

154. C

Markovnikov's rule is followed in the addition of HBr to Compound I and Compound II. Hence, the following carbocation is formed:

$$CH_3CH_2\underset{+}{C}H-CH_3$$

Br⁻ then adds to this carbocation to produce 2-bromobutane; choice C is therefore correct. Choice D is wrong because Markovnikov's rule is only disobeyed when radical initiators such as peroxides or ultra-violet light are present. Choice A is wrong because internal, more highly substituted double bonds are stabilized by their alkyl groups. Thus the double bond in Compound I is more stable than the double bond in Compound II. Choice B is also wrong because if the double bond in Compound I is more stable, it will be less reactive.

Passage IV (Questions 155–160)

155. A

All viruses have a protein coat consisting of protein subunits. Since all viruses are so closely related, there will be homology between the viral genes coding for the protein coats of different viruses. This means that probes specific for proteins present in the protein coats of almost all viruses can be created. By hybridizing the unknown infectious agent with probes specific for the few major variants of viral protein coats, the nature of the infectious agent can be determined. If the probes hybridize with the genes of the infectious agent, the agent must be a virus. If the probes do not hybridize with the genes, this means that the infectious agent does not contain the viral genes coding for the protein coat, which means that the agent must be bacterial.

Choice B is wrong because, while viruses do not have any photosynthetic pigments, only some bacteria do have them. Only the cyanobacteria, or blue-green algae, are photosynthetic, and cyanobacteria are not infectious agents in humans. Choice C is wrong because although most viruses are DNA viruses, RNA viruses also exist. And since all bacteria have RNA, if the infectious agent was an RNA virus, both would stain positive for the presence of RNA. Choice D is wrong because all bacteria and all viruses have proteins and so both would stain positive for the presence of proteins.

156. A

Since all four of the microbes are bacteria, you're looking for the structure not found in bacteria. Bacteria are prokaryotes—unicellular organisms characterized by the lack of a true nucleus as well as the absence of all other membranous organelles. Bacteria have a single circular chromosome located in a region of the cell known as the nucleoid. So, choice A is correct and choice B can be eliminated. Choice C is wrong, since bacteria have cell walls. Likewise, bacteria contain all the necessary machinery for protein synthesis and reproduction, such as RNA, enzymes, ribosomes, and proteins, which is why choice D is wrong. For your information, prokaryotic ribosomes are structurally different from eukaryotic ribosomes, and this difference is often exploited in the development of effective antibiotics.

157. B

By culturing the four strains of bacteria on different nutrient plates, the epidemiologist was able to determine the nutritional requirements of each strain. A strain can only grow on those plates that contain all of the amino acids essential to that strain; if any of these amino acids are lacking, growth will not occur. Microbe Q grew on Plate 1 and Plate 3, both of which contain threonine and cysteine. Microbe Q did not grow on Plate 2 or Plate 4. Plate 4 is identical to Plate 1, except that tryptophan has been substituted for cysteine. Plate 2 is identical to Plate 3, except that phenylalanine has been substituted for threonine. Since growth occurred when threonine and cysteine were both present and was prohibited when either of them was absent, it can be deduced that both threonine and cysteine are essential amino acids for Microbe Q. Therefore, choice B is correct.

Choice A and choice C can be eliminated because neither of these amino acids is present in Plate 3, which supported Microbe Q growth. Choice D is wrong because proline can not be an essential amino acid for Microbe Q because it is missing from Plate 1, which also supported growth.

158. A

The phrase "pathogenic microbes" refers to Microbe Q and Microbe T only, since Microbes R and S were found to be non-pathogenic. To test whether the strains were affected by the antibiotics, the experimenter needed to use a medium that the strains could definitely grow on in the absence of antibiotics. With this in mind, you should have translated the question to read: Which of the four nutrient plates is capable of sustaining colonies of both Microbe Q and Microbe T? According to Table 1, Microbe Q grew on Plate 1 and Plate 3, while Microbe T grew on Plates 1, 2, and 4. Plate 1 is therefore the only plate that the epidemiologist could have used in the experiment illustrated in Figure 1. Thus, choice A is correct and choice B, choice C, and choice D are wrong.

159. C

An effective antibiotic is one that inhibits, if not completely prevents, bacterial growth. According to the passage, shaded areas in Figure 1 represent regions of good bacterial growth, and as can be seen, Microbe Q growth is inhibited by both Antibiotic Y and Antibiotic Z, while Microbe T is inhibited only by Antibiotic Z. Since Antibiotic Z inhibits both strains of bacteria, it makes sense that this drug would be the most effective in treating patients simultaneously infected with Microbe Q and Microbe T. Thus, choice C is correct and choice A, choice B, and choice D are wrong.

160. C

The best way to approach this question is by the process of elimination. Choice A can be eliminated, since centrifugation separates substances on the basis of density and would therefore be of little use here, since all bacteria are so close in density that they would sediment into the same layer. Choice B sounds like a good idea—especially if you determined from Table 1 that cysteine and threonine are essential for Microbe Q, and that phenylalanine is essential for Microbe T. You might therefore expect only Microbe Q to grow on the nutrient plate containing cysteine, and only Microbe T to grow on the nutrient plate containing phenylalanine. However, Microbe Q requires both cysteine and threonine for growth, and while Microbe T would grow on the phenylalanine plate, Microbe Q would not grow on either one. So choice B is wrong. Choice C is similar to choice B, except that one of the plates has all of the amino acids except cysteine, and the other has all of the amino acids except phenylalanine. This means that Microbe Q would grow on the plate lacking phenylalanine, but not on

the plate lacking cysteine. Likewise, Microbe T would grow on the plate lacking cysteine, but not on the plate lacking phenylalanine. In this way, Microbe Q could be isolated from Microbe T, and so choice C is correct. Choice D is obviously wrong, since clearly, a mechanism for isolating the two microbes does exist. By the way, the easiest way to isolate these microbes would be to use the original Plate 3 and Plate 4. As can be seen in Table 1, Plate 3 sustained only Microbe Q, and Plate 4 sustained only Microbe T.

Discrete Questions

161. A

Calcitonin lowers blood Ca^{2+} by promoting the incorporation of calcium ion into bone. A way to remember this is as follows: Calcitonin tones down the Ca^{2+}. Parathyroid hormone (PTH), on the other hand, increases blood Ca^{2+} concentration by promoting its removal from bone and its release into the bloodstream. PTH also decreases the excretion of Ca^{2+} from the kidneys and converts vitamin D3 into its active form, which stimulates the absorption of Ca^{2+} in the intestines.

Choice B is wrong because prolactin is a hormone synthesized by the anterior pituitary gland, and stimulates the secretion of milk from female mammary glands. Choice C is incorrect because the function of ACTH, also synthesized and secreted by the anterior pituitary, is to stimulate the production of hormones from the adrenal cortex. Choice D is wrong because thyroxine (T_4) is a thyroid hormone involved in regulating metabolism.

162. A

The partial pressure of CO_2 in the blood is highest in those vessels carrying deoxygenated blood. Deoxygenated blood is returned to the right atrium of the heart via the inferior vena cava and the superior vena cava. From the right atrium the deoxygenated blood drains into the right ventricle, where it is pumped into the pulmonary arteries. The pulmonary arteries deliver the blood to the capillary beds surrounding the alveoli, which is where gas exchange occurs: CO_2 is traded for O_2. The now oxygenated blood is returned to the heart via the pulmonary veins, which empty into the left atrium. The left atrium drains into the left ventricle, which pumps the oxygenated blood into circulation via the aorta. In addition, the heart is delivered its own supply of oxygenated blood via the coronary arteries which branch off the aorta. Thus, choices B, C, and D are wrong, since these vessels carry oxygenated blood.

163. C

The three primary germ layers, which arise during the gastrulation stage of embryonic development, and from which all organ systems and structures are derived, are endoderm, mesoderm, and ectoderm. Endoderm is the innermost layer of cells, from which the following structures arise: the lining of the digestive tract, the lining of the respiratory tract, the liver, the thyroid, the pancreas, and the bladder. Mesoderm is the middle layer of cells, from which the following structures arise: skeletal muscle, dermis, bone, blood, the gonads, the kidneys, and the circulatory system. Ectoderm is the outermost layer of cells, from which the following structures arise: epidermis (including nail, hair, and the outer layer of skin), the lens of the eye, the pituitary gland, the lining of the mouth and nose, nervous tissue, and the adrenal medulla.

164. B

Blood type is determined by the antigens expressed on the surface of the red blood cells (RBCs). Type A blood has RBCs with the A antigen and will produce anti-B antibodies when exposed to the B antigen. Type B blood has RBCs

with the B antigen and will produce anti-A antibodies when exposed to the A antigen. Type AB blood has RBCs with both the A antigen and the B antigen and will not produce anti-A or anti-B antibodies upon exposure to either antigen. Type O blood has RBCs with neither the A antigen nor the B antigen and will produce anti-A antibodies when exposed to the A antigen and anti-B antibodies when exposed to the B antigen. The Rh antigen is another RBC antigen. Rh^+ blood has the antigen and Rh^- blood does not. Rh^- blood produces anti-Rh antibodies only upon a second exposure to the Rh antigen. Rh^+ blood does not produce antibodies against Rh^- RBCs. The ideal blood transfusion is one where donor and recipient blood types are a perfect match. The worst blood transfusion is one where donor and recipient blood types are a complete mismatch, resulting in severe agglutination and blood clotting.

Choice A is wrong because it would be a fairly good match, though not ideal, because donor and recipient are both type B, and the donor RBCs lack the Rh antigen. Choice B is correct because this blood type would cause severe agglutination in the recipient. Although they are a match in terms of the Rh antigen, the presence of A^+ RBCs would elicit an attack by anti-A antibodies produced by the recipient's immune system. Since type O blood is known as the "universal donor" in the world of blood transfusions, it won't elicit antibody production against the A antigen or the B antigen, so choice C and choice D are wrong.

165. B

The most important factors determining the rate at which a compound diffuses through a membrane are the compound's size and its polarity, assuming there is no facilitated diffusion. Since Compound A and Compound B are the same size, and since there is no facilitated diffusion occurring, only polarity needs to be considered. Cell membranes are nearly impermeable to polar compounds because polar compounds are insoluble in the membrane's hydrophobic lipid bilayer. In contrast, nonpolar compounds (e.g., O_2) diffuse easily through the cell membrane. This implies that the transmembrane diffusion rate of a polar compound is likely to be fairly low and essentially independent of its concentration, which corresponds to the rate depicted by curve B. Likewise, the transmembrane diffusion rate of a nonpolar compound is likely to be fairly high and strongly dependent on its concentration, which corresponds to the rate depicted by curve A. Thus, Compound A is most likely a nonpolar compound and Compound B is most likely a polar compound, so choice B is correct.

Passage V (Questions 166–170)

166. B

The contractile unit of a muscle fiber is called a sarcomere, and is composed of actin, myosin, troponin, and tropomyosin. When acetylcholine binds to receptors on the surface of a muscle fiber, it triggers the depolarization of the muscle sarcolemma, which in turn triggers the release of calcium ions from the sarcoplasmic reticulum. The calcium ions bind to troponin, causing a conformational change within the sarcomere that causes the tropomyosin strands to shift and expose the myosin-binding sites on actin. Myosin binds to actin and the sarcomere contracts. So, choice B is correct. Choice A and choice D are wrong since the calcium ions do not bind to either the sarcolemma or to actin. Choice C is wrong since the formation of permanent actin-myosin crossbridges occurs only in the absence of ATP and leads to the development of rigor mortis.

167. D

According to the passage, an incoming action potential triggers the release of acetylcholine via exocytosis, which means that the synaptic vesi-

cles fuse with the membrane of the nerve terminal and release their contents into the synapse. Exocytosis is not a passive process and so requires ATP. The abundance of mitochondria in the nerve terminal supply the ATP.

Choice A is wrong because it doesn't account for the particularly high concentration of mitochondria in the nerve terminal. Also, choice A is not true; not all eukaryotic cells contain mitochondria, as in the case of red blood cells. Choice B is wrong because while the fact that neurons are aerobic cells does account for the presence of mitochondria, it fails to explain why there is a high concentration of mitochondria in the nerve terminal. Choice C is wrong because diffusion is a passive process, which means that ATP is not required.

168. A

If the student's receptors for hot pain (the free nerve endings in the skin) had been severed, then the student would not have felt any pain and would not have withdrawn his hand from the hot plate. Thus, choice A is right and choice B is wrong. The sensation of pain is the result of an impulse being transmitted to the brain's sensory cortex via a sensory receptor and a sensory neuron. If one of these pathways were severed at any point, the impulse would not be sent to the brain, and the sensation of pain would not be felt. Thus, choice C and choice D must be wrong. By the way, though the sensation of pain is also conveyed to the sensory cortex via a different pathway, this pathway also begins with the stimulation of the hot pain receptors in the skin. So if these receptors were severed, the message would not be sent to the brain by this route either.

169. D

Touching a burning hot plate is more painful and dangerous than touching uncomfortably warm water. Thus, it's beneficial to withdraw a limb more rapidly from the hot plate than from warm water. The difference in reaction time corresponds to two factors: the distance the impulse must travel and the number of synapses the impulse must cross. The withdrawal reflex in response to hot pain is a reflex arc of two synapses: a sensory neuron synapses with an interneuron and the interneuron synapses with a motor neuron. Since this action is faster than the response to warm water, the nerve impulse triggered by the stimulation of the skin's "uncomfortably warm" receptors most likely travels through more than two synapses and does not bypass the brain by synapsing in the spinal cord. This makes sense, since there isn't any real threat of injury.

Choice A is incorrect because an action potential is an all-or-nothing response; the quantity of acetylcholine released does not affect its magnitude. Choice B is incorrect because the withdrawal reflex in response to intense heat bypasses the sensory areas of the brain, synapsing directly in the spinal cord. In addition, the passage tells you that the sensation of pain is transmitted more slowly to the sensory cortex than to a motor neuron. Choice C is incorrect because, while it's true that epinephrine secretion does trigger the "fight-or-flight" response, acetylcholine is the only neurotransmitter secreted at the neuromuscular junction.

170. C

Since you're told that when one limb is withdrawn the opposite limb extends, the correct answer must have the left arm extending. According to the passage, to move the arm towards the shoulder, the biceps contract and the triceps relax. From this, it can be inferred that to straighten the arm, the biceps relax and the triceps contract. So, choice C is correct, since when the left biceps relax and the left triceps contract, the left arm extends.

Choice A is incorrect because this would cause the right arm to extend, not to withdraw. Choice B, in which both the right biceps and the right triceps contract, is wrong because it's impossible. The muscles of the arm work in antagonistic pairs, so that when one muscle contracts the other muscle relaxes. Choice D is wrong, because if the left biceps contract, then the left triceps relax, which means that the left arm would be withdrawn. Likewise, the relaxation of the right biceps dictates the contraction of the right triceps, which would lead to the extension of the right arm, which is the opposite of what actually occurs.

Passage VI (Questions 171–175)

171. D

Chlorination of butane results in the formation of 1-chlorobutane and 2-chlorobutane, since butane possesses two types of hydrogen that can be substituted. 1-Chlorobutane is achiral, so Statement III is correct. On the other hand, 2-chlorobutane possesses a chiral carbon, so Statement I is correct:

$$CH_3CH_2 \overset{\overset{\displaystyle H}{|}}{\underset{\underset{\displaystyle Cl}{|}}{C}} CH_3$$

Choice D is the only choice that contains both Statements I and III so it is the correct response. Statement II is also correct because the reaction occurs through a free radical intermediate; the halogen can add to either side of the molecule forming a racemic mixture, which has no observed optical rotation.

172. A

The passage tells you that the order of reactivity of the halogens is fluorine, then chlorine, then bromine, then iodine. Bromine produces five times as much tertiary product than primary product, so it seems to be selective about which hydrogen it reacts with. However, with fluorine, equal amounts of product form, so it must be pretty unselective. Therefore, choice A is correct: fluorine is the most reactive halogen, but it is the least selective, so there is an inverse relation between reactivity and selectivity. Choice B is wrong because fluorine is more reactive than bromine, so it will be a better halogenating agent. Choice C is also wrong because fluorine is simply more reactive than bromine: It doesn't matter which sort of hydrogen it is substituting. Choice D is true in that fluorine forms stronger bonds to primary carbons than bromine, but it doesn't account for the different products that are formed.

173. B

In free radical substitution reactions, only a small amount of initiator is required because a halogen radical is produced in the propagation step which can drive the reaction without the help of the initiator (resulting in a chain reaction). Therefore, the reaction can be started by light of low intensity to produce a small concentration of halogen radicals; so choice B is the correct response. Choice A is wrong because these reactions have high activation energies. Choice C is wrong because halogen-halogen bonds are quite strong. Finally, choice D is wrong because alkanes are extremely unreactive molecules.

174. B

A chain termination step is one that ends the reaction chain. The chain in this reaction is kept going by the presence of free-radicals: To terminate the chain, the number of radicals must be reduced. This is shown in choice B, where two radicals combine to form a neutral molecule. Choice A and choice D are wrong because these

are propagation steps; bromine radicals are generated which assist in the reaction, not terminate it. Choice C is wrong because no radicals are shown here at all. This is actually the overall reaction which occurs between bromine and the alkane.

175. D

The passage states that the most reactive type of hydrogen toward substitution is a tertiary hydrogen. Substitution of the tertiary hydrogen in 2-methylpropane will result in the formation of 2-bromo-2-methylpropane, choice D. Choice B is wrong because it names the molecule as a butane and the longest carbon chain has three carbons, not four. Choice A names the molecule as 2-bromomethylpropane. If this were true, propane would have a bromomethyl substituent, not a bromo and a methyl substituent. Choice C is wrong because it states that the product has a 1-bromo substituent, not a 2-bromo substituent. This product would only be formed if the less reactive primary hydrogen was substituted.

Passage VII (Questions 176–181)

176. D

According to the passage, eukaryotic cells contain genes known as proto-oncogenes, which normally code for proteins involved in the regulation of growth. If any of these proto-oncogenes become transformed into an oncogene, then that cell is said to be tumorigenic. A tumorigenic cell is one that gives rise to a tumor, and unlike normal cells, tumor cells don't obey the rules of normal cell growth and divide indefinitely. Thus, in a tumorigenic cell, you would expect to see an increase in all of the activities and processes associated with cell growth and division, such as mRNA synthesis (transcription) and ribosomal assembly. Likewise, cell division would also increase, since tumor cells replicate at an accelerated rate.

177. A

A point mutation is the replacement of one nucleotide base pair with another pair of nucleotides in double-stranded DNA. A point mutation is also referred to as a base-pair substitution. Thus, a cellular oncogene activated by point mutation differs from the proto-oncogene from which it was derived by a single base-pair.

178. C

In order for a proto-oncogene to transform a cell, oncoproteins must be produced from proto-oncogene transcripts. But if there are complementary nucleic acid sequences present, the proto-oncogene mRNA will base pair with the nucleic acids before it can be translated and produce oncoproteins.

According to the passage, cellular proto-oncogenes often become tumorigenic via a point mutation that leads to the formation of a defective protein, so choice A is wrong. Choice B is wrong, since you're told that a mutation that causes a proto-oncogene to produce an excess of its protein product, such as a chromosomal translocation, will convert the proto-oncogene into a tumorigenic oncogene. Choice D is wrong, since you're told that a mutation that causes the proto-oncogene to undergo gene amplification would also cause an excess of protein product and convert the proto-oncogene into a tumorigenic oncogene.

179. C

A c-onc (proto-oncogene) is a cellular gene found in an organism's own genome. A v-onc is a gene found in the genome of transforming viruses. The v-onc is not normally part of the viral genome; it was incorporated into the viral genome from c-onc genes formerly found in a eukaryotic host cell. If the v-onc gene was captured from a host cell in the form of c-onc RNA, the v-onc gene will have a sequence similar to the sequence of c-onc RNA. The v-onc gene will be similar to the exons the c-onc gene spliced together. So choice C is the correct answer.

Choice A is wrong, since if the v-onc gene contained only c-onc introns, the v-onc gene would code for nonsense, since it's the exons that contain the coding sequences. Choice B is wrong, because although it is true that a v-onc gene has a greater level of expression than its corresponding c-onc gene, expression level is independent of gene sequence. Choice D is wrong because although the v-onc RNA could be spliced after it had transcribed inside a eukaryotic host cell, it would not explain why the v-onc gene itself resembled the mRNA sequence of the c-onc gene.

180. D

The binding of a compound to a growth-factor receptor on the cell surface triggers a series of reactions that activate the protein *ras,* which in turn triggers another cascade of reactions. The end result is the activation of specific transcription factors and the expression of select genes. This is an example of signal transduction. Likewise, the second messenger system (as utilized by peptide hormones) is put into action by the binding of a molecule to a receptor on the outer surface of the cell membrane. This event triggers a cascade of events in which a signal is transmitted to the interior of the cell. On receipt of a signal from outside the cell, other reaction cascades are initiated inside the cell that result in a specific change in cellular activity. Typically, second messenger systems involve G proteins and cyclic AMP.

Choice A is wrong since formation of an antibody-antigen complex occurs within the vessels of the circulatory and lymphatic systems, and involves the binding of proteins expressed on the surface of the antigen to the antibody-binding sites of the antibody itself. Choice B is wrong since the sodium-potassium pump transports sodium and chloride ions across membrane without any signal transduction. Choice C is wrong because the Krebs cycle, which is a part of cellular respiration, is regulated via a negative feedback mechanism. The synthesis of citrate from oxaloacetate and acetyl CoA is an important control point in the cycle. ATP inhibits citrate synthase, the enzyme that catalyzes citrate synthesis. As ATP levels increase, citrate synthesis is inhibited.

181. B

A promoter is a region of DNA involved in the binding of RNA polymerase to initiate transcription. The promoter region is located approximately 10–35 base pairs before the first coding base of the gene. The strength of a promoter describes the frequency at which RNA polymerase initiates transcription and appears to be related to the closeness with which its sequences conform to the ideal consensus sequences. So, a strong promoter increases the frequency with which RNA polymerase binds to the region and transcribes the gene. Based on this, choice B is the correct answer.

Choice A is wrong since promoters are involved with transcription, not translation. Choice C and choice D must be wrong since translocation and mutation typically lead to abnormal gene product, not to an excess of normal gene product.

Passage VIII (Questions 182–187)

182. A

An animal's immune system produces antibodies in response to the presence of antigens—sub-

stances that are recognized by the animal as being "foreign," or "nonself." Healthy animals do not normally produce antibodies against their own circulating hormones. Since mice and rabbits are not normally exposed to human hormones, injecting them with extract from the human endocrine gland that synthesizes a particular hormone will elicit the production of antibodies specific for that hormone. The antibodies are then isolated from a blood sample for use in an RIA. Thus, choice A is the correct answer.

Choice B is wrong because human endocrine gland cells produce hormones not antibodies; the B-cells of the immune system produce antibodies. Furthermore, if human endocrine cells could produce antibodies, then they would be able to produce them in vivo. Choice C is wrong because it implies that human hormones will only elicit an immune response in mice and rabbits. Human hormones would do the same in most other mammals, too. Rabbits and mice are commonly used as test animals in laboratories because of certain similarities they share with humans, and because they are fast breeders. (For your information, exposing chimpanzees to a human hormone extract might not elicit antibody production by the chimp because both species share approximately 96 percent of their DNA.) Choice D actually describes the principle behind vaccinations. Vaccination with a weakened or killed form of a pathogen elicits a mild immune response in the organism. This primary exposure to the pathogen results in B-cell proliferation and antibody production. Upon subsequent exposure to the pathogen, the immune response is typically faster and more efficient. What's wrong with choice D is that immunization with a hormone extract will not cause an infection. Viruses and bacteria cause infections.

183. D

ADH, or antidiuretic hormone, is the hormone secreted by the posterior pituitary gland in response to low blood volume or high plasma osmolarity. ADH restores plasma osmolarity or blood volume to normal levels by increasing water reabsorption in the kidneys. Therefore, you would expect the concentration of circulating ADH to be higher in a person suffering from severe blood loss than in a healthy person. Since the RIA for ADH in a healthy person yielded an ADH concentration of 3 pg/mL, then the only possible answer is 5 pg/mL, which is the only choice higher in value than the ADH RIA of a healthy person.

184. D

According to the passage, labeled and unlabeled hormones compete for binding sites on the antibody. If there is little unlabeled hormone in the sample, the percentage of antibody-bound radiolabeled hormone will be high; if there is a lot of unlabeled hormone, the percentage of antibody-bound radiolabeled hormone will be low. FSH (follicle-stimulating hormone) stimulates the maturation of an ovarian follicle during a typical menstrual cycle. During pregnancy however, the menstrual cycle is inhibited because progesterone, which is secreted by the corpus luteum during the first trimester of pregnancy and secreted by the placenta during the remainder of the pregnancy, inhibits FSH secretion. So, the concentration of FSH is very low during pregnancy. If an RIA for FSH were done on a woman before pregnancy and again in her 16th week of pregnancy, you would expect the percentage of antibody-bound radiolabeled FSH to be higher during pregnancy since the concentration of FSH in her body will be low. Thus, on Figure 1, the point that corresponds to the before pregnancy state must have a higher FSH concentration on the x-axis than does the pregnancy state. Therefore, choice D is the correct answer.

Choice A, choice B, and choice C all show the FSH concentration to be greater during pregnancy than before pregnancy, and so are incorrect. Since all of the answer choices except for choice D have a higher FSH concentration at the second

point, you could have concluded that choices A, B, and C all imply the same thing, and therefore must be wrong.

185. B

So long as the antibody binds to the radiolabeled hormone and the unlabeled hormone with equal affinity, then the concept of competition for the binding sites is valid, and so is the RIA. If the antibody preferentially bound the radiolabeled hormone, then the percentage of antibody-bound radiolabeled hormone would always be high, regardless of the concentration of unlabeled hormone in the blood sample being assayed. The standard curve generated from such data would be invalid, and therefore useless for calculating hormone concentrations. Thus, choice B is correct and choice A is wrong.

Choice C is wrong because if there was enough antibody in the solution to completely bind all of the radiolabeled hormone and unlabeled hormone, then the two couldn't compete for antibody binding sites. This competition is essential to RIA because the percentage of each of the hormones that binds to the antibody is directly proportional to its concentration in the solution. Choice D is wrong because there is no evidence in the passage to support it. Antibodies can only bind to antigens at their antigen-binding sites.

186. B

Insulin is the pancreatic hormone that lowers blood glucose concentration mainly by stimulating the conversion of glucose into its storage form, glycogen. In response to high blood glucose, the pancreas secretes insulin, and blood glucose concentration decreases. Thus, one hour after an infusion of glucose, you would expect to find a higher concentration of insulin in a blood sample taken from the subject than before the infusion. And, in an RIA in which the concentration of unlabeled hormone is expected to be high relative to the concentration of radiolabeled hormone, the percentage of antibody-bound radiolabeled hormone is expected to be low. Thus, if Figure 1 were the standard curve for insulin, the point representing insulin after the glucose infusion must correspond to a higher hormone concentration than the point representing insulin concentration before glucose infusion.

187. C

That the precursor and active forms of a hormone are chemically and structurally similar implies that an antibody developed against either form of the hormone would be capable of binding to both, and would do so with equal affinity. The question stem states that the researcher wanted to measure the concentration of the active form of the hormone, since it's the active form that circulates and acts on target cells. However, the researcher used the precursor form to develop the antibodies and generate the standard curve used for the RIA. If the sample to be assayed contained only the active form, the results of the RIA would be valid. However, if the sample of unlabeled hormone to be assayed were somehow contaminated with the unlabeled precursor form, then the antibody would bind to both forms. Now there would be three competitors vying for the antigen-binding sites on the antibodies: the radiolabeled precursor form, the unlabeled precursor form, and the unlabeled active form. This means that the percentage of antibody-bound radiolabeled hormone would be atypically low. And since the percentage of antibody-bound radiolabeled hormone is inversely proportional to the concentration of unlabeled hormone in the sample, the calculated concentration of the active hormone would be greater than its actual concentration. Thus, choice C is correct and choice D is wrong.

Choice A is wrong for two reasons. First, the standard curve generated using the precursor

form of the hormone would be valid, but only for calculating the concentration of either form of the hormone in a sample containing only that form. Second, according to the question, the researcher is looking to measure the concentration of the active form of a particular hormone, not its precursor form. Choice B is wrong since it proposes that the percentage of antibody-bound radiolabeled hormone would be greater than normal, while in actuality, it would be less than normal.

Discrete Questions

188. A

Osmosis is the tendency of water to flow from regions of lower solute concentration to regions of higher solute concentration. Freshwater fish tend to gain water because of osmosis, and marine fish tend to lose it. If water is flowing into the freshwater fish, then the fish's environment must be hypotonic to its blood; that is, the freshwater has a lower concentration of dissolved solutes than the fish's blood. The marine fish is losing water to its surroundings, which means that its aqueous environment must be hypertonic to its blood. In both cases, the water is flowing from hypotonic regions to hypertonic regions. The term isotonic means that there is no difference in osmolarity between two regions; there is no net osmosis between isotonic regions.

189. D

Hemoglobin has four subunits, each with its own heme group, while myoglobin has only one unit and therefore one heme group. The sigmoid, or S-shape of hemoglobin's O_2-dissociation curve reflects the fact that the saturation of hemoglobin depends not only on the concentration of O_2 in blood, but also on the number of subunits that are occupied with O_2 molecules. Cooperative binding means that the binding of the first O_2

molecule to one of hemoglobin's subunits makes it easier for the second O_2 to bind. And the binding of the second makes it easier for the third, and so on. In other words, when the partial pressure of O_2 in the blood is low, it is more difficult for that first O_2 to bind, but because of the cooperativity after the first one does bind, it becomes much easier for the other O_2 molecules to bind, which is why the curve rises steeply. Since myoglobin does not have multiple subunits, O_2 cannot bind to it in a cooperative fashion, which is the reason why myoglobin's O_2-dissociation curve is not S-shaped. Its curve reflects the fact that the saturation of myoglobin is directly proportional to the concentration of O_2 in the blood. Thus, choice D is correct and choice B is wrong. Choice A is wrong because the Bohr effect is the term used to describe hemoglobin's decrease in O_2 affinity at high plasma concentrations of CO_2 and low pH. Choice C is wrong because while the difference in the partial pressure of O_2 between muscle tissue and arterial blood is the factor accounting for the diffusion of O_2 into O_2-depleted muscle tissue, it does not account for the difference in the shapes of the two curves.

190. B

All *meta*-directors have a positive charge on the atom directly bonded to the ring or can be polarized to have a partial positive charge there. Most *ortho* and *para* directing groups have at least one pair of nonbonding electrons on the atom directly bonded to the ring. Choice B is correct because the nitrogen possesses a pair of nonbonding electrons. The carboxyl group in choice A will certainly be a *meta* director since the carboxyl carbon is positively polarized. The same thing applies to the ketone group in choice C: The carbonyl oxygen polarizes the bond so that the carbon has a slight positive charge. Choice D is also a *meta* director, since the electron withdrawing nature of the oxygens ensure that the sulfur atom is positively polarized.

191. A

When an amino acid reaches its isoelectric point, it is in the form of a zwitterion. In this state, the molecule is electrically neutral: The carboxylate group is negatively charged and the ammonium group is positively charged. As a result, it will not migrate toward either the cathode or the anode when placed in an electric field. Since the amino acid migrates to the anode at pH 8.5, it must have a net negative charge. To attain neutrality and hence reach the isoelectric point, the ammonium group has to be protonated, which can be achieved by lowering the pH. Therefore, the isoelectric point must be lower than 8.5.

192. C

Both LH and FSH are released by the anterior pituitary under the influence of their respective hypothalamic gonadotropin-releasing factors. However, male and female hormones differ in their pattern of release and physiological function. In males, the release of LH and FSH is relatively constant because they stimulate two continuous processes: testosterone synthesis and spermatogenesis. In females, the release of LH and FSH is strictly cyclic. Prior to ovulation, FSH and LH secretion continuously increase; the increase in FSH stimulates follicle development and the increase in LH stimulates the development of the corpus luteum following ovulation. The secretion of both hormones drops sharply following ovulation and does not begin to rise again until the onset of the next menstrual cycle. Therefore, the switch from cyclic production of gonadotropin-releasing factors to acyclic production during reproductive development would most certainly affect the release patterns of both of these hormones, and so choice C is correct.

Passage IX (Questions 193–198)

193. D

Bacteria are often classified and named on the basis of their shape, of which there are three: spherical, rod-like, and helical (spiral). Spherical bacteria are know as cocci; rodlike bacteria are know as bacilli; and helical bacteria are known as spirochetes, or spirilla. Thus, if a sample from a CF patient infected with *Staphylococcus* were cultured and viewed under a microscope, the bacteria would appear spherical in shape. So, choice D is the correct answer.

Helical bacteria are the least common of the three groups; rod-shaped bacteria include the common *E. coli,* as well as those bacteria responsible for causing lockjaw, diphtheria, and tuberculosis. So, choice A and choice C are wrong. Choice B is wrong since sickle-shaped bacteria do not exist; however, those individuals with the genetic disease sickle-cell anemia have red blood cells with an abnormal sickle shape.

194. C

CF patients suffer from pancreatic insufficiency because of abnormally viscous mucus secretions that block the ducts linking the pancreas to the small intestine. The pancreas synthesizes and secretes the following enzymes: trypsinogen, chymotrypsinogen, carboxypeptidase, amylase, and lipase. Lipase digests fats; amylase digests carbohydrates; carboxypeptidase, trypsinogen, and chymotrypsinogen all digest proteins. Trypsinogen and chymotrypsinogen are secreted into the small intestine, where enterokinase, an enzyme secreted by the glands of the small intestine, converts trypsinogen to its active form, trypsin. Trypsin then converts chymotrypsinogen to its active form, chymotrypsin. Choice C is therefore correct, since enterokinase—a product of the small intestine—would not be lacking in a CF patient. On the other hand, lipase, trypsin, and chymotrypsinogen would be included in an enzyme supplement administered to CF patients.

195. B

According to the passage, the gene for cystic fibrosis is autosomal recessive. Let F = the normal gene and f = the cystic fibrosis gene. Those individuals with CF have the genotype ff; those who are carriers have the genotype Ff; and normal individuals have the genotype FF. So in a cross between two heterozygotes: Ff × Ff, 25 percent of the offspring will have the genotype FF and will be normal; 50 percent will have the genotype Ff and will thus be carriers; and 25 percent will have the genotype ff and will have cystic fibrosis. Therefore, in a cross between two carriers, there is a 25 percent chance that their child will be affected by CF, and choice B is the correct answer.

196. D

Since the CF gene codes for a defective transmembrane chloride channel, it would seem that this is the cause of the increased chloride and sodium in the sweat of CF patients. The chloride channel coded for by the CF gene must be unable to transport chloride from the sweat ducts into the surrounding epithelial cells. And due to the principle of electroneutrality, sodium would follow suit.

Choice A is incorrect because transporting less chloride into the sweat ducts would produce a lower concentration of chloride in the sweat. Choices B and C are wrong because they suggest that the defective channel in CF patients transports sodium, contradicting the information in the passage.

197. B

The pancreas secretes trypsinogen, chymotrypsinogen, and carboxypeptidase, which are

 347

all involved in protein digestion; pancreatic amylase, which is involved in carbohydrate digestion; and lipase, which is involved in fat digestion. So, you might expect a CF patient to suffer from malabsorption of proteins, fats, and carbohydrates. However, it is fat absorption that is the most severely impaired because lipase is the only enzyme that digests fat (in conjunction with bile). Carbohydrates, on the other hand, are digested by salivary amylase, maltase, sucrase, and lactase, in addition to pancreatic amylase. Likewise, proteins are digested by pepsin, aminopeptidases and dipeptidases, in addition to the pancreatic enzymes. Therefore, choice B is correct and choice C is wrong. Although pulmonary obstruction is also a symptom of CF, it is caused by the thick mucus secretions of the respiratory epithelial lining, which often become infected by bacteria of the *Staphylococcus* family. So, choice A is wrong. Choice D is wrong because although the passage implies that CF patients are susceptible to penicillin-resistant bacteria, this is not the result of pancreatic exocrine insufficiency.

198. A

According to the passage, CO_2 remains in the blood of CF patients longer than in the blood of healthy individuals. The CO_2 produced by cellular respiration diffuses out of the tissues and into plasma, where it reacts with water to form H_2CO_3, which dissociates into HCO_3^- and H^+. Most of the H^+ binds with hemoglobin. So, though there is an increase in plasma H^+ as a result of normal cellular function, the binding of the H^+ to hemoglobin maintains blood pH to within a fairly constant range. When the blood reaches the capillaries of the lungs, the reactions reverse: The H^+ and HCO_3^- reassociate to form H_2CO_3, which is then converted back into CO_2 and water, both of which are exhaled. However, in CF patients, the sticky, thick mucus interferes with normal gas exchange in the alveoli, causing the CO_2 to

remain in the blood for a longer period of time in the form HCO_3^- and H^+ before they reassociate back into H_2CO_3. An increase in plasma H^+ decreases blood pH, since the two are inversely related. Since a decrease in blood pH is just another way of saying an increase in acidity, choice A is the correct answer.

Passage X (Questions 199–203)

199. D

In Figure 2, H^+ bonds with the oxygen of the carbonyl group. It is then lost in step 4 to regenerate H_3O^+ and the α-halo ketone. A catalyst is a material that increases the rate of a reaction but remains unchanged itself, so the hydrogen ion does fit this definition.

On the other hand, the hydroxide ion is a reactant. In Figure 1, the hydroxide abstracts an a-hydrogen from the ketone in the first step to produce water and the enolate ion. Since the hydroxide anion is used up, and not regenerated, it is a reactant and not a catalyst. Therefore, choice D is the correct response.

200. A

Tautomers are compounds which differ in the arrangement of their atoms, but exist in equilibrium with each other. The most common type of tautomerism is that in which molecules differ in the attachment of a hydrogen and the placement of a double bond; namely keto-enol tautomers. In Figure 2, the reactant, acetone, is in its keto form. It becomes protonated by acid to form an intermediate which then slowly isomerizes to produce the enol form of acetone.

Enantiomers are a subdivision of stereoisomers, so they differ in their spatial arrangement, not their atomic connectivity. The product and reactant in Step 2 do differ in their atomic connectivity, so choices C and D are wrong. Geometric isomers are also another type of stereoisomer and are defined as compounds that differ in the position of groups around a double bond. The product and reactant do not fit this definition either, so choice B is wrong.

201. A

Alpha halogenation in basic solution usually doesn't stop at the mono-halogenated product stage because the halogen on the alpha carbon is highly electronegative: It pulls electron density towards it, so the two remaining protons are highly acidic. Since the conditions are basic, these hydrogens can be easily abstracted and the anion that is formed can attack the positively polarized region of another halogen molecule, resulting in multiple halogenations. Therefore, choice A is the correct response. Choice B is true in that the base is strong and will abstract protons, but it is not the reason why multiple halogenations occur. Choice C is incorrect because α-halo ketones are not unstable compounds; they can be isolated quite easily. Choice D is wrong because abstraction of a proton will result in the formation of a carbanion not a carbocation, and a halogen would destabilize a carbocation, not stabilize it.

202. C

This question can be interpreted as, "What reactants are involved in the rate limiting step?" Remember that the rate-limiting step is the slow one. Therefore, in Figure 1, the rate depends upon the abstraction of an α-proton from acetone. The two species involved in this reaction are acetone and OH⁻, roman numerals I and III, making choice C correct. Bromine has nothing to do with the slow step; it is only involved with the fast step, which does not affect the rate. Hence, choices B and D are wrong. Choice A is wrong

because the rate of the reaction does not solely depend upon the concentration of acetone.

203. B

In this reaction, a ketone reacts with a Grignard reagent to form an alcohol:

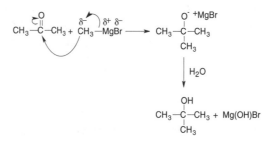

Therefore, the molecule formed is *tert*-butyl alcohol, choice B. Choice A, choice C, and choice D can be eliminated because none of these functionalities are formed in the reaction. In addition, choice A and choice D do not contain the *tert*-butyl group.

Passage XI (Questions 204–209)

204. C

Synapses are neural junctions that transmit depolarization waves from one neuron to another. Once a depolarization wave has reached the presynaptic knob, vesicles containing a neurotransmitter, in this case acetylcholine, merge with the presynaptic membrane and diffuse across the synaptic cleft to bind with receptors of the postsynaptic membrane. This results in depolarization of the postsynaptic membrane and thus initiates the transmission of another nerve impulse. After depolarization, acetylcholine remains bound to the postsynaptic receptors, and thus no more neural impulses can be transmitted unless acetylcholine is removed from the receptors. Acetylcholinesterase restores the excitability of the postsynaptic membrane by cleaving acetylcholine; therefore, choice C is the correct answer. Choice B is wrong since the passage states that acetylcholinesterase doesn't work until after acetylcholine has been released by the presynaptic membrane. Choice D is wrong because a plausible mechanism to restore full excitability to the presynaptic knob would be to replace acetylcholine. However, ACE breaks down acetylcholine, so it does cannot affect the activity of the presynaptic membrane. Choice A is true in that the reaction of ACE with acetylcholine will prevent the transmitter being reabsorbed by the presynaptic membrane, but it is the reactivation of the receptors which is the most important consequence of the action of ACE.

205. B

Since a carboxylate group (designated as CO_2^-) is negatively charged, and the quaternary nitrogen atom of acetylcholine is positively charged, they will be attracted by electrostatic interaction; choice B is correct. Choice A is wrong because there is no hydrogen in the carboxylate group or the quaternary nitrogen which can take part in hydrogen bonding. Choice C is wrong because a hydrophobic interaction is an attraction between nonpolar groups. However, the attraction between the carboxylate group and the quaternary nitrogen is the opposite of this: It is a polar interaction. Choice D is wrong because London forces are weak attractive forces between instantaneous and induced dipoles occurring in nonpolar molecules.

206. D

In the imidazole ring, the double bonded nitrogen has five valence electrons, three of which are used in bonding. The remaining lone pair of electrons are donated to form an N-H bond, leaving a positive charge on the nitrogen. A Lewis acid is an electron pair acceptor and a Lewis base is an electron pair donor. Nitrogen, therefore, acts as a

Lewis base by donating its electrons to form a bond to hydrogen; choice D is therefore the correct answer. Choice A and choice B are wrong because they give the wrong definitions for Lewis acids and bases. Choice C is incorrect because nitrogen doesn't have any room in its valence shell to accept electrons, so it definitely won't act as a Lewis acid.

207. D

In Figures 1 and 2, the tyrosine residue of the enzyme donates a proton which becomes bonded to the carbonyl oxygen in acetylcholine. This gives the ester carbon a positive charge. In Figures 2 and 3, an esterification reaction occurs: the oxygen in the serine group nucleophilically attacks and adds to the positively charged carbon in acetylcholine to form an ester (acetylserine) and an alcohol (choline). Therefore, protonation of the carbonyl oxygen in acetylcholine results in an increased positive charge on the carbon attached to it, increasing its susceptibility to nucleophilic attack. The increased positive charge on the carbon causes it to be attracted more strongly to the negative charge on serine's hydroxyl oxygen so it will diffuse towards serine more quickly, and the reaction will proceed at a faster rate. Therefore, choice D is correct. ACE is a catalyst, whose function is to increase the rate of reaction, not to affect the equilibrium or the extent of the reaction, so choice B is wrong. Protonation does not effect the leaving ability of the choline group, so choice A and choice C are wrong.

208. B

Acetylcholine undergoes nucleophilic attack by the hydroxyl oxygen of serine. Since the carbon-oxygen single bond of acetylcholine is broken (resulting in the loss of choline) and replaced by a new carbon-oxygen single bond to serine, the reaction is a nucleophilic substitution. The oxygen of serine attacks the positively charged carbon while at the same time, the choline group leaves. This is characteristic of an S_N2 reaction, so choice B is the correct answer. Choice A, S_N1, is wrong, since the first step in an S_N1 reaction is loss of the leaving group to form a carbocation. In this reaction loss of the leaving group would place a double positive charge on the central carbon atom, making it a very unfavorable step. Choice D is wrong because if serine was a better leaving group than choline, the reaction would not proceed. Although Choice C is true, there is nothing in the passage or the diagrams that state this. In addition, none of the reactions involve competition between OH⁻ and CH_3^-.

209. A

Just as esterification occurs in Figures 2 and 3, so the ester that is formed can be basically cleaved by OH⁻. This is exactly what happens in Figures 6 and 7:

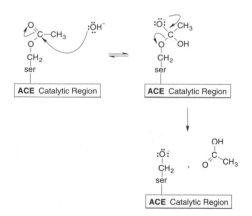

This process fits the definition of an ester being hydrolyzed by a base, the only key difference being that in this situation, the ester is not free—it is attached to the ACE catalytic region. Therefore, choice A is correct. Choice B is incorrect because acetylserine does not contain an ether functionality. Choice D is incorrect because a carboxylic acid is formed, not reacted. Choice C is wrong since there is no alcohol functionality present to oxidize.

Discrete Questions

210. A

Lysosomes are membrane-bound organelles containing hydrolytic digestive enzymes, which work best at a pH of 5—well below the pH of the cytosol. Lysosomes fuse with endocytotic vesicles and digest their contents; also, lysosomes recycle the cell's own organic material by engulfing an organelle or chunk of cytosol, dismantling it, and returning the organic monomers to the cell for reuse. Thus, choice A is correct. Choice B is wrong because peroxisomes are organelles that contain enzymes that transfer hydrogen from various substrates to oxygen, producing hydrogen peroxide. Through these reactions, peroxisomes detoxify alcohol and other harmful compounds in the liver, and break down fats into smaller molecules that can be used for cellular respiration. Choice C is wrong since rough endoplasmic reticulum is the network of interconnecting channels continuous with the outer nuclear membrane. Rough endoplasmic reticulum is studded with ribosomes on its outer surface and functions in the synthesis of membrane and proteins. Choice D is wrong since ribosomes are the organelles responsible for translating messenger RNA into polypeptides.

211. C

The four bases found in DNA are adenine, thymine, guanine, and cytosine. The four bases found in RNA are adenine, uracil, guanine, and cytosine. Adenine binds with uracil or thymine and guanine always binds with cytosine. In double-stranded nucleic acid, the quantity of adenine equals the quantity of thymine (if it's DNA) or the quantity of uracil (if it's RNA). In single-stranded nucleic acid, the quantity of base does not matter, as long as they add up to 100%. The viral genome is most likely single-stranded RNA, since the amount of adenine does not equal the amount of uracil and the amount of cytosine does not equal the amount of guanine. So, choice C is correct and choice D is wrong. Choice A and choice B are wrong since DNA doesn't contain uracil.

212. C

Choice C is correct for two reasons. First, $(CH_3)_3COH$ will form a tertiary carbocation: $(CH_3)_3C^+$. Here, there are three alkyl groups which, by electron donation through sigma bonds, can stabilize the positive charge. Second, the polar protic solvent H_2SO_4 is used. This drives the formation of the carbocation, since it can stabilize the transition state that forms. Choice B is wrong because even though $(CH_3CH_2)_3COH$ would form a tertiary carbocation, acetone is a polar aprotic solvent which would not be able to stabilize the transition state as effectively as a polar protic solvent. Choice A and choice D would form secondary and primary carbocations, respectively. These are not as stable as the tertiary carbocation, since they possess fewer alkyl groups to stabilize the positive charge on the carbocation.

213. B

Pepsin is the protein-digesting enzyme secreted by the gastric glands of the stomach. The environment of the stomach is very acidic; it has a pH of approximately 2, due to the continuous secretion of HCl by the stomach's parietal cells. In contrast, the lumen of the small intestine is alkaline, due to the secretion of bicarbonate ion from the pancreas. Pepsin requires the highly acidic environment of the stomach for optimal function. Therefore, a graph representing the optimal activity of pepsin as a function of pH would be centered around and have its peak at a pH of 2, and so choice B is correct and choice A, choice C, and choice D are wrong.

214. D

Mammalian fetal circulation differs from mammalian adult circulation in a number of very important ways. The ductus arteriosus and the foramen ovale are the two shunts in fetal circulation that divert blood away from the lungs, and the ductus venosus is the shunt that diverts blood away from the liver. In the fetus, gas exchange occurs in the placenta, not in the lungs, which are nonfunctional prior to birth. The combined effect of these factors is that there is a mixing of oxygenated and deoxygenated blood in a majority of the blood vessels of the fetal circulatory system; this mixing stops at birth, when the lungs become functional. Likewise, with two atria and only one ventricle in the amphibian heart, there is a mixing of oxygenated and deoxygenated blood.

Choice A is wrong since gas exchange in the fetus occurs in the placenta, and gas exchange in the adult amphibian occurs in its lungs when it's on land, and in its gills when it's in water. Choice B is wrong because placentas are unique to mammals. Choice C is wrong because the amphibian heart has only three chambers, while the mammalian fetal heart always has four.

How Did We Do? Grade Us.

Thank you for choosing a Kaplan book. Your comments and suggestions are very useful to us. Please answer the following questions to assist us in our continued development of high-quality resources to meet your needs. Or go online and complete our interactive survey form at **kaplansurveys.com/books**.

The title of the Kaplan book I read was: _____

My name is: _____

My address is: _____

_____

My e-mail address is: _____

What overall grade would you give this book?   Ⓐ Ⓑ Ⓒ Ⓓ Ⓕ

How relevant was the information to your goals?   Ⓐ Ⓑ Ⓒ Ⓓ Ⓕ

How comprehensive was the information in this book?   Ⓐ Ⓑ Ⓒ Ⓓ Ⓕ

How accurate was the information in this book?   Ⓐ Ⓑ Ⓒ Ⓓ Ⓕ

How easy was the book to use?   Ⓐ Ⓑ Ⓒ Ⓓ Ⓕ

How appealing was the book's design?   Ⓐ Ⓑ Ⓒ Ⓓ Ⓕ

What were the book's strong points? _____

How could this book be improved? _____

Is there anything that we left out that you wanted to know more about?

Would you recommend this book to others?   ☐ YES   ☐ NO

Other comments: _____

_____

_____

Do we have permission to quote you?   ☐ YES   ☐ NO

Thank you for your help.
Please tear out this page and mail it to:

Managing Editor
Kaplan, Inc.
1440 Broadway, 8th floor
New York, NY 10018

Thanks!

KAPLAN®

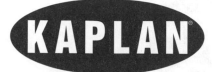
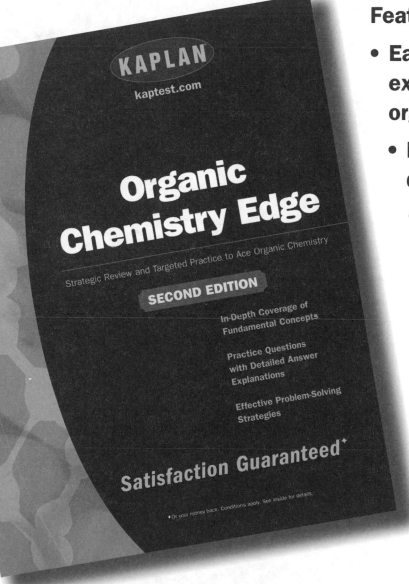
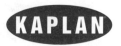

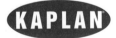